not curr ud d
10/7/2021
am

THE COMPLETE NATURAL MEDICINE GUIDE
to
BREAST CANCER
A Practical Manual
for Understanding,
Prevention & Care

SAT DHARAM KAUR
Naturopathic Doctor

Preface by Dr. Carolyn Dean, ND, MD

Robert
ROSE

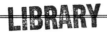
Dedication

To three women who used their disease to change the world –
Rachel Carson, Bella Abzug, and Nicole Bruinsma,
Thank you for your efforts.

And to the women of the world, the guardians of life and growing things,
may we create a revolution to heal ourselves and the earth.

The author gratefully acknowledges permission to reprint and reproduce the following information: Greenpeace for the chlorine pie chart and the alternatives to PVC chart.

The publisher acknowledges the financial support of the Government of Canada through the Book Publishing Industry Development Program.

The nutritional, medical, and health information presented in this book is based on the research, training, and professional experience of the author, and is up to date and complete to the best of the knowledge of the author. However, this book is intended only as an informative guide for those wishing to know more about health, nutrition, and medicine; it is not intended to replace or countermand the advice given by the reader's personal physician. Because each person and situation is unique, the author and the publisher urge the reader to check with a qualified healthcare professional before using any procedure where there is a question as to its appropriateness. A physician should be consulted before beginning any exercise program. The author and the publisher are not responsible for any adverse effects or consequences resulting from the use of the information in this book. It is the responsibility of the reader to consult a physician or other qualified healthcare professional regarding his or her personal care.

National Library of Canada Cataloguing in Publication

Kaur, Sat Dharam
The complete natural medicine guide to breast cancer : a practical manual
for understanding, care and prevention / Sat Dharam Kaur.

Includes bibliographical references and index.
ISBN 0-7788-0083-0 (bound).—ISBN 0-7788-0080-6 (pbk.)
1. Breast—Cancer—Alternative treatment. 2. Breast—Cancer—Prevention. 3. Naturopathy. I. Title.

RC280.B8K38 2003   616.99'449   C2003-902878-X

Edited by Bob Hilderley, Senior Editor, Health.

Design and page composition by PageWave Graphics Inc.

Printed and bound in Canada.

Published by Robert Rose Inc., 120 Eglinton Ave. E., Suite 800, Toronto,
Ontario Canada M4P 1E2 Tel: (416) 322-6552.
1 2 3 4 5 6 7 GP 09 08 07 06 05 04 03

Contents

Preface

A grand statement made by Marshall McLuhan in his *Interior Landscape* keeps coming back to me when I think about women and cancer. "Must we continue to mow down the Kennedys," McLuhan asked in 1969, recognizing that we are living in a collective society where everything you do affects me and everything I do affects you. We are all responsible, all culpable. The same can be said about the cancer dilemma. We are the cause of the present state of affairs but we are also the cure.

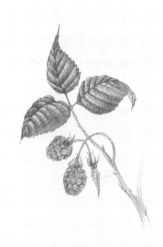

Cancer is a very expensive illness, an 'industry' whose treatment costs have almost reached the five billion dollar mark annually in North America. Cancer is big, big business and access to the 'market' — in other words, our bodies — is fiercely fought over. Yet over the past 40 years, treatments have barely improved and survival rate is no better. And the greatest and most recent increase is in hormone-dependent cancers of the breast, prostate, and testicles. Every 12 seconds a woman dies of breast cancer.

This realization was brought home to me during two conferences on breast cancer held during 1999, the Second World Conference on Breast Cancer in Ottawa and another in Hamilton. The common theme of both conferences was that our current social and economic system is the ultimate cause of cancer. Thirty years ago the World Health Organization declared that up to 90% of all cancers are caused by pesticides, radiation, and other toxic chemicals in our environment. Dr Samuel Epstein, whose research was key to banning DDT, pointed out that all of us now carry more than 500 different compounds in our cells, none of which existed before 1920, and that "there is no safe dose for any of them." For Sandra Steingraber, special advisor on cancer prevention to the President of the United States and author of the best selling *Living Downstream*, cancer has "become a human rights issue" which can only be tackled with "old fashioned political organization." That is why "scientists are now going directly to the public" in order to expose "the deception at the heart of the chemical industry, namely that these pesticides are necessary."

Although the earth has been made "chemically addicted" and all life is being poisoned, Steingraber states there are signs of change. For example, drycleaning fluid, which can cause many cancers, including bladder cancer, may be completely phased out in the foreseeable future. And organic farming has become a multi-billion dollar business.

Another sign of change is the growth in the popularity of alternative and complementary medicine offering a different approach to the cancer dilemma through prevention. *The New England Journal of Medicine* reported in 1993 that one-third of American citizens were using alternative medicine and annually spending over 10 billion dollars out of pocket on visits to alternative medicine practitioners. A follow up survey in 1998 in the *Journal of the American Medical Association* reported that between 1990 and 1997 Americans increased their visits to alternative medicine practitioner by 43%. The total visits were 427 million in 1990, 629 million in 1997.

Among alternative and complementary health care practices, naturopathic medicine has gained wide-spread respect. When I practiced as a Naturopathic Doctor in Ontario for 13 years, I taught my patients how to take responsibility for their own health — to ask their doctors questions about their health and to work with practitioners who followed the seven principles of naturopathic medicine, whether they were medical or naturopathic doctors.

There are now several naturopathic colleges training in these principles. One such doctor educated at the Canadian College of Naturopathic Medicine is Sat Dharam Kaur, who has applied her skills in an exceptional way by writing this definitive text on breast cancer prevention using the naturopathic model.

The Complete Natural Medicine Guide to Breast Cancer is not a book you can skim in one session; you might have to sit with it a dozen times to grasp all the information and the scope of the book. But starting with the first chapter you can begin to put your health in order and prevent breast cancer. The medical information and advice for prevention found throughout the book make this an indispensable resource and companion for all women, in poor or good health. I also love the fact that Dr Kaur is spearheading Rachel Carson Day on May 27th each year, honoring the woman that alerted us to the poisoning of our environment. She never lets us lose site of our need to clean both our bodies and our environment. Focusing on only one or the other will never be enough.

Fully aware that her book is asking a great deal from you in terms of taking on personal responsibility for your own breast health, Dr Kaur uses an extremely gentle and loving approach. You can see her smiling through the lines on the page and embracing you when you read a particularly difficult passage. These things are palpable through the whole text and make me weep just thinking about her care and concern for her readers and for the planet. And weep we must if we are to get in touch with our feelings for ourselves and for others. For the pain we have caused ourselves and our children and grandchildren. Weeping is not a sign of weakness but a sign of caring. A call to action. A call to women.

I am often drawn to the Greek play *Lysistrata*, written by Aristophanes in the fifth century BC, about the role women played in ending the Peloponnesian War by withholding sex from their men folk. Women of our new millennium may establish a similar victory in the war against cancer by withholding our considerable buying power. Stop rewarding industry that pollutes our air, soil, and water and begin to reward clean and pure products, organic goods, and companies that care for the environment. Involve yourself with simple acts of activism and kindness that will ripple across the planet. That is how I see our larger mission as modern-day warriors. I know Dr Sat Dharam Kaur has the same vision. And I trust you will be amply rewarded by participating in her Healthy Breast Program.

— DR CAROLYN DEAN, ND, MD

PRINCIPLES OF NATUROPATHIC MEDICINE
1) Identify and Treat the Causes
2) First Do No Harm
3) Doctor as Teacher
4) Treat the Whole Person
5) Emphasize Prevention
6) Support the Healing Power of the Body
7) Physician Heal Thyself

Introduction

A Call to Women

10 ACTIONS FOR PREVENTION

The following 10 suggestions summarize the components of a natural medicine program for prevention of breast cancer and breast care. Each suggestion will be discussed in greater detail chapter-by-chapter. Further 'actions for prevention' appear throughout the book. Read these first, if you wish, before digging into the text for more information.

1) Breast Cancer Risk Factors: Determine your hereditary, reproductive, lifestyle, hormonal, environmental, dietary, psychological, and spiritual risks for developing breast cancer. Complete the Breast Health Risk Balance Sheet provided in Chapter 7.

2) Breast Examinations: Get to know your breasts through self-examination and mapping. If you have high risk factors for breast cancer or suspect a problem during self-exams, use thermography, ultrasound, and other diagnostic procedures annually to ensure that no cancer is present. Use mammography biannually after the age of 50, and before age 50 when there is suspicion of cancer.

In the fall of 1996 I began teaching the Healthy Breast Program because I felt it was necessary for women to become proactive in the prevention of breast cancer. From my studies of naturopathic medicine, I had some knowledge to share, and while I was a student, I had watched one friend in her early thirties die of breast cancer. My inability to help her at the time stimulated the writing of this book years later.

As I read more articles about breast cancer, I was not only astounded by the connection between the deteriorating environment and cancer development in our age but also angered by the cover-up of this knowledge. My passion to communicate this knowledge grew. I started to visualize women all over the world getting together in small groups — supporting each other, educating each other, claiming their identities, preventing the disease in themselves, and taking an active role in preserving the environment. I felt inter-species grief resonating in my heart. The grief of mothers unable to nurse their young and unable to nurture themselves because the soil, the air, and the water have become inhospitable to life. The grief of bald eagles who see the shells of their offspring shatter unnaturally beneath their weight; the grief of St. Lawrence beluga whales dying of cancer, their carcasses hazardous waste because of the chemicals they contain. I heard the painful cries of future generations robbed of children because their hormones have been tampered with. It is the feminine principle, the right to raise offspring, that is being violated. The waters of life have been poisoned along with the earth and breath of Gaia. Breast cancer is the call to arms. Arms of action, arms of prayer, arms of holding and joining, arms held up in resistance to complacency, convenience, and denial, arms united. We each have two arms. Together we are one body.

This call to arms has many facets. Breast cancer reminds us that we must be honest with ourselves and in our relationships — that we speak our truth and follow our inner guidance. Breast cancer draws the anger out of us — anger at God, anger at ourselves for having surrendered pieces of our wholeness we must now retrieve, anger at the political, corporate, and industrial forces that have got us in to such an insane environmental mess, anger at the unconscious ease of convenience. The breast cancer epidemic offers us a path of purification that we sorely need. Each of us must choose when to plant our feet upon that path — before or after a diagnosis. I believe that the only way out of the global breast cancer epidemic is through a path of purification. To me this includes honoring the soul and our unique abilities, being mindful of what and how we eat, releasing toxic emotions, cleansing the body, adopting a spiritual practice which is suited to our individual make-up, and realizing that it is our duty to make the environment safe and sacred once again.

It became clear to me as I was writing this book that we must shift from our present attitude of domination to cooperation and facilitation. We have been trying to dominate nature with our agricultural practices and it is making us, wildlife, and the planet sick. We have been trying to dominate the body with the overuse of antibiotics, the birth control pill, hormone replacement therapy, chemotherapy, and invasive treatments. The body has its own intelligence. It is much more fruitful to work with, rather than against, the body's processes: assist the liver in detoxification; enhance elimination with fiber and probiotics; balance the glands with herbs and meditation rather than cut them out, shut them down, or replace them with drugs; fortify the immune system with nutrition, herbs, visualization, and yoga before we immobilize it with chemotherapy and radiation. This is a naturopathic medical approach which recognizes the inherent ability of the body to heal itself when given the means to do so.

We have been trying to dominate each other with marketing hype and consumerism. The driving force behind domination is greed. Greed is destroying the Earth, our home, and destroying us. We must move from greed to living simply, realizing the consequences of our actions. What we do to the Earth, we do to ourselves. Breast cancer is evidence of that. Governments are not acting in the best interests of planetary ecology. We cannot rely on 'them' to take care of us or the earth. Industry continues to spew out billions more tons of chemicals each year into the environment while insisting that it does no harm. Countries explode nuclear weapons and nuclear power plants malfunction. There is no other Earth but the one we live on. Is there anywhere safe? Where can my children go?

Before we buy a product, we can consider how the air, earth, water, and wildlife were affected in the production of it, if it can be recycled or not, and whether it is safe to burn or bury. Most of the things we use are not. As our population expands, so does our toxic landfill. Before we eat our food, drink our water, and flush our toilets, we can ask these same questions. Then we do what we can to create positive change. We can accomplish a lot together. We are the guardians of the fertility of the Earth. All of us.

I feel a responsibility to do what I can in my own lifetime and to help others do the same. And so this book has been born. My prayer is that you will take it, use it yourself, share it with your daughters, sons, husbands, partners, friends, and lovers, teach someone else and perhaps start your own Healthy Breast Program. And that all over the world women will say no to food that is not organic, to plastic, to nuclear power, to chlorine, to anything that nature cannot take back into herself to nurture something else. We have broken the cycle of creation with our toxic waste. We must mend it.

Our immune systems resonate with the health of the planet. The planet is our collective body — if she is sick, so are we. She is in our blood, our bones, our muscles, our organs. When I had my first child, I felt the earth split as my daughter entered the world. I felt the oceans in my breasts as they filled with milk. I was initiated into the mysteries of the earth. I have not forgotten. She is my mother. I

3) Hormone Balance: Gain an understanding of your endocrine or hormone system, especially the link between estrogen and breast health. Monitor your hormone levels yearly, checking estradiol, estrone, estriol, the ratio of C2 to C16 estrogen, serum IGF-1 and 2, testosterone, insulin, progesterone, TSH, T4, T3, reverse T3, cortisol and melatonin using saliva testing.

4) Environmental Toxins: Decrease your exposure to known carcinogens and toxins. Become active in your home and community in protecting yourself from environmental toxins and in restoring the health of our environment. Use non-toxic body and home care products.

5) Detoxification: Do a liver cleanse for at least six weeks, once or twice a year, or on an ongoing basis if you have breast cancer or live in a particularly polluted area. Do a parasite cleanse for three months, once or twice a year, while simultaneously cleansing the intestines with a fiber formula or enemas and using probiotics (good bacteria). Make saunas a part of your life, having at least one each week (two 20-minute periods with a cool shower in between). Do a sauna detoxification program with supervision every 1-5 years.

6) Lymphatic and Immune Systems: Activate your lymphatic and immune systems. Exercise at least four hours a week and rebound daily for from 5-30 minutes. Practice the exercises for lymphatic cleansing at least three times weekly. Use one of the herbal formulas for lymphatic cleansing for at least three months twice yearly, or continuously if you have breast cancer. Practice skin brushing and have alternating hot and cold showers daily. Activate your immune system with one of the immune herbal formulas each winter, as needed, or continuously if you have breast cancer.

7) Diet: Follow a preventative dietary regime, including increasing your consumption of foods with high phytoestrogen content. Try following the Healthy Breast Diet.

8) Nutritional Supplements: Supplement your diet with vitamins, minerals, and other nutrients in consultation with your health care professional. Develop a daily supplement schedule.

believe that as conscious women, we can and must act as the white blood cells of the planet. Our bodies' immune systems are not separate from the earth's self-protective functions. We have loaded our Earth matrix with debris of every description that does not belong in her body — nuclear fallout, plastics, plutonium, organochlorines, pesticides, chemical hormones, non-biodegradable landfill — just as we must recognize and rid our bodies of toxins, so must she. The earth is our body too. Our bodies arise from the 'mater' of the earth and to the earth they will return. There is no separation.

Mankind has become the cancer of the earth as cancer has become the scourge of humanity. Where are the white blood cells of the earth? We find them in the environmentalists, the activists, the educators, the naturopaths and herbalists, the organic gardeners, the builders of windmills and solar energy units, the clean-up crews of environmental disasters. We are the 'cure' for this cancer. I invite each of you to become one of the white blood cells of the earth as you activate your own immune systems. Answer this call to women to act against the breast cancer epidemic by using some of your renewed energy to participate in healing the planet. We need one another to survive. We are the guardians of life and growing things.

I believe that women can turn things around. We stand united. We say no. We shall remain conscious rather than bowing to convenience. We hear the voices of the beluga whales, the polar bears, the Lake Apopka alligators, the Baltic seals, the bald eagles, Great Lakes salmon, and the voices of each other pressing us on, asking us to please help and act now. We act with the welfare of future generations of all species in our minds and hearts. We can and must make a difference.

A Program for Prevention and Care

Make your health a priority today, so that you can enjoy your family, work, and leisure time tomorrow. Develop a positive relationship with your body and breasts and put your well-being ahead of family and job responsibilities. Simplify your life, consume less, enjoy more. Throughout this book, various mental, emotional, physical, and spiritual exercises encourage this process.

This book was written to be used by you as an individual or in a group. You can read the information and apply it to your own health, making the changes in your life that are possible at this time. The content may take some time and considerable effort to absorb, but this information is comprehensive, authoritative, and thoroughly grounded in contemporary scientific research. Skim through the book, glancing at the glossary of terms to begin, then review the "Facts" and "Prevention" information in the margins. Move on to the referenced information section-by-section, chapter-by-chapter. Stop and take breaks. Try out the exercises and complete the charts and checklists. Drink some water. Focus on positive changes to your lifestyle. Do the best you can, but don't stress yourself about completing the book and following the program immediately. This is only a guide — it is up to you to feel comfortable with it and adapt it to your particular set of circumstances.

You may want help in understanding this information and adopting this program for breast cancer prevention. Find support.

Join or form a breast cancer awareness and prevention group. The program will be more powerful this way, and the group support will make the information easier to digest. Go through the chapters together. You don't have to cover all the details in each chapter. Focus on enough to get an overview, on the experiential exercises, and on group sharing. Keep the momentum going. If you are in a group, please take action on the environmental links to breast cancer in your area. Figure out what you can do together. Make waves. Let us bring about a tidal wave of personal and global transformation.

Exercises and Worksheets

The book is interactive, in that each chapter features exercises, charts, checklists, and worksheets for you to study and complete. Here is a list of the most important worksheets. Complete them in the book or photocopy these sheets. Revise them periodically to self-monitor your breast health and present them to your health-care professional for advice and action. The final chapter in the book, 'Working with Healthcare Professionals,' offers a set of guidelines and a 'Breast Health Data Sheet' for diagnosis and ongoing care you can share with your physician.

- ❑ Breast Health Balance Sheet (p. 29)
- ❑ Breast Map Worksheet (p. 44)
- ❑ BBT (Basal Body Temperature) Chart (p. 82)
- ❑ pH Balance Chart (p. 152)
- ❑ Weekly Diet Diary (p. 238)
- ❑ 14-Day Diet Routine Worksheet (p. 239)
- ❑ Daily Therapeutic Amounts of Vitamins and Minerals Chart (p. 261)
- ❑ Daily Supplement Schedule Worksheet (p. 264)
- ❑ Exploring Your Beliefs Exercise (p. 270)
- ❑ Letting Go Exercise (p. 271)
- ❑ Communication Style Worksheet (p. 274)
- ❑ Assertive Behavior Worksheet (p. 276)
- ❑ Meaning Mandala Worksheet (p. 289)
- ❑ Breast Health Data Sheet (p. 323)

9) Emotions and Spirit: Develop assertiveness and release anger. Practice imagery and visualization. Live your life in harmony with your true nature, making the most from your gifts and doing what makes you feel happy and fulfilled. Make time for play and being. Practice a relaxation, meditation, or breathing exercise 1-5 times daily, including before bed. Develop a spiritual practice that suits you and helps you stay in touch with your soul. Include prayer in your life.

10) Healthcare: Monitor your program daily and yearly. Make adjustments as necessary. Consult regularly with healthcare professionals. Maintain with your physician a Breast Health Data Sheet.

Keeping Abreast

This program is continually evolving. As I work with patients and groups to understand the implications of breast cancer research, I add and subtract information, always looking for new, authoritative studies and clinical evidence. You can keep abreast (!) of changes by attending conferences, workshops, and training courses. Link up with women worldwide who are following this Healthy Breast Program by contacting my website at www.healthybreastprogram.on.ca. or by consulting the 'Resources Directory' at the back of this book. The better we understand the medical basis of breast cancer, the better our ability to prevent this disease.

Glossary

adaptogen: a substance that helps us adapt to stressors of all kinds.

adrenal gland: a gland that sits on top of the kidneys and secretes various hormones, some of which help us adapt to stress.

angiogenesis: the process of blood vessels growing, sometimes to feed cancer cells.

antibacterial: inhibits or kills bacteria.

antibiotic: a substance used to kill bacteria.

anti-cancer: prevents or stops the initiation, promotion or progression of cancer.

antifungal: prevents or stops fungal growth.

anti-inflammatory: prevents or stops inflammation.

antioxidant: substances that protect the body from free radical (oxidative) damage. These include vitamins A, C, E, the carotenes, selenium, co-enzyme Q10, grape seed, milk thistle, gingko biloba, amla and many others.

antiviral: prevents or stops viral infections.

areola: area of pigment around the nipple.

atypical cells: cells that are slightly abnormal and could progress to cancer.

axilla: armpit.

benign: not cancerous

Biomedical Center: the Mexican clinic that uses the Hoxsey Formula as a standard treatment for cancer.

biopsy: removal of tissue from the body for diagnostic purposes, usually through aspiration or surgery.

bone marrow: the soft, inner core of the bones where blood cells are made.

bone scan: a test using radiation to look for metastases in the bones.

brassicas: the vegetable family that includes broccoli, cauliflower, Brussels sprouts, kale, Swiss chard, etc.

BRCA1: gene linked to high risk of breast cancer.

breath of fire: a breathing exercise commonly used in kundalini yoga as taught by Yogi Bhajan.

C-2 metabolite (2-hydroxyestrone): a breakdown product of estrogen metabolism that is inactive and harmless. Also known as 'good estrogen'.

C-4 metabolite (4-hydroxyestrone): a breakdown product of estrogen metabolism that is increased by environmental chemicals and may cause breast cancer.

C-16 metabolite (16-hydroxyestrone): a breakdown product of estrogen metabolism that is recycled, active and possibly harmful. Women with breast cancer have nearly five times more of the C16 metabolite than women without.

calcifications: small calcium deposits visible in a mammogram that are occasionally indicative of breast cancer.

carcinogen: substance that can cause cancer.

cell: basic unit of biological growth in an organism.

chemotherapy: use of drugs to kill cancer cells in the body.

chromosomes: found in the cell nucleus and contain the genes made of DNA.

clinical study: a review of the records of people with a particular disease.

complementary medicine: a group of substances and practises that are natural, have been used historically and can be used alongside drug treatments.

contraindicated: not to be used.

cortisol: hormone produced by the adrenal gland.

coumestrol: phytoestrogen found in high quantities in mung bean sprouts.

cyst: a fluid-filled sac or growth.

daidzen: phytoestrogen found in soy and other foods.

DDT: an organochlorine pesticide now banned in the United States but still used in Mexico and third world countries.

DES: diethylstilbestrol, a synthetic form of estrogen previously given to pregnant women to lower the risk of miscarriages. Now linked to increased reproductive organ and breast cancers.

DNA: deoxyribonucleic acid, which contains genetic information in a double spiral configuration and is found in the nucleus of each cell.

doubling time: how long it takes a group of cells to double in number.

duct: a narrow tube through which fluid passes.

carcinoma in situ: a group of atypical cells with a clear boundary, which is reversible without invasive treatment but may at some point progress to cancer.

edema: swelling caused by fluid build up between the cells.

eczema: skin ailment characterized by itching, redness, soreness.

endometrium: the tissue lining the uterus which fills with blood during the menstrual cycle, to be released during the menstrual period.

estrogens: hormones made by the ovaries, adrenals, fat cells and placenta which tend to promote breast cancer. Certain environmental chemicals and plant chemicals can also act as estrogens.

estrogen metabolism: bodily processes which make, use and eliminate estrogen.

estrogen receptor: special site in a cell to which estrogen attaches, allowing it to be active within the cell.

fibroadenoma: fibrous tumor of the breast.

fibrocystic breast disease: benign lumps in the breasts that fluctuate with the menstrual cycle.

free radicals: oxygen molecules with unpaired electrons which interfere with normal cellular functions. They are produced in the body from radiation, cigarette smoke, cooked and rancid oils, smog, chemicals and pollutants, and normal bodily processes. Antioxidants help to eliminate them.

FSH: hormone from the pituitary gland that stimulates the ovary to produce estrogen.

genes: cellular material composed of DNA that control physical and biochemical traits in all living things.

genistein: a phytoestrogen found in high amounts in soy, clover sprouts and the herb baptisia, among others.

Gerson Therapy: an alternative cancer therapy utilizing vegetable juices, extra potassium and iodine, coffee enemas and a vegetarian diet.

glucuronic acid: a substance to which estrogen binds in the liver.

glucuronidation: the process of estrogen binding to glucuronic acid.

glucuronide conjugate or complex: the substance formed when estrogen binds to glucuronic acid.

homeopathy: a system of healing based on the principle of "like cures like" which utilizes very diluted amounts of herbs, minerals and other substances as remedies.

hyper: too much, overactive.

hypothalamus: area in the brain that controls hormonal functions and stimulates the pituitary gland.

hypo: too little, underactive.

immune system: network of organs, glands and specialized cells and proteins that defend the body from bacteria, viruses, fungi, parasites and cancer.

immunoglobulins: IgA, IgD, IgE, IgG, and IgM are antibodies active throughout the body.

indole-3-carbinol: a plant chemical found in the Brassica family that is able to decrease the amount of the C-16 metabolite formed from estrogen.

initiation: the process of beginning something, such as damage to the DNA that turns on oncogenes, and starts cancer.

interferon: a protein produced by the immune system that inhibits viruses and activates T-cells.

intraductal: within the duct.

intraductal carcinoma: cancerous tumor within the breast duct.

invasive breast cancer: cancer growing beyond the original site into the surrounding tissue.

isoflavones: plant estrogens found in soy and other foods.

isothiocyanates: a group of plant chemicals found in the brassica family that have anti-cancer activity.

kidneys: organs which filter waste from the blood.

kundalini yoga: a system of teachings which include physical postures, breathing exercises and mantras that is thousands of years old. It was brought to North America in 1969 by Yogi Bhajan.

liver: the body's main organ of detoxification and hormone breakdown.

lignan: a type of plant fiber that decreases breast cancer risk, found in flaxseeds.

lobules: milk-producing breast tissue.

lumpectomy: breast surgery to remove a lump.

lymphatic fluid: clear fluid that circulates among the cells and through the lymphatic vessels.

lymph nodes: cleansing stations packed with white blood cells that filter lymph; the major ones are found in the armpits, groin, neck, and abdomen. Metastatic cancer cells can sometimes be found in the lymph nodes.

lymphatic system: a complex array of capillaries, vessels, ducts, cells, nodes and organs that maintain the fluid environment and cleanse cellular debris.

lymphatic vessels: small tubular structures that carry lymph to and from lymph nodes.

lymphedema: swelling caused by the build up of lymphatic fluid, usually caused by damage to or removal of lymph nodes.

lymphocytes: specialized white blood cells that target viruses and cancer cells.

macrobiotic diet: an eating plan which focuses on brown rice, soy products, vegetables, occasional fish and excludes meat, dairy products and eggs.

macrophage: a large cell that can surround and digest foreign substances in the body. Found in the liver, spleen and elsewhere.

malignant: cancerous

mastitis: breast infection.

mammogram: picture of the breasts taken with an X-ray.

mass: a group of cells.

mastectomy: surgical removal of a breast.

melatonin: a hormone produced by the pineal gland that has an anti-cancer effect. It is produced in the dark and proximity to electromagnetic radiation decreases production.

menopause: when the menstrual periods stop permanently.

metabolism: natural biochemical processes that occur in the body, liberating nutrients and energy.

metastasis: cancer of the same type as the original cancer but which is located in a distant part of the body. Typical sites for breast cancer metastases include the liver, lungs, bone and brain.

methylxanthine: chemical found in coffee, tea, chocolate that causes cystic changes in the breasts.

naturopathy: a medical system based on helping the body to heal itself through detoxification, strengthening areas of weakness and the use of natural substances and non-invasive therapies.

oncogene: a normal gene that initiates cancer when it is damaged or activated. We know of about 100 of them at present.

oncologist: a medical doctor who specializes in treating cancer.

osteoporosis: loss of bone density that is common in postmenopausal women.

pectoralis major: muscle beneath the breasts.

phagocytes: cells that surround, eat and digest cell waste, toxins, and small organisms.

phyto-: from a plant.

phytochemical: natural chemical made by a plant. Many phyochemicals protect us from cancer. phytoestrogen: plant substance that mimics estrogen but is generally protective from breast cancer.

pituitary gland: a gland in the brain behind the eyes that secretes hormones to regulate the other glands.

platelets: components of the blood that stop bleeding and repair blood vessels.

progesterone: hormone produced by the ovaries that acts in partnership with estrogen.

prognosis: a medical doctor's prediction of the probable outcome of a disease.

protocol: a particular program used in treating a specific disease.

recurrence: return of a cancer after it had disappeared.

remission: shrinkage of a tumor or disappearance of cancer.

side effect: undesirable result of using a substance for healing.

soy products: include tofu, tempeh, soy milk, soy sauce, tamari, Bragg's liquid aminos.

species: different genetic variations of the same organism.

spleen: an organ that is part of the immune system and houses red and white blood cells.

synergistic: a group of 2 or more substances working together in a way that is greater than the sum of each of the individual substances.

T-cells: specialized white blood cells that protect the body from viruses and cancer and are activated by the thymus gland.

tamoxifen: a hormonal drug which blocks the uptake of estrogen, used in breast cancer treatment.

tissue: group of cells of the same type that make up a particular body part.

tonify: strengthen, improve the function of a particular organ or body system.

tumor: a benign or malignant mass of abnormal cells.

virus: a very small organism that can only survive in the cells of another species and can cause disease.

white blood cells: lymphocytes, basophils, eosinophils, monocytes, and neutrophils that destroy bacteria, parasites, viruses, toxins, and damaged or abnormal cells.

xenoestrogen: non-natural substances that mimic estrogen, which include many environmental chemicals.

CHAPTER ONE

What Is Your *Risk* of *Developing Breast Cancer?*

CONTENTS

EXERCISES, CHARTS, CHECKLISTS & WORKSHEETS

BREAST CANCER is a multifaceted disease with many contributing causes and a complex array of interactions between these causes. It would be convenient if we could say with certainty that an individual woman's breast cancer was caused by exposure to a particular chemical or to radiation, by an excess of dietary fat or increased estrogen levels, by an emotional turmoil or grief. Most of the time we do not know the cause. We do know, however, numerous contributing factors that predispose a woman to breast cancer. Many of these factors are within our control. And while there is no specific 'cure' for breast cancer, just as there is no one cause, we can do much to prevent the disease by changing our diet and lifestyle, cleaning up our environment, and participating in various regimes for healing.

There are many factors that help to protect us from breast cancer. With educated determination, women can decrease their risk factors. We can take our breast health into our own hands and help to heal our sisters and our planet at the same time. The growing incidence of cancer among women, especially in North America, makes this an urgent task.

Incidence Rates

Among women worldwide, breast cancer is the most common cancer and the leading cause of cancer deaths.[1] The age-standardized incidence of breast cancer is almost three times higher in industrialized nations than it is in developing countries (63.2 vs. 23.1 per 100,000 women). However, incidence rates are now rising more rapidly in developing countries like Africa and India than they are in the developed world.[2]

The Netherlands and the United States lead the world in the breast cancer epidemic, with Denmark, France, Australia, New Zealand, Belgium, Canada, and Sweden following close behind. Breast cancer is much less common in other parts of the world, indicating that dietary, environmental, and lifestyle factors play a large role in its occurrence. Countries with a low incidence include most of Africa, Haiti, Mongolia, Korea, China, India, Costa Rica, and Japan.

Present statistics suggest that approximately one woman in nine in Canada and one in eight in the United States will develop breast cancer at some point in her life. In the 1920s a woman's risk was one in 20.[3] Women with no identifiable risk factors have a lifetime risk of breast cancer of about one in 16 through to the age of 80.[4] The estimated number of new cases of breast cancer in Canada and the United States in 2003 was 21,200 and 212,600, respectively, while the estimated number of deaths from breast cancer in Canada and the United States in 2003 was 5,300 and 40,200.[5,6,7] Breast cancer is a leading cause of death for women ages 35-50 living in these two countries.

Looking at the differences in rates between countries, we can speculate as to why some score low or high in breast cancer incidence. Third world countries may experience a risk reduction due to women having their children at an earlier age, having more of them, and breastfeeding for longer periods of time. Women in third world countries are also much less likely to use the birth control pill or hormone replacement therapy, reducing their risk. Exposure to radiation through nuclear power, the use of x-rays, and nuclear weapons testing is less common in third world countries, as is chronic exposure to strong electromagnetic fields and light at night, which both depress melatonin production and increase risk.

The diets of women in the non-industrialized world are likely to contain more fiber, less fat, less animal protein, less dairy, and more legumes. Equatorial countries tend to have a lower incidence, possibly linked to higher consumption of fruits and vegetables and increased sunlight and numbers of receptors for vitamin D in breast tissue, which confer protection. There is a striking correlation between global dairy consumption and global breast cancer incidence, probably related to milk fat. Chinese and Japanese women consume more soy products which are beneficial, particularly when introduced in infancy and before puberty. The Japanese are the world's largest consumers of sea vegetables, rich in iodine that protects the breasts. The turmeric present in the Indian diet has been found to deter breast cancer.

Cancer Incidence Rates Worldwide, 2000 [2]

Countries with the Highest Breast Cancer Incidence

Country	Incidence per 100,000 Women
Netherlands	91.6
USA	91.4
Denmark	86.2
France	83.2
Australia	82.7
New Zealand	82.6
Belgium	82.2
Canada	81.8
Sweden	81.0
Barbados	79.5
Israel	79.1
Finland	78.3
U.K.	75.0
Germany	73.6
Ukraine	73.2
Ireland	71.6
Iceland	70.2
Norway	68.5

Countries with the Lowest Breast Cancer Incidence

Country	Incidence per 100,000 Women
Haiti	4.7
Gambia	5.9
Mongolia	6.6
Korea	12.5
El Salvador	12.9
Thailand	15.9
China	16.4
India	19.1
Bolivia	26.6
Costa Rica	28.3
Japan	31.4
Spain	47.9

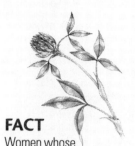

Causes of Breast Cancer

Any 'cure' for breast cancer must treat the causes of this disease, not simply eliminate the cancerous tissue through surgical intervention or chemotherapy, though these procedures may be necessary once the cancer has advanced to a critical stage. From an understanding of the causes, we can devise strategies to reduce the risk of developing cancer. These risks can be placed in several categories, ranging from hereditary through environmental to spiritual factors. A brief overview of these factors is presented here, with a more comprehensive discussion of hereditary, reproductive, lifestyle and healthcare risks given in this chapter. Subsequent chapters will focus on understanding and addressing hormonal, environmental, dietary, psychological, and spiritual risks.

Once you have read this overview, complete the 'Breath Health Balance Sheet' at the end of the chapter to assess your personal risk of developing breast cancer and to discover ways to protect yourself. Many natural therapies are described in this book to prevent breast cancer and to assist in recovery from it. These remedies can be used to complement surgery, chemotherapy, radiation, and pharmaceutical treatments.

Hereditary Risk Factors

We cannot change our genes but we can influence gene expression through lifestyle and environment. Inheriting the genes linked to breast cancer accounts for approximately 5% of cases of the disease. Avoiding other risk factors wherever possible, actively participating in environmental reform, strengthening immunity, and adopting a health-promoting lifestyle can prevent breast cancer, even when the genetic predisposition exists. By following the breast health program described in this book, you can significantly decrease the likelihood of breast cancer even if you have the genes associated with the disease.

Mother or Sister with Breast Cancer

Having a mother or sister with breast cancer is probably the risk factor most overestimated by women, increasing risk 1.5 to 3 times above the average one in 8 susceptibility.[8,9] Increased age of the mother when diagnosed reduces the risk for the daughter.[10,11] The influence of heredity decreases as a woman grows older.[12]

Genetic mutations are most common in Ashkenazic Jewish, Icelandic, Finnish and Russian populations.[13,14] Generally women with inherited genetic mutations have a 59% chance of developing the disease by age 50 and an 80% chance by age 65. The predominant genes connected with the expression of breast cancer are BRCA-1 and BRCA-2. Only 0.5% of all women have these genetic weaknesses.[15]

Female Relatives with Ovarian or Endometrial Cancer

If you have a first, second, or third degree relative with ovarian or endometrial cancer, then you are at greater risk for breast cancer.[16] Women with BRCA-1 and BRCA-2 gene mutations are more susceptible to both breast and ovarian cancer. If these women develop breast cancer before the age of 40, they are at higher risk of developing ovarian cancer later on.[17] Unfortunately, ovarian cancer is difficult to detect until it is fairly advanced. Early symptoms may be a vague discomfort, similar to indigestion, in the pelvic region. Later on, the ovaries may become enlarged, with fluid accumulation in the abdomen. The CA125 is a useful blood test for monitoring the progression or remission of ovarian cancer.

One of my patients was diagnosed with ovarian cancer three months after her breast cancer diagnosis. She underwent surgery, chemotherapy, and radiation for both diseases, and combined these treatments with a diet overhaul, health promoting supplements, and a dramatic lifestyle shift. She immersed herself in yoga and meditation throughout her year of transformation, addressed family issues revolving around her husband and children, and maintained a positive attitude throughout. She had minimal side effects from her treatments, maintained good energy levels, and continues to be well several years later.

Brother or Father with Prostate Cancer

Studies show up to a fourfold elevated risk when a brother or father is diagnosed with prostate cancer.[18] Plausible theories for this include inherited genetic mutations, similar dietary histories, or siblings who have common exposures to environmental toxins, which can initiate both prostate and breast cancer.[19] Another link may be the blood levels of insulin-like growth factors 1 and 2 (or IGF-1 and IGF-2), which when elevated dramatically increases risk of both breast and prostate cancer.[20] Or siblings may be exposed to similar environments in utero, when hormone-related cancers may originate, only to develop decades later.[21]

Light-Skinned Women

Light-skinned women are slightly more likely to develop breast cancer than women with dark skin, although black women are more likely to die from it.[22,23] The reasons for the higher mortality rate in black women are at least partially due to lower socioeconomic status and inferior quality of treatment.

Body Length and Head Circumference at Birth

Girls who are born weighing more than 8.8 pounds are 3.5 times more likely to develop breast cancer before menopause than girls weighing less than 6.7 pounds at birth.[24] This effect is magnified in infants with a longer length at birth, larger head circumference, and a shorter gestation time. Infants measuring longer than 51.5 cm at birth were more likely to develop breast cancer than infants measuring less than 50 cm.[25]

PREVENTION
If you are pregnant, consume a primarily organic vegetarian diet with supplemental calcium, zinc, and iron throughout pregnancy to decrease hormonal influences that may increase breast cancer risk in your daughters later in life. Avoid dairy that contains bovine growth hormone.

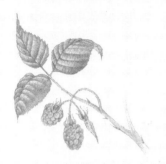

Girls who had the highest fetal growth rate are more prone to the disease later in life. Most likely hormonal influences related to diet, environmental exposures, and genetic predisposition stimulate a faster growth rate in fetuses. The mammary gland begins to develop in utero, and exposure to higher amounts of saturated fat, meat, dairy foods, estrogen, insulin, IGF-1, and growth hormone during pregnancy will have a stimulating effect on both the breasts and body of the fetus.[26,27,28,29] Exposure to chemical estrogens present in pesticides, plastics, foods and fish may have an augmenting effect on breast development in utero. The fetus is ultra-sensitive to the levels of hormone-like substances because of its small body mass. Women eating a vegetarian diet tend to give birth to children with a lower birth weight.[30]

Tallness, Obesity, and Body Mass Index

Weight management is a necessary component of a breast cancer prevention and recovery program. Larger women who are over 5 feet 6 inches tall and weigh more than 154 pounds are 3.6 times more likely to get the disease.[31] The more body fat we have, the more estrogen we will produce. Our fat cells convert adrenal hormones into estrogen and this process becomes more efficient as we grow older, particularly after menopause.[32] Obesity is also

Body Mass Index

Calculate your Body-Mass Index (BMI) using this chart.

Height (inches)	Weight (pounds)													
58	91	96	100	105	110	115	119	124	129	134	138	143	167	191
59	94	99	104	109	114	119	124	128	133	138	143	148	173	198
60	97	102	107	112	118	123	128	133	138	143	148	153	179	204
61	100	106	111	116	122	127	132	137	143	148	153	158	185	211
62	104	109	115	120	126	131	136	142	147	153	158	164	191	218
63	107	113	118	124	130	135	141	146	152	158	163	169	197	225
64	110	116	122	128	134	140	145	151	157	163	169	174	204	232
65	114	120	126	132	138	144	150	156	162	168	174	180	210	240
66	118	124	130	136	142	148	155	161	167	173	179	186	216	247
67	121	127	134	140	146	153	159	166	172	178	185	191	223	255
68	125	131	138	144	151	158	164	171	177	184	190	197	230	262
69	128	135	142	149	155	162	169	176	182	189	196	203	236	270
70	132	139	146	153	160	167	174	181	188	195	202	207	243	278
71	136	143	150	157	165	172	179	186	193	200	208	215	250	286
72	140	147	154	162	169	177	184	191	199	206	213	221	258	294
73	144	151	159	166	174	182	189	197	204	212	219	227	265	302
74	148	155	163	171	179	186	194	202	210	218	225	233	272	311
75	152	160	168	176	184	192	200	208	216	224	232	240	279	319
76	156	164	172	180	189	197	205	213	221	230	238	246	287	328
Body Mass	19	20	21	22	23	24	25	26	27	28	29	30	35	40

linked to higher levels of another hormone, insulin, which when present in the blood can both increase breast cancer risk and contribute to easy weight gain. Post-menopausal women who are more than 50 pounds overweight are 1.5 times more likely to develop breast cancer.

Researchers have found that the avoidance of weight gain and accumulation of central body fat during adulthood decreases the risk of both endometrial and post-menopausal breast cancer. The risk of breast cancer is lowest in lean women (BMI or body-mass index <22.8) who exercise at least four hours per week in their leisure time and are active in their work. In premenopausal women, a BMI >31 can increase risk by 54%, while in postmenopausal women, a BMI >28 increases risk 126%. A 2002 study demonstrated that 30-50% of deaths from breast cancer in postmenopausal women can be attributed to obesity.[33,34]

Waist Circumference and Waist-to-Hip Ratio

Body shape and fat distribution influence risk, particularly in postmenopausal women. Women with a larger waist circumference are more at risk than those who are slim.[35] Chronic high levels of insulin in the blood cause fat to be deposited around the waist and is directly related to increased risk of breast cancer.

Waist : Hip Ratio Calculation

Divide your Waist circumference _____ : _____ by your Hip circumference

= _____

If your waist-to-hip ratio is greater than .81, you have a sevenfold increase in likelihood of getting breast cancer. A ratio under .73 is protective. If you are over 50 and your waist-to-hip ratio is greater than .81, start exercising to decrease risk.[36,37,38]

Reproductive Risk Factors

Reproductive factors refer to questions of whether we have children and how many children we have and whether we nurse them or not. Many women find that they do not have a lot of control over if and when they have a child, nor should we have children simply for the sake of breast health. We must consider our emotional health, relationship stability, financial security, and life circumstances. Having a child is not a guarantee against developing breast cancer, although it helps. Earlier childbearing will have positive biological effects for mother and child.

Having Children Early

Breast cells complete their maturation process only with a full-term pregnancy, when they stabilize. They become less affected by menstrual cycle hormones, developing greater resistance to breast cancer until menopause. Partially matured breast cells have unstable DNA that is more susceptible to the process of cancer.[39,40,41]

During pregnancy, the hormone estriol (a weak, short-acting,

Having children before the age of 20 or even 30 is protective against breast cancer.

FACT

The longer the period of breast-feeding, the lower the risk of breast cancer for the mother but the higher the risk for the child.[43,44] Considering the high toxicity of organochlorines towards breast tissue and their presence in human breast milk, breast-feeding is one way of diminishing the concentration of these chemicals in our bodies.[45] Protection is given to the mother but the chemicals are passed on to the child.

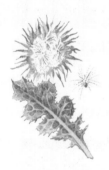

protective estrogen) is secreted by the placenta at about 1000 times the level that exists in the body before pregnancy. After a first pregnancy, there continues to be an elevated ratio of estriol to estradiol. Serum estriol concentration may be increased 14-25% for many years following a first pregnancy. Estriol is able to bind to estrogen receptors in breast cells and competitively prevent the stronger estrogens, estradiol and estrone, from binding where they would promote cell division and tumor growth.[42]

Recently a 17-year-old young woman came to see me for help with an autoimmune disorder. Her parents came in with her, and her father carried a car seat holding a beautiful baby girl. It was only half way through the interview that I realized the child was the daughter of the 17-year old, being raised by the whole family. It also turned out that the young woman was especially susceptible to breast cancer with the genetic link present on her father's side. Her grandmother had died of breast and ovarian cancer and five of her father's sisters had the disease. I couldn't help but marvel that the early pregnancy, difficult as it was, would offer her significant protection.

Breast-Feeding Dilemma

I have thought much about this very sobering issue. On the one hand, breast-feeding is good for the mother and good for the baby as it introduces beneficial bacteria to the intestinal tract, decreases allergies, provides superior nutrition, immune strength, emotional bonding, and security. On the other hand, we release our toxic inventory of environmental chemicals into our children's small bodies when we nurse, particularly the first child.

Breast Milk Toxicity

Breast milk contains about 3% fat, and as it is made, the blood carries pollutants to the breasts from fat reserves throughout the body. Contaminants in breast milk can affect the development of our children's kidneys, liver, central nervous system, and immune system.[46,47] Exposure to DDT and DDE is linked to behavioral changes in children. In 1976, 25% of samples of breast milk in the U.S.A. were found to contain PCB concentrations exceeding the legal limit, above 2.5 parts per million. Had it been bottled and sold as food it would have been banned as being too contaminated. In only six months of breast-feeding, an infant in Canada, the United States, and Europe receives the maximum recommended lifetime dose of dioxin and five times the allowable limit of PCBs set by international standards for a 150-lb adult.[48] In the Arctic, infants take in seven times more PCBs (spread by wind and water currents and ending up in animal fat) than southern Canadian or American babies and are suffering from chronic ear infections and weakened immune systems.[49]

Generally, the concentration of organochlorine chemicals in breast milk increases with the age of the mother and the amount of sport fish consumed, and decreases dramatically the longer a woman breast-feeds and the more children she nurses.[50] A 1998 study by David Josephy, Professor of Biochemistry at the University of Guelph, found that all samples of breast milk from 31 nursing mothers living near Guelph, Ontario contained aromatic amines capable of causing breast cancer in rats. These toxic substances are present in plastics, dyes, pesticides, pharmaceutical drugs, industrial waste, air, water, tobacco smoke, and some foods.[51] Guelph lies in the 'golden triangle' in southwestern Ontario, less than a hundred miles from Lake Ontario. The dioxin level in the Great Lakes was zero in the 1920s, while today it is upwards of 3200 parts per trillion.[52,53] Our breast milk contains dioxin, one of the most toxic substances known, and a potent endocrine disruptor.

Detoxifying Our Breast Milk

One way of releasing these chemicals before we conceive is through the regular, intensive use of saunas. The Finnish people have used these for many generations and have significantly lower breast cancer rates than surrounding Scandinavian countries.[54] We could eliminate most of the body's burden of toxic chemicals before having a child. Subsequent generations would not accumulate the toxins from the previous generation, which have been found to persist for five generations in animal studies. Surely this is prevention. Other ways to release toxins stored in fat tissue may be through using homeopathic preparations or chelation therapy.

While we breast-feed, we can express as much milk as possible between nursings in the first few months and discard it. Most of the fat in milk is supplied at the end of a feeding, with a higher sugar content present in the milk at the beginning of a feeding. We could express a little milk after we nurse our infants, then throw it away. We can protect ourselves and our children by eating organically grown food, limiting animal products, filtering our water, using unbleached paper, using non-freon refrigerators, and using glass containers for food and water storage rather than plastic ones. We should aim to detoxify weekly and annually with saunas, homeopathic preparations, and liver and bowel cleansers.[55]

Greater Number of Children

Having a greater number of children may reduce breast cancer risk.[56,57] Women who have five or more children have a 50% less risk of breast cancer than women with no children.[58]

Lifestyle and Healthcare Risk Factors

Lifestyle and healthcare factors linked to breast cancer are also under our control. Usually we have a little room in our lives to develop a relaxation program of some kind, to create an exercise routine, and to do annual cleansing. The challenge for many women is to put themselves first, making these goals a priority in the face of family, social, or work demands.

FACT
Women who nurse for at least six months after the age of 20 reduce their risk by 25%, while nursing for just two months offers some protection. However, breast milk has been found to contain at least 17 pesticides, 13 furans, 65 PCBs, 10 dioxins, and 30 other organochlorines. All of these chemicals contain chlorine and are hormone disruptors.

PREVENTION
Adopt a chemical free lifestyle (including reducing animal fat consumption) as early as possible in life and cleanse the body before conceiving. Breast-feed your children for at least six months. For more information on environmental risk factors, see Chapter 4, 'Environmental Impact on Breast Health.'

PREVENTION
To slow down the aging process and protect your DNA from damage take antioxidant supplements, such as vitamins C and E, or get them from your food. For more information on antioxidants, see Chapter 8, 'Nutritional Supplements for Breast Health.' Sleeping in a dark room maximizes levels of melatonin, the anti-aging hormone. See Chapter 3, 'Understanding the Hormone Puzzle,' for more information on melatonin.

Age

The risk of breast cancer increases with age. In the United States between 1994-1996, the incidence of breast cancer in women was 1 in 235 for women younger than 39 years; 1 in 25 for women 40-59 years old; 1 in 15 for women ages 60-79; and 1 in 8 over a woman's lifetime.[59]

Increased Breast Density

Breast density is evaluated and quantified most commonly through mammography. Women whose mammograms show extensive areas of dense breast tissue have a risk of breast cancer that is 1.8-6 times that of women of the same age with little or no breast density.[60]

Genetic, hormonal, and dietary factors determine breast density. A 2002 study on several hundred sets of twins from Canada, the U.S.A., and Australia determined that 63% of breast density is determined by additive genetic factors.[61] Hormones linked with increased breast density are estradiol, estrone, prolactin, and IGF-1, while progesterone and melatonin contribute to decreased breast density and offer protection.[62] Hormone replacement therapy increases breast density in post-menopausal women and should not be used by any woman interested in protecting her breasts.[63] Dietary factors that correspond to increased breast density are meat consumption, increased saturated fat and dietary cholesterol, and alcohol intake.[64,65] Breast density can be reduced with a diet low in total and saturated fat, low in cholesterol, low in animal protein, high in fiber, and high in the carotenes (present in many orange fruits and vegetables, sea weeds, and tomatoes).[66,67]

Exercise

Exercise is a protective factor against breast cancer. This effect is more pronounced among pre- rather than post-menopausal women.[68,69]

One study found that if girls engaged in any one of four specific activities, they were less likely to be diagnosed with breast cancer later in life. These activities included walking to school, biking to school, competitive training, or vigorous household chores.[70]

Long-term exercise decreases estradiol and progesterone secretion, lowers the blood levels of glucose, insulin, and IGF-1 (all of which promote breast cancer growth when they are high), delays the onset of menstruation in girls, and can prevent ovulation.[71] Exercise also enhances the metabolism of estrogen.

Prescription Drugs

Among prescription drugs that may increase the risk of breast cancer are Beta-blockers (such as Atenolol), the antidepressants Prozac, Paxil and Elavil, the antipsychotic drug Haldol, and steroids.[72,73] The tricyclic antidepressants Amoxapine (Asendin), Clomipramine (Anafranil), Desipramine (Norpramin), and Trimipramine (Surmontil) increase breast cancer risk.[74] Reserpine, a drug commonly used to lower blood pressure, increases the blood concentration of prolactin, which can stimulate breast cancers to develop.

Women who take the blood pressure lowering drug Hydralazine, also known as Apresoline, for more than five years can double their risk of breast cancer.[75] Other blood pressure lowering drugs known as calcium channel blockers increased risk in postmenopausal women, particularly in those who were simultaneously using hormone replacement therapy. These drugs include verapamil, diltiaxem, nifedipine, and nonnifedipine dihydropyridines.[76] Spironolactone (Aldactone) and Furosemide are diuretics used to lower blood pressure which may increase breast cancer risk. Two different antibiotics may increase risk — Metronidazole (Flagyl), which is used as an antifungal agent, and Nitrofurazone, used to treat skin wounds and stomach ulcers.[77,78]

The tranquilizers Valium and Xanax increase prolactin levels, which stimulates the growth and development of invasive breast cancer.[79] Unfortunately, these two medications are commonly given to cancer patients to decrease anxiety. Actual anti-cancer drugs may elevate breast cancer incidence 15 or more years after their use. Nitrogen mustard, vincristine, acronycine, cytembena, isophosphamide, and procarbazine have been linked to increased future risk of breast cancer.[80,81] Cholesterol-lowering drugs consisting of fibrates and statins, such as Pravachol (pravastatin), have been found to cause breast cancers in rodents; one study found that women taking pravastatin had 12 times the rate of breast cancer than women who were not taking the drug.[82] Tagamet, a drug commonly used to treat indigestion and ulcers, can cause breast enlargement in men who use it and is linked to increased breast cancer risk.[83] Antihistamines, such as Claritin and Atarax, may promote the growth of already existing cancers.[84]

Dental Problems

Many medical doctors and alternative health practitioners, particularly in Germany, are aware of chronic degenerative diseases being linked in part to problems with the teeth. Each tooth is associated with an acupuncture meridian and organ. The teeth most directly related to the breasts are the two teeth to the front of the wisdom teeth on both sides of the upper jaw. If there is a low-grade infection, mercury toxicity, or root canal associated with a particular tooth, it may manifest as a problem in another area of the body. The teeth are commonly sites of bacterial or parasitic infections.

Root canals in particular may harbor bacteria and toxins that enter the lymphatic system and bloodstream from the tooth root. These circulate through the body, causing depressed immunity and potentially infecting or producing inflammation in another body part. Practitioners who use electrodermal screening, thermography, or applied kinesiology can sometimes determine whether this is a problem, while dentists can scan the teeth and jaw with a sophisticated ultrasound device called a 'Cavatat' or, less effectively, with a panoramic x-ray. Treatment may include the use of homeopathic remedies, extraction of the infected tooth, or removal and replacement of mercury amalgam fillings with ceramic or porcelain fillings, followed by mercury detoxification. The plastic replacement fillings can act as weak estrogens, as they usually include phthalates and bisphenol-A. I believe they should not be used.

Body Terrain Imbalance

Just as certain vegetables or flowers require different minerals, organic matter, water, and a specific soil pH to flourish, so do our bodies.

If this 'terrain' is normalized, disease retreats. We now have several methodologies to analyze biological terrain, used by naturopathic doctors, medical doctors, and other health practitioners. You can seek out a well-trained practitioner who uses Darkfield Microscopy and/or Biological Terrain Analysis (BTA) to help assess your body's willingness to harbor cancer cells. These tests will not tell you if you have cancer, but they will suggest whether your body presents the kind of terrain conducive to the growth of cancer. An unhealthy terrain would be one with low minerals, an excessive production of free radicals, an overly acidic or overly alkaline pH of various body fluids, the presence of toxic metals and/or chemicals, an overload of bacteria, fungus, parasites and/or viruses, low oxygen, and sluggish 'sticky' blood.

It is not too difficult to alter the biological terrain with liver, bowel, kidney, lymphatic, and sauna detoxification, a cleaner diet, digestive enzymes, antioxidant and mineral supplementation; and the use of specialized formulas such as the German Sanum remedies.

Chronic Inflammation

Chronic inflammatory diseases occur in an unbalanced terrain and are the result of a cascade of biochemical reactions in the body, which culminate in the production of harmful hormone-like substances. These substances promote heart disease, arthritis, allergies, asthma, colitis, dermatitis, Alzheimer's, and cancer.

Inflammation can be the product of toxic overload, poor liver and bowel function, faulty diet, antioxidant deficiency, injury, stress, allergy and/or chronic infection. The inflammatory hormones are set off by two different enzyme pathways, the cyclooxygenase pathway (COX-2) or the lipoxygenase pathway (LOX). Luckily there are simple, effective natural ways to intercept these pathways and prevent excessive formation of the harmful end products. Some natural substances that decrease inflammation are fish oils and flaxseed oil, small amounts of evening primrose oil or borage oil, the minerals magnesium and zinc, the antioxidant vitamins A, C, and E, as well as vitamin B6. Particularly good inhibitors of COX-2 and LOX are curcumin (which gives the golden color to turmeric), bromelain (from pineapple), green tea, grapes, quercetin, ginger and the Ayurvedic herb Boswellia. Herbal inhibitors of COX-2 that show promise in cancer treatment include the Chinese herbs Scutellaria baicalensis, Tripterygium wilfordii Hook.f., and Isatis

FACT
The pH or acid/alkaline balance of our bodily fluids, the ability of our red blood cells to take up oxygen, the amount of free radical activity, the 'stickiness' of our blood, and our mineral balance influence the kinds of organisms and diseases that can live within us.

FACT
Drugs or nutritional supplements which block the production of certain inflammatory hormones (called prostaglandins, thromboxanes, and leukotrienes) have been found to cut the risk of breast cancer in women who use them regularly. [33]

PREVENTION
Reduce breast cancer risk with the regular use of green tea, pineapple, grapes, turmeric, and ginger in your diet to decrease harmful prostaglandins, leukotrienes, and thromboxanes.

tinctoria, and the western herb, white willow bark.[85,86,87,88]

Researchers at Ohio State University found that postmenopausal women who took a single ibuprofen tablet at least three days a week for a decade or more reduced their breast cancer risk 49%. Ibuprofen is an anti-inflammatory drug commonly known as Advil or Motrin. Women who used aspirin (acetylsalicylic acid) several times a week saw their risk drop by 28%. Tylenol or 'baby aspirin', on the other hand, had no effect.[89] The dietary substances listed above work in a similar way without side effects.

Immune Deficiency and Allergies

Persons with illnesses suggestive of immune deficiency, such as allergies or chronic viral infections, have a greater susceptibility to breast cancer. Specific conditions can be treated effectively with naturopathy, homeopathy, and Chinese medicine to improve immune function.

Constipation

Women who do not have at least two bowel movements per week increase their risk of breast cancer. One study has shown that women with two or less bowel movements per week had 4.5 times the risk of pre-cancerous breast changes than other women who had bowel movements more than once daily.[90] Part of a breast cancer prevention program, therefore, includes encouraging at least two bowel movements daily.

Monthly Breast Self-Exams

Approximately 90% of all breast cancers are found by women who notice changes in their own breasts.[91] Women who practice breast self-exams detect their cancers earlier with less likelihood of finding positive lymph nodes and have smaller tumors than women who do not perform breast self-exams.[92] Monthly breast self-exams are able to reduce breast cancer deaths by 20-30%, by providing early detection before the cancer has become invasive.[93]

Cigarette Smoking

Common sense tells us that cigarette smoking is harmful and can increase breast cancer risk. Several studies demonstrate that girls who begin to smoke before age 17 and continue for several decades are slightly more likely to develop the disease.[94] There may be a weak association between chronic second-hand smoke exposure and breast cancer, but the research is divided.[95] We do know that women who are smokers are prone to infection and require a longer healing time after breast cancer surgery.[96]

Hair Dyes

Roughly 40% of American women between the ages of 18 and 60 dye their hair every month or two, and may continue this practice for decades. Chemicals from permanent and semi-permanent dyes are easily absorbed through the scalp. Some of the carcinogenic substances found in hair dyes, detergents, and preservatives include

PREVENTION
To increase regular bowel movements, drink 8-10 glasses of water daily. Use wheat bran, psyllium, flaxseeds, and legumes, and eat 6-9 servings of fruits and vegetables daily to increase your fiber content. For more information on dietary fiber, see Chapter 7, 'Eating Right for Breast Health.'

PREVENTION
Perform monthly breast self-exams. Teach your daughters to do the same. For a complete discussion of breast self-examination techniques, with breast mapping exercises, see Chapter 2, 'Getting to Know Our Breasts.'

PREVENTION
Stop smoking and avoid second-hand smoke. Consult an acupuncturist, naturopathic doctor, or self-help group to help you stop smoking.

FACT
Women who start to use hair dyes in their twenties are more at risk of developing breast cancer than women who begin to dye their hair in their thirties or forties.

PREVENTION
Avoid hair dyes containing carcinogenic substances. Use henna or natural dyes instead.

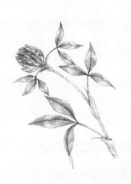

PREVENTION
Avoid breast implants and consider surgical removal if you already have them.

FACT
Women who wear their bras more than 12 hours a day increase their risk of breast cancer by a factor of 6.

PREVENTION
Don't wear a bra unless you have to; take it off as soon as you are able to; use a cotton stretchy bra without underwires if you can.

diaminotoluene, diaminoanisole, 4-ethoxy-m-phenylene sulfate (4-EMPD), para-phenylenediamine, artificial colors (C1 disperses Blue 1, D&C Red 33, HC Blue No. 1), dioxane, diethanoloamine, triethanolamine, ceteareth, laureth, polyethylene glycol, DMDM-hydantoin, imidazolidinyl urea, quarternium 15, nitrosamines, and formaldehyde.

Hair dyes represent a cumulative toxicity. Darker shades of dyes contribute most to increased breast cancer risk. Hairdressers who apply these dyes have higher than normal rates of bladder cancer as well.

In the last several years there has been a movement towards safer hair dyes. Some lines that are safe include Igora Botanic, VitaWave from California, and Paul Penders hair coloring products.[97]

Breast Implants

There are two main types of breast implants that have been in use since the late 1960s — one uses silicone gel wrapped in either a seamless silicone outer envelope or casing made of polyurethane foam; the other uses a saline solution injected into a silicone pouch that has been surgically inserted into the breast. Silicone gel implants were banned in the United States in 1992, while saline filled implants are still readily available.

Some of the problems associated with silicone gel implants include rupture and leakage of the silicone into the body, an increase in autoimmune and rheumatoid diseases, and a higher breast cancer incidence in women with the implants. Polyurethane foam, used for the casings of many implants, degrades in breast tissue as it releases a potent carcinogen, 2, 4-toluene diisocyanate (TDI), which then is converted into another carcinogen, 2, 4-diaminotoluene (TDA). Both TDI and TDA are able to induce breast cancer in rodents. TDA is found in the urine, blood, and breast milk of women with implants containing polyurethane foam.[98]

Wearing a Bra

Wearing a bra, especially an underwire bra, increases our risk of cancer. The lymphatic system is one of the body's mechanisms that protects our breasts by removing cellular debris. For it to function properly, there needs to be movement of the breasts. Tight bras restrict movement and collapse the lymphatic vessels, while going braless increases lymphatic circulation and offers protection.

Hormonal Risk Factors

There are many hormonal links to breast cancer and profound interactions between the environment and our glands. We have a degree of control over hormonal links through the choices we make about using birth control pills, fertility drugs, and hormone replacement therapy. We also need to do more subtle, routine testing of glandular function, specifically monitoring the estrogen quotient, C2 and C16 estrogen ratio, IGF-1 and IGFBP-3 ratio, fasting insulin, a.m. and p.m. cortisol, progesterone, testosterone, melatonin, and thyroid function, including reverse T3. We need to acknowledge the profoundly debilitating effects our chemically toxic environment is having on our glandular health and work to eliminate these toxins from our bodies and from our environment. See Chapter 3, 'Understanding the Hormone Puzzle,' for a complete discussion of the endocrine system and breast health.

Environmental Risk Factors

The links between our environment and breast cancer are overwhelmingly evident, though for many years I could not bear to know this intellectually and emotionally. I believe our culture is in a collective state of denial about what we have done and continue to do to the environment. The only way we will heal ourselves and the earth is by shaking off that denial and taking personal responsibility. We must each look at how we contribute to the environmental crisis, clean up our little corner of the earth, and take a stand together against the chemical, plastic, pulp and paper, and nuclear industries — and the political machinery that support them. See Chapter 4, 'Environmental Impact on Breast Health,' for a complete discussion of environmental risk factors and strategies for avoiding them.

PREVENTION
Complete the 'Breast Health Balance Sheet' and revise it periodically as you reduce your risk factors and increase your protective factors by following the actions for prevention in this book.

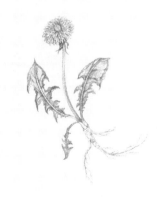

Dietary Risk Factors

Here is where we can make a great deal of difference to our breast health. We now know which foods promote breast cancer and which ones prevent or even reverse it. Foods can be medicine. There is a growing trend supporting organic farming methods, and as this continues, breast cancer may decline somewhat. For our physical and spiritual health, it is important that we make a connection to the soil that grows our food — plant a garden, use window boxes, link up with an organic farm and work in the fields. Part of our sickness is due to our alienation from nature and our broken link to the creative cycle. We have become uprooted from the soil that nourishes us. We can utilize and develop farming methods that replenish the soil rather than trying to dominate and control nature with chemicals. See Chapter 7, 'Eating Right for Breast Health,' and Chapter 8, "Nutritional Supplements for Breast Health," for a complete discussion of the role of diet and nutrients in the causes and prevention of cancer.

Psychological and Spiritual Risk Factors

Psychological factors linked to breast cancer are mostly about denying who we really are, ignoring or bottling up our true feelings, and assuming the role of the 'pleaser' in our attempts to feel loved. Healing comes from connecting to our deepest desires and callings, courageously creating our own path and honoring our intuition. Healing also comes from developing assertiveness, releasing anger, and resolving conflict.

I think of serious illness as a path of purification so that eventually we'll relate to our soul. Illness is sometimes the messenger sent to wake us up, asking us to choose to live or to die. Our spiritual selves need to be nourished just as our minds, emotions, and bodies do. No longer can we separate these parts of ourselves, feed one or two occasionally, and hope to stay healthy. They all need to be taken care of. We take care of our spiritual self when we connect to what is meaningful for us, live with a sense of purpose, express our creativity, laugh and have fun, and develop some sort of regular checking-in process. We can call this a spiritual practice. It may consist of prayer, meditation, yoga, dreamwork, martial arts, writing, creative activity, or walking in the woods. Mostly it's a listening process — paying attention to the inner voice that guides our life and actions day to day. See Chapter 9, 'Psychological and Spiritual Means for Preventing Breast Cancer,' for a discussion of these related risk factors and how to use psychological and spiritual strategies to overcome them.

Breast Health Balance Sheet

This 'balance sheet' summarizes the risk factors for breast cancer explained throughout the book. It also outlines those factors that protect us from breast cancer. Make checkmarks beside the risk factors and protective factors that are true for you. The bracketed numbers to the right of some entries refer to how much that risk factor increases your likelihood of having breast cancer; that is, (+2) means your risk doubles, (+3.6) means it increases your risk over three and a half times. If the number is beside a protective factor, it means that it decreases your risk by that amount. Mark these high risk and highly protective factors with a highlighter.

Come back to the balance sheet at least once a year to see what progress you have made in adopting a breast health/cancer prevention program. If you feel overwhelmed on your first read through, put it aside and come back to it another day. Things you may not understand initially will be explained in later chapters of this book in their appropriate section.

To calculate your 'body-mass index', take your weight in kilograms or pounds and divide by the square of your height in meters or feet — or use the chart above. To determine your waist-to-hip ratio, divide your waist measurement by your hip measurement, using the calculation above.

RISK FACTORS	*PROTECTIVE FACTORS*
HEREDITARY	**HEREDITARY**
☐ Mother or sister with breast cancer (+2)	☐ No family history of cancer
☐ Relative with ovarian or endometrial cancer	☐ No family ovarian or endometrial cancer
☐ Brother or father with prostate cancer (+4)	☐ No family prostate cancer
☐ Light-skinned	☐ Dark-skinned
☐ Body mass index > 28	☐ Body mass index < 22.8
☐ Birth weight > 8.8 lbs (+3.5)	☐ Birth weight < 6.7 lbs
☐ Birth length > 51.5 cm	☐ Birth length < 50 cm
☐ Over 5' 6" tall	☐ Under 5' 6" tall
☐ Weight > 154 lbs. (+3.6)	☐ Appropriate weight; weight < 153 lbs.
☐ Waist to hip ratio >.81 (+7)	☐ Waist to hip ratio < .73
REPRODUCTIVE	**REPRODUCTIVE**
☐ No children or children after 30	☐ Gave birth before age 20 or 30
☐ No children	☐ More than one child (-.5 with 5 kids)
☐ No breast-feeding	☐ Breast-fed kids for at least 6 months (-2.5)

RISK FACTORS	PROTECTIVE FACTORS
LIFESTYLE AND HEALTHCARE	**LIFESTYLE AND HEALTHCARE**
☐ Aging	☐ Use antioxidants and anti-aging supplements
☐ High breast density (+1.8 - +6)	☐ Low breast density
☐ Lack of exercise	☐ Regular exercise (4 hours weekly) (-.60)
☐ < 2 bowel movement per week (+4.5)	☐ 2 or more bowel movements daily
☐ Use prescription drugs: beta-blockers (Prozac, Paxil, Elavil); tricyclic antidepressants (Amoxapine, Clomipramine, Desipramine and Trimipramine, Haldol); steroids (Reserpine, hydralazine, Tagamet, metronidazole, vincristine, Nitrofurazone, Valium, Xanax, nitrogen mustard, procarbazine); cholesterol-lowering drugs; Claritin, Atarax, the diuretics Spironolactone and Furosemide, and the anti-cancer drugs (vincristine, acronycine, cytembena, and isophosphamide)	☐ Use herbal, nutritional, homeopathic, and naturopathic recommendations when possible instead of prescription drugs. Educate yourself on the side effects of medications before taking them.
☐ Dental problems: mercury fillings, root canals, chronic infection	☐ Replace mercury fillings with ceramic, remove root canal teeth, clear infection
☐ Imbalanced biological terrain	☐ Normalize biological terrain
☐ Chronic inflammation use curcumin and bromelain regularly	☐ Vegetarian, no dairy fat in diet,
☐ Immune deficiency, allergies	☐ Follow immune-strengthening program
☐ Underactive thyroid; iodine deficiency	☐ Correct thyroid function; use seaweeds
☐ Annual mammograms (from radiation exposure) (+.5)	☐ Monthly breast self exam; annual thermograms, use AMAS test to find cancer early (-.2)
☐ Cigarette smoking increases risk	☐ No smoking; avoid secondhand smoke
☐ Alcohol increases risk (> 3 drinks/week)	☐ Avoid alcohol or have minimally
☐ Use commercial hair dyes	☐ Use henna or natural hair dyes
☐ Have breast implants	☐ No breast implants; have them removed
☐ Wear a tight-fitting bra	☐ Go braless or use looser cotton bra
☐ Mineral and enzyme deficiency	☐ Eat organic, replace minerals and enzymes
☐ Parasitic infection	☐ Do parasite cleanse once or twice yearly
☐ Liver toxicity	☐ Do liver cleanse once or twice yearly
☐ Bowel toxicity	☐ Do bowel cleanse once yearly; replace flora
☐ Use of antibiotics	☐ Avoid antibiotics, deal with candidiasis
☐ Chemical toxins accumulate in fat tissue	☐ Use saunas regularly or sauna detox yearly
☐ Poor lymphatic circulation	☐ Use skin-brushing, rebounding, exercise

RISK FACTORS	PROTECTIVE FACTORS
HORMONAL	**HORMONAL**
☐ Estrogen quotient is .5-.8	☐ Estrogen quotient is >1.2
☐ Low ratio of C2 to C16 estrogen	☐ High ratio of C2 to C16 estrogen
☐ Low ratio of C2 to C4 estrogen	☐ High ratio of C2 to C4 estrogen
☐ Early onset of menstruation (<11) (+2)	☐ Late onset of menstruation (>14)
☐ Late menopause (>52) (+2)	☐ Early menopause (<45)
☐ Menstrual cycle <25 days (+2)	☐ Menstrual cycle 26-28 days
☐ Low progesterone (+5.4)	☐ Normal progesterone
☐ Fibrocystic breasts (+1.8)	☐ Healthy breast tissue
☐ Increased testosterone	☐ Normal testosterone
☐ Increased prolactin	☐ Normal prolactin
☐ Increased growth hormone	☐ Avoid dairy with bovine growth hormone
☐ Increased insulin	☐ Normal insulin levels
☐ Women whose mothers had high estrogen levels during pregnancy	☐ Protect self/fetus from high estrogen in pregnancy
☐ Unbalanced thyroid; iodine deficiency	☐ Correct thyroid function; use seaweeds
☐ High blood levels of IGF-1 (+7)	☐ Normal blood levels of IGF-1
☐ Unbalanced cortisol	☐ Normal cortisol
☐ Decreased melatonin levels	☐ High melatonin; meditation practice
☐ Sleep with light on at night: exposure to light at night decreases melatonin production, increases risk	☐ Sleep in a dark room; meditate shortly before bed
☐ Birth control pills used before age 20 or for more than 5 years before age 35 (+3)	☐ Natural fertility methods such as sympto-thermo or Justisse method, condoms, Luna
☐ Use of fertility drugs in past year	☐ Avoidance of fertility drugs
☐ Post-menopausal and >50 lb. overweight	☐ Post-menopausal and not overweight
☐ Estrogen replacement therapy, especially when used for more than 5 years	☐ No estrogen replacement therapy, or have stopped for > 5 yrs.
☐ Former use of the drug DES or your mother took it while pregnant (+.4)	☐ No DES; avoid drugs in pregnancy
ENVIRONMENTAL	**ENVIRONMENTAL**
☐ Exposure to radiation	☐ Seaweeds daily, miso and lentils 3x weekly
☐ Fly frequently	☐ Fly seldom
☐ Live within 50 miles of a nuclear reactor	☐ Live > 50 miles from a nuclear reactor
☐ Continuous exposure to electricity and electromagnetic fields	☐ Live in the country with few electrical devices

RISK FACTORS	PROTECTIVE FACTORS
❑ Work in the electrical trade (+.7)	❑ Work away from excess electricity
❑ Install, repair telephones (+2.2)	
❑ Sleep within 2' of electrical devices	❑ Sleep >3' away from electrical devices
❑ Sit < 2' from front, < 4' from sides of computer video display terminals	❑ Sit further from computer video display terminals and use them < 20 hours weekly
❑ Use an electric blanket	❑ Use cotton, wool, down blankets
❑ Have worked on a farm (+9)	❑ Never worked on a farm, or worked on organic farm
❑ Exposure to pesticides: food, lawn, farm, golf courses, public areas	❑ Eat organic, avoid pesticides
❑ Live in industrialized area	❑ Live away from industry & chemical exposure
❑ Exposure to petrochemicals, gas stations	❑ Use car less, use full serve gas station
❑ Exposure to formaldehyde	❑ Choose products without formaldehyde
❑ Exposure to benzene	❑ Avoid benzene
❑ Exposure to organochlorines	❑ Recognize and avoid organochlorines
❑ Use of chemical or industrial cleansers	❑ Use of non-toxic cleansers
❑ Exposure to carcinogens	❑ Recognize and avoid known carcinogens
❑ Live near a hospital incinerator	❑ Live away from a hospital incinerator
❑ Live near a PVC recycling plant	❑ Live away from a PVC recycling plant
❑ Use plastics	❑ Avoid plastics, use glass, wax paper, cardboard, butcher paper
❑ Live near a chemical plant	❑ Live away from a chemical plant
❑ Live near a toxic waste site or dump	❑ Decrease waste; live away from a toxic waste site or dump
❑ Live near a sewage treatment plant treatment plant	❑ Use a composting toilet, live away from a sewage
❑ Use chlorine bleach	❑ Use non-chlorine bleach
❑ Drink chlorinated water	❑ Drink filtered water
❑ Dry-clean clothing	❑ Avoid dry-cleaning; use natural detergents

DIETARY	DIETARY
❑ High fat consumption: > 30% total calories	❑ Low fat consumption: < 15% total calories
❑ Low fiber: < 10 grams daily	❑ High fiber: >30 grams daily (-.30)
❑ Eat meat weekly	❑ Vegetarian (-.30)
❑ Use dairy products	❑ Use soy milk, organic goat milk, or low fat org. dairy
❑ Eat sweets, sugar products	❑ Have 2 or more fruits daily, avoid sweets
❑ Use processed food	❑ Use whole, unrefined foods
❑ Use bread products regularly	❑ Use beans, whole grains

RISK FACTORS	PROTECTIVE FACTORS
❑ Drink coffee	❑ Drink herbal teas, e.g., red clover, dandelion
❑ No soy products	❑ Soy products daily
❑ No orange fruits and vegetables	❑ Use 2 foods high in vitamin A daily
❑ Use vegetable oils, animal fat, margarine and cooked oils; have low essential fatty acids	❑ Use unheated flaxseed and olive oil, clean fish oil
❑ Minimal fruits and vegetables	❑ Use 6-9 servings of fruits and vegetables/day
❑ Eat mostly cooked food	❑ 50-85% raw food
❑ No brassicas (cauliflower, cabbage, broccoli)	❑ Raw brassicas daily
❑ High salt intake	❑ Low sodium / high potassium
❑ Overly acidic body	❑ Keep pH of urine and saliva at 6.4 -7.2
❑ Use of plastic food containers and wraps	❑ Use glass, ceramic or stainless steel containers

PSYCHOLOGICAL | **PSYCHOLOGICAL**

❑ Deny, bury, repress or hold on to anger	❑ Express anger constructively and let it go
❑ Ignore one's own needs; please others	❑ Define your needs; become assertive
❑ Feel alienation	❑ Find or create your community
❑ Death of a loved one or loss of a relationship within the previous one to five years	❑ Express your grief; find reasons for living, find something or someone to love
❑ Stress and the inability to relax	❑ Regular relaxation breaks
❑ Living a life following someone else's script rather than one's own	❑ Follow your deep desires and callings; create your path

SPIRITUAL | **SPIRITUAL**

❑ Hopelessness, despair	❑ Spiritual counseling, therapy, prayer, yoga
❑ Lack of a sense of purpose	❑ Develop a meaningful life, find your passion
❑ Lack of joy	❑ Laugh, play, have fun
❑ Loss of faith	❑ Create a relationship with your soul
❑ Foiled creative fire	❑ Express your creativity
❑ Ignored intuition	❑ Awaken and follow your intuition
❑ Lack of support	❑ Find at least one supportive person, support group or spiritual group

OTHER RISK FACTORS | *OTHER PROTECTIVE FACTORS*

Summary

Many practical actions for avoiding or ameliorating the risk of developing breast cancer from hereditary, reproductive, and lifestyle or healthcare risks are within our immediate control. Strategies for preventing cancer arising from hormonal, environmental, dietary, psychological, and spiritual factors will be presented in the following chapters. As we develop our understanding, we can return to the "Breast Health Balance Sheet" and choose to eliminate risk factors while gradually incorporating protective strategies.

For now, look at some of the lifestyle and healthcare links to breast cancer we've discussed and choose one or two that you can implement right away.

1) How can you include 35 minutes of exercise in your day? Can you walk to work instead of driving, or get up a half hour earlier in the morning and use the treadmill, go to the gym or find a neighbor to walk with near your home?
2) If you are not having at least two bowel movements a day, it is time to increase your fiber intake or see a health practitioner to guide you to a solution.
3) Wear your bra less often, or find one that fits a little looser.
4) Talk to your health food store or hair dresser about alternatives to chemical dyes, or use henna to hide your gray.
5) See a biological dentist who can advise you about porcelain fillings and whether you may have a low-grade infection from a root canal that needs to be addressed.

CHAPTER TWO

Getting to *Know* *our* Breasts

CONTENTS

*I*NTIMATELY LINKED with nurturing, sexuality, and motherhood, our breasts are perhaps the part of our body that we have the most feelings about, positive and negative. Many of us ignore those feelings and don't understand how our breasts work and what affects them. We are often ignorant about the conditions that show up as lumps or pain at different times in our lives and are hesitant to perform breast self-exams because of what we may find. We can become familiar with our breasts by understanding their anatomy and physiology through breast exploration and self-examination. We can recognize the symptoms of various breast ailments and diseases, including cancer. We also need to understand the diagnostic tests for breast cancer and become fully aware of these procedures so we can make informed choices.

Breast Anatomy and Physiology

The normal function of our breasts is to secrete milk, providing food for our infants after they are born. They are also a source of sexual attraction and stimulation. Found between the second and sixth ribs, and extending from the sternum to the axilla, or armpit, the breasts rest upon the pectoralis major muscles. Each breast has a nipple located at its tip and a surrounding circular area of pigmented skin called the areola.

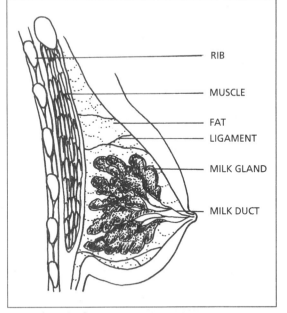

RIB

MUSCLE

FAT

LIGAMENT

MILK GLAND

MILK DUCT

The mammary glands found in each breast are specialized tissue, being modified sweat glands surrounded by adipose (fatty) tissue. It is the amount of fatty tissue that determines breast size and shape. During puberty the ovaries produce estrogen which initiates the growth of the mammary glands and adipose tissue.

Resembling the branches of a tree, each mammary gland is composed of 15-20 lobes. The lobes are subdivided into smaller lobules, which contain the glandular alveoli. After pregnancy and delivery, the hormones of prolactin (luteotropin) and oxytocin, secreted by the pituitary gland, stimulate the mammary glands in the breasts to secrete milk. The milk is carried from the lobes through ducts to the nipple. Breast cancer most commonly occurs in these ducts and lobes.

I think of this 'tree' in our breasts as being a hidden tree of life. Breast milk is its fruit. Normally breast milk sustains life. Today chemical pollutants and radiation poison the fruit, just as our air, water, soil and many planetary life forms are poisoned. The breast cancer epidemic is but a symptom and symbol of our planet in crisis. The tree of life is poisoned and dying.

Breasts and Our Body Systems

The health of our breasts is intimately linked and dependent upon the health of our other body systems. If we have breast cancer, healing depends on accurately assessing imbalances in each of these systems, and then correcting them. To prevent breast cancer, we must optimize the functioning of each of these guardians of our health.

The Lymphatic System

The lymphatic system is composed of lymphatic vessels, lymph nodes located along these vessels, lymphocytes (or white blood cells) housed in the nodes, and specialized lymphatic organs (thymus, spleen, tonsils). The circulation and efficiency of the lymphatic system is dependent upon exercise, deep breathing, and freedom from constrictive clothing.

The lymphatic system is the house-cleaner for the body's circulatory system. Every 24 hours, the heart pumps over 5 gallons or about 20 liters of fluid from the network of capillaries belonging to

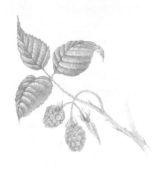

the circulatory system into the tissues of the body, bathing them with oxygen and nutrients. About 85% of this fluid returns to the capillary network of the circulatory system, carrying carbon dioxide and metabolic waste back to the lungs and heart. Fifteen percent of the fluid is left behind in the spaces between the cells.

The job of the lymphatic system is to return this residual 15% of fluid to the heart and circulation, after filtering it and removing dead cells, cancer cells, bacteria, fungi, viruses, and toxic debris. This amounts to about one half cup of fluid every hour. If this fluid were not removed, the swelling would destroy surrounding tissues and we would eventually die. Along with the cleaned up fluid, the lymphatic system delivers its own army of lymphocytes into the blood to fight cancer, infection, and unwanted organisms.

The many lymph nodes and lymphatic vessels present in the underarm area, beneath and above the collar bone, and deep in the breast tissue are there to protect us from breast cancer. If we exercise regularly, move our armpits daily, breathe deeply, and don't compress our lymphatic vessels with a tight bra, these nodes and vessels will work stupendously for us. For more tips on reconditioning your lymphatic system, see Chapter 6, 'Activating Our Lymphatic and Immune Systems.'

The Endocrine System

The glands of the endocrine system — ovaries, liver, thyroid, pineal, pituitary, thymus, adrenals, pancreas — are like an orchestra whose players have a score in front of them, but the performance is always slightly different. The glands are the various musical instruments and the hormones they produce are the notes we hear. They are dependent upon and responsive to one another, each with a separate task, and the music is their simultaneous expression.

Our glands have an amazing communication system between them — and their interactive hormonal expression has a profound effect on our breasts, positive and negative. We can evaluate this expression using blood, urine, and saliva tests, and re-tune the glands through diet, specific nutrients, balancing regimens, adjustments in our environment, and shifts in our thoughts and feelings. With these tools we gain confidence in managing our breast health.

The Digestive System

What we eat, how we eat, when we eat, how we absorb, and how we eliminate our food strongly affects the vitality of the liver, how our hormones express themselves, and ultimately our breast health. Digestion begins before we even sit down to eat, with salivary enzyme secretion in the mouth occurring at the mere thought of a delicious bite. Complete chewing, relaxation, conscious food choices and the timing and size of each meal all play a role in maximizing digestive, hormonal, and whole body health.

The digestive organs include the mouth and salivary glands, esophagus, stomach, liver, gallbladder, pancreas, small intestine, and large intestine. If we don't take the time to relax and chew our food, digestion will be impaired. If the stomach is unable to produce enough hydrochloric acid, protein and mineral absorption will suffer, leading to deficiencies in iodine, zinc, selenium, magnesium, and calcium, which can negatively affect our breasts. If the large intestine is sluggish and we have few bowel movements each week, liver function suffers, we hold on to more estrogen, and breast cancer risk increases. We need to practice eating to live rather than living to eat.

The Liver or Hepatic System

At the center of digestion and breast health is the liver. One of the primary jobs of the liver is to filter the blood – almost 30% of our entire blood supply goes through the liver each minute. Most of that blood has come from the stomach, spleen, pancreas, and small and large intestine through the portal vein en route to the liver to be detoxified. A small amount of blood comes into the liver via the hepatic artery.

The liver has two detoxification systems that act in sequence to neutralize chemicals and break down hormones. These systems manage our estrogens for us, converting the potentially harmful ones into safer estrogens. The liver can only do this well when it is not overwhelmed with chemicals and waste from the external and internal environment, dumped into it through the portal vein and hepatic artery.

The liver also adjusts blood sugar levels – it stores glycogen and releases it to be utilized as glucose for energy. The liver is responsible for making the hormone IGF-1 when stimulated to do so by dietary and other hormonal signals – this hormone is strongly associated with increased breast cancer risk. The liver makes some nutrients for us, like coenzyme Q10, and vitamin D. Both of these nutrients protect our breasts. Bless your liver each day by limiting your intake of coffee and alcohol, eating organic food whenever possible, and using a sauna regularly to lighten the burden of chemicals that need to be deactivated in the liver.

The Cardiovascular/Pulmonary System

The cardiovascular system refers to the heart and blood vessels — the role of the arteries is to distribute oxygenated blood to the rest of the body, supplying energy and nutrients, while the veins return the blood, carrying carbon dioxide back to the heart and lungs for re-oxygenation. Efficiency in this task is dependent upon the strength of the heart as a muscle, the openness of the arteries, the fluidity of the blood, and lack of local constriction of the blood vessels.

Several things will improve blood circulation. Regular aerobic exercise tonifies the pumping action of the heart, a diet low in saturated fat, cholesterol, sweets, refined carbohydrates, and meat and high in anti-oxidants helps to keep the arteries clean. Vitamins B3, C, and E as well as Omega 3 oils such as flaxseed and fish oils increase the fluidity of the blood. Daily alternating hot and cold showers enhance local circulation.

The amount of oxygen carried by the red blood cells is dependent in part upon the quality of our breathing, for after the blood returns to the heart it is circulated to the lungs where the red blood cells pick up a new supply of oxygen.

FACT

If we have been exposed to chemicals, pollutants, and carcinogens, if we have inefficient digestion or a toxic bowel, if we drink coffee or alcohol, take pharmaceutical medications, or eat food sprayed with pesticides, added stress will be placed on the liver and its detoxification systems.

PREVENTION

Develop daily and seasonal rituals to cleanse the liver, kidneys, lymph, and large intestine to improve long term liver function, protecting your breasts as you do so. More strategies for improved liver performance are presented in Chapter 5, 'Detoxifying Our Bodies.

FACT

Cancer thrives in tissues that are low in oxygen, so the more effectively we deliver oxygen and nutrients to our cells, the better. With a regular practice of breathing exercises we can improve tissue oxygenation and discourage the possibility of cancer.

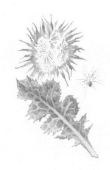

Befriending Our Breasts

Many of us feel vulnerable around our breasts. We may have celebrated their gentle expansion during puberty or felt shame and discomfort. We may perceive them as being too large or too small, too noticed or not noticed enough. We often judge our bodies based on the images that television, film, and advertising gives us, causing many women to reshape their breasts through implants or surgery. We may feel that they are touched too much or want them to be touched more. We may be uncomfortable with the way they move when we exercise or their tenderness before menstruation. We may lament the fact that we could not or did not breast-feed our children long enough or we may have disliked the breast-feeding experience. Our breasts are intimately connected to our capacity to nurture others and ourselves and to the nurturing we received from our mothers.

Most of us experience an element of fear connected to our breasts because of the risk of breast cancer. Many women consider their breasts a liability. Often this fear causes us to cut ourselves off from our breasts psychically. Our fear prevents us from touching our breasts and from befriending them. In its wisdom, our mind sometimes expresses symptoms in parts of our bodies we deny in order to gather our attention. This can be the catalyst that moves us towards wholeness and integration.

Breast Self-Examinations

Once we have developed a healing tactile relationship with our breasts, we can begin to perform regular breast self-exams. Many women experience fear at the thought of a breast self-exam and are reluctant to perform them on a regular basis. Other women have a hard time distinguishing between various kinds of lumps and feel confused and frustrated. The key to success is familiarity through repetition. Each of you will have your own unique 'breast topography'; once a familiarity with what is normal for you is gained, variations from the norm are more easily noticed. Be patient and persist.

The self-exam involves two stages: a visual exam and a palpation exam. Women who include a thorough visual exam of their breasts are twice as likely to find tumors smaller than 2 cm at the time of diagnosis. Several studies have shown that women who do not palpate their breasts are twice as likely to have lymph node involvement at the time of a breast cancer diagnosis. Although breast self-exams do not reduce the risk of breast cancer, they can reduce the risk of dying from breast cancer as tumors are detected sooner and treatment can begin earlier in the course of the disease.[1]

Breast Lumps

During your BSE you may encounter breast lumps. Eighty percent of all breast lumps are benign for cancer but may indicate other breast conditions. The lumps that are non-tender, irregular, hard, and fixed are the ones most likely to be breast cancer. However, there are exceptions. Follow-up testing might include an ultrasound, a mammogram, thermography, fine needle aspiration, the

FACT
A monthly breast self-exam is usually best performed a few days after your period begins or at the same time each month if your periods have stopped.

PREVENTION
Bring any lump to your doctor's attention for further investigation. Be particularly attentive to lumps that persist for more than two menstrual cycles and do not disappear after your period.

Exploring Positive and Negative Associations with Our Breasts

Let's explore the positive and negative associations you have with your breasts. Lie down in a comfortable place. Imagine you are relating to your breasts as though they were close friends. Bring compassion and acceptance to your fingers.

1) With one hand, begin to touch your breasts in a loving, exploring way, leaving your analytical mind out of it. Allow the quality of touching to welcome your breasts to the rest of your body. Invite them in. Reclaim them.

2) Explore their topography, being sensitive to the different textures beneath your fingers. Notice how it feels when you dance lightly over the surface of your breasts, and when you press in deeply. As you press deeply, trace the boundaries of your ribs beneath. Move your breasts around, squeezing or massaging them as you do so. Touch your nipples and notice their sensitivity. As you touch one breast and then the other, notice any emotional differences you experience between them.

3) Be aware of your breathing as you continue to explore your breasts, allowing it to slow down and deepen. Release the tension you might be holding in your abdomen. Let go of any fear you experience and bring your awareness to the present moment and to the sensitive exploration of your breasts. Spend an equal amount of time on either side. Go slowly, for 10 minutes.

4) Now, using an unlined sheet of paper, about 18 x 24 inches, or using the space below, draw a picture of your breasts as you experience them. Use colored markers, pastels, or crayons to express feelings you have about your breasts, including emotions or past traumas you associate with them. Include cysts, scars, tumors, and sensations you feel within them.

5) Beneath the drawing divide the page in two. On the left hand side, write all the positive associations you have with your breasts. On the right hand side, write the negative associations you have. If you are in a group, share your drawings and experiences with one another. Sit in a circle and let each group member speak about some of the ways she has related to her breasts in the past or present. If there are more than 15 women, break into small groups of five to do this.

Positive Associations	Negative Associations

Breast Self-Examination Directions (BSE)

Breast self-examination consists of two stages: a visual exam and a palpation exam.

VISUAL EXAM

Stand before a mirror. With each of the following positions, observe your breasts in the mirror. Each position highlights a different part of your breast. Be watchful for any dimpling, puckering, bulging irregularities, or changes in size. Look for any changes in your nipples such as nipple inversion or displacement to one side. Notice any changes in skin texture or color. Take the time to be thorough and bring tenderness to it. The positions are as follows:

1) Place your hands on your hips and apply pressure. Examine the contour of your breasts, noticing any irregularities.

2) Slowly raise both arms over your head, stretching them up high. Examine your breasts and the underarm area, or axilla.

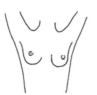

3) With your arms above your head, clasp your hands together and bring them down behind your head. Pull your elbows back and squeeze your hands together. Look for any changes in the appearance of your breasts and the axilla.

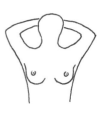

4) Bring your palms flat together in front of your forehead with your elbows out to the sides. Press your hands together. Examine your breasts.

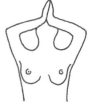

5) Bend forward from your hips until your nipples point down, resting your hands on your knees. In the mirror, observe the contour of your breasts for any irregularity.

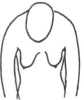

AMAS blood test, an MRI, or a biopsy. We'll discuss these procedures after reviewing various breast conditions.

Common Breast Conditions

From your self-examination, you may discover some common breast conditions.

Since there is an association between some benign breast diseases and breast cancer, it makes sense to improve our breast health should any of the following conditions be present. Understanding and treating these ailments may prevent cancer. Protective and therapeutic nutrient supplement regimes are mentioned here and fully explained in Chapter 10, 'Breast Disease Treatments.'

Premenstrual Breast Pain and Swelling

During a breast self-exam, your breasts may feel swollen and tender. Roughly 35% of all pre-menopausal women experience swollen, tender breasts one to two weeks before their periods. If you are one of these women, you may also experience weight gain,

PALPATION EXAM

The second stage of BSE is palpation — gently but firmly feeling the breasts to detect any unusual thickening or lumps. There are a number of accepted palpation methods. The three most commonly used are illustrated as follows.

Spiral   Clock

Zig zag

1) Hold the first two or three fingers of one hand close together. Use the pads of those fingers to palpate the opposite breast. Make small circles with your fingers as you press towards the ribcage, moving the skin with your fingers. Use three levels of pressure on your breast so that you may detect lumps at various depths. For each position, start with gentle pressure, followed by moderate pressure and then press deeply enough so that you can feel the ribs beneath your breasts. Follow one of the patterns diagrammed above and use it consistently. Keep your breathing slow and relaxed.

2) Some women prefer to do their breast examination while in the shower, placing the hand of the examined side behind the head. If you have larger breasts, you may find it more efficient to lie down for a BSE. Place a towel or pillow under your shoulder to support and stabilize the breast that you are examining; the hand of the examined side rests behind your head. The opposite hand is then used to palpate your breast. Following either of the patterns above, slowly and thoroughly palpate each breast, being aware of any lumps or changes in lump size from your previous breast self-exam.

3) Breast tissue extends from the collarbone to just below the fold of skin under your breast, and from the middle of your chest to your side and armpit, so be sure to palpate this whole area. Also palpate the area above the collarbone, known as the supraclavicular area. Occasionally, breast cancer may be detected through persistent swollen lymph nodes in this area or in the nodes in the armpit. As you complete your exploration of each breast, squeeze your nipple to notice any discharge. Any unusual or bloody discharge warrants further examination with your medical doctor. A persistent nipple discharge on only one side may be due to cancer 4-21% of the time, particularly if it is bloody.[2]

abdominal bloating, and swelling of the face, hands, and ankles. The symptoms are caused by an increase secretion of the adrenal hormone, aldosterone, which can be triggered by stress, excess estrogen, and a deficiency of dopamine, a brain neurotransmitter.

Dopamine levels in the brain are depleted when there is a deficiency of magnesium and B6. Vitamin B6 promotes the production of dopamine in the hypothalamus, which then inhibits the release of the hormone prolactin. Increased prolactin causes breast swelling.

Low magnesium in the body causes the adrenal glands to release more aldosterone, resulting in increased fluid retention and weight gain.

Low vitamin B6 levels decrease the kidney's ability to get rid of sodium, causing water retention. Sufficient B6 helps to increase progesterone levels, which reduces breast swelling. Excess sugar results in water retention due to the increased secretion of insulin from the pancreas. Other causes of premenstrual breast pain and swelling include thyroid imbalance, iodine deficiency, and an overgrowth of intestinal yeast.

The liver is the organ most vulnerable to stress. Repressed

FACT

In Traditional Chinese Medicine, breast swelling is believed to occur due to 'stagnation of liver energy and blood'. The energetic function of the liver is to allow for the free flow of energy outward in all directions.

Breast Map Worksheet

It is difficult to detect from month to month what changes have occurred in our breasts, particularly if we have fibrous and lumpy breasts to begin with. If we map our breast topography with notations about size of lumps, location, texture, shape, mobility, and tenderness, we provide ourselves with a comparative study. We can take our maps to our health practitioners and more accurately describe our concerns or ask questions. Take time to explore and befriend your breasts at least once weekly. Become an expert at performing monthly breast self-exams and mapping their topography.

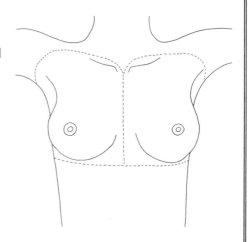

1) Photocopy this drawing, map your breast topography on it monthly, and record any changes. Palpate the area within the doted lines on your own breasts and draw what you find using the notations provided. Check your map each month, making changes as needed.

2) Using the following key with abbreviated notations, draw the topography of your breasts as you perceive it from your breast self-exam. As your breasts change in time, or as you become more proficient at breast self-exams, change your map accordingly. Use a small ruler to estimate the size of any lumps. Superimpose an imaginary clock over your breasts to describe the location and specify in which quadrant you find the lump — upper right (URQ), upper left (ULQ), lower right (LRQ) or lower left (LLQ).

3) Draw any lumps and document beside them the following characteristics:

SIZE: size of lumps in cm, both length and width.

LOCATION: where it is located on the imaginary clock (i.e. 2:00); how far outward from the nipple (i.e. 6 cm); and in which quadrant of which breast (i.e. upper left quadrant ULQ of the left breast LB).

TENDERNESS: tender (T), non-tender (NT), and describe the quality and severity of the pain (achy, bruised, needle-like, cramping, pulling, tearing, burning, throbbing).

SHAPE: regular shape with smooth edges (R), irregular (I).

TEXTURE: hard (H), soft (S). Circle which of the following best describes the overall texture of your breasts:

      smooth   granular   lumpy   cystic   fibrous

MOVEABILITY: freely moveable (FM), fixed (F).

For example, if you find a small, tender, regular shaped, soft, freely moveable lump, you would draw its location and write beside it: "1 cm, 3:00, T, R, S, FM.".

LYMPH NODES: underarm: L R   supraclavicular swelling   hardness   # of nodes palpable.
Circle which area of nodes has swelling or hardness and indicate the number of nodes you are able to feel.

NIPPLE DISCHARGE: no yes   L R   nonbloody bloody

4) Now map your breast topography monthly, as you do your breast self-exams, using additional copies of this breast map to record what you find.

anger, depression, frustration, excess stress, alcohol, too much meat and unhealthy fats are some of the things that disturb the liver's ability to circulate energy and blood, which may result in breast swelling. Aerobic exercise, expressing emotions, regular deep breathing, and relaxation are ways to relieve liver stagnation.

Fibrocystic Breast 'Disease'

Fibrocystic breast disease represents a wide variety of breast conditions, mostly benign, and is better described as a 'condition' rather than a 'disease'. It is associated with changes in breast physiology related to diet and hormonal fluctuations. If you notice soft, tender, moveable cysts in your breasts that are predominant one to two weeks before your period and diminish after your period, you may have this condition. Fibrocystic changes, like breast cancer, are increasing in frequency. In 1928 an autopsy series reported a 3% incidence, while in 1973 an autopsy report quoted an 89% incidence.[3,4] Women whose breast cyst biopsies reveal ductal or lobular proliferation, or atypical hyperplasia (33% of biopsied patients) have a risk of developing breast cancer four times higher than age-matched controls.[5] Otherwise, women with cystic breasts have a subsequent breast cancer risk of 1.8.[6,7,8]

The cysts are cyclic, vary in size, and are often painful, freely moveable and multiple, occurring in both breasts. Twenty percent of women with this condition are able to feel swollen lymph nodes in the underarm area as well.

Causes

The condition is more severe before the menstrual period and is thought to be due to an increased estrogen to progesterone ratio. Some researchers have also suggested it is linked to an upset in the ratio between estrone and estriol, or an underactive thyroid.[9] Yet others suggest that it may be due to high estradiol and low testosterone. Clearly it is related to hormonal imbalance. It may also relate to nutritional deficiencies in vitamins E and B6, iodine, coenzyme Q10, or essential fatty acids. Sluggish bowels, an overburdened liver, and a diet too high in meat and fat are also implicated.

Low thyroid function may cause an increase in prolactin levels. Interestingly, the thyroid gland may be underactive due to a deficiency of iodine, and supplementation with one of several forms of iodine has been shown to improve fibrocystic breast disease.[10,11,12]

Women having fewer than three bowel movements per week have a risk of fibrocystic breast disease four to five times greater than women having at least one a day, for two reasons. First, certain intestinal bacteria linked to high fat and meat based diets can break apart an estrogen complex (called a glucuronide conjugate) formed in the liver that would ordinarily be excreted in the stools. Estrogen is then reabsorbed through the wall of the large intestine and becomes active in the body. High fiber, plant-based diets which increase the frequency of bowel movements prevent this from occurring. Second, fecal bacteria can make three types of estrogen from dietary cholesterol, the precursor of estrogen hormones.

FACT

Cystic breasts commonly affect up to 50% of pre-menopausal women between the ages of 20 and 50 years. Fibrocystic breast disease can sometimes be a precursor for later breast cancer.

PREVENTION

You can reverse fibrocystic breast disease with natural medicines. For detailed guidelines, see Chapter 10, 'Breast Disease Treatments.'

FACT

There is a strong association between methylxanthine consumption and fibrocystic breast disease. Methylxanthine is found in coffee, black tea, green tea, cola, chocolate, and caffeinated medications and has been shown to promote the growth of cancer cells in the mammary gland of rats. Fibrocystic breast disease often improves when women stop using foods or drugs containing methylxanthines.[13,14]

These three estrogens (estrone, estradiol, and 17-methoxyestradiol) can be absorbed back into the body.[15] Fatty foods (particularly in meat) promote the growth of harmful bacteria in the large intestine that accomplish these two tasks and will also slow down bowel transit time. This partially explains the link between fatty foods, fibrocystic breast disease, and breast cancer.

Fibroadenomas

Fibradenomas are the third most common breast disease, and are usually found in younger women, between 20 and 35 years of age. Unlike a fibrocystic condition, the tumor is not cyclic, but is constantly present. Although not malignant, its presence indicates a higher possibility of breast cancer later in life. The lump is firm, smooth, round, and moveable, with a rubbery texture, like a marble under the skin.

Mastitis

Mastitis is an inflammation of the breast and milk duct systems, usually due to infection caused by bacteria entering a fissured or cracked nipple. It most often occurs in a first-time mother after childbirth and during breast-feeding. A duct becomes blocked with thick milk that then encourages bacterial growth, usually of the organisms staphylococci or streptococci. Symptoms include breast pain with heat and redness, a hard swelling, fever, and possibly swollen cervical and/or axillary lymph nodes. It may occur due to poor nipple preparation in the final two to three months of pregnancy, a small fissure in the nipple, breast engorgement due to incomplete emptying, excessive suckling by the newborn, dehydration or stress. The infection spreads in the breast through the lymphatic vessels and ducts.

Mastitis can progress to form an abscess that requires surgical drainage, or to chronic mastitis. As mastitis heals, a bit of scar tissue may form, which can feel hard and similar to a cancerous tumor. In the acute phase when the breast is red, hot and swollen, it may be difficult to differentiate this condition from inflammatory breast cancer.

Intraductal Papillomas

Intraductal papillomas are relatively uncommon, small, benign tumors occurring on the lining of the nipple ducts of the breast, most frequently noticed in women between the ages of 30 and 50. Often they are too small to feel. The main symptom is a watery, pinkish, or bloody discharge from the nipple. Surgical removal of the affected ducts is the standard treatment. The tissue must be biopsied since a bloody discharge from the nipple, especially if it occurs in only one breast, can be due to malignancy.

Breast Calcifications

Calcifications in the breast are felt as small, hard, regular shaped tumors. They may have originated from old fibroadenomas that you had as a teenager which have calcified. They may also be calcifica-

FACT

If a fibroadenoma breaks down on its own, it can develop into calcifications or microcalcifications, which may be associated with the development of cancer. A mammogram or biopsy is necessary to differentiate a fibroadenoma from breast cancer.

FACT

I have healed my own mastitis in 24-48 hours several times with increased fluid intake, warm compresses, and frequent nursings, along with the supplements listed in Chapter 10, 'Breast Disease Treatments'.

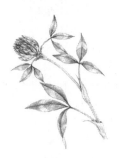

tions in a blood vessel that occurs with aging. As we age, calcium leaves our bones and may collect in other tissues such as the joints and arteries, particularly if our bodies are overly acidic. For a discussion on testing and resolving hyperacidity, see Chapter 7, 'Eating Right for Breast Health.'

Eighty percent of calcifications are not linked to breast cancer. If they are clustered close together, are very small, and don't seem to be in other parts of the breast, they are more likely to be pre-cancerous; however, if there are many spread evenly throughout both breasts, this is less likely.[16] A biopsy will tell.

Breast Cancer

Most often breast cancer is felt as a hard, irregular-shaped, non-tender lump that feels as though it is attached to the underlying tissue. There may be puckering of the skin near the lump site, bloody nipple discharge, and/or changes in nipple size and shape.

Cancer Cells and Tumors

Cancer cells are often present 10 years before a mass is finally detectable, having grown to a size one centimeter in diameter and consisting of one billion cells. The time required for one cell to divide into two cells is called doubling time, and the rate varies between about 21 and 188 days, depending on breast cancer type and age. Aggressive cancers have a faster doubling time.

Ordinarily the cell has the capacity to repair its DNA, bolstered by a healthy diet and lifestyle. Cells from our immune systems also constantly survey the body, on guard for disfigured, pre-cancerous cells. When DNA repair is unable to keep up with genetic damage, the cell repeats or accentuates the damaged DNA as it divides and reproduces itself. Several hormones — excess estrogen, insulin, prolactin, IGF-1 and growth hormone — contribute to the faster multiplication of breast cells and accelerate the rate at which damaged cells form a tumor, though they may not have caused the original genetic defect.

When the clump of aberrant cells spreads out from the tissue of origin to the surrounding area, it is classified as invasive cancer. Nutritional substances, such as beta carotene and all the carotenoids, zinc, iodine and flaxseed oil, help to protect the epithelial lining of the breast ducts and lobules to be more resistant to invasion by cancer cells. This growth phase of the tumor is kept in check by melatonin and possibly progesterone and thyroid hormone. Many foods and nutrients, such as garlic, fish oil, lycopene (in tomatoes), ellagic acid (in red raspberries), and IP6 (in beans and bran) help to slow down this growth phase.

When the tumor reaches a critical size of about 2 millimeters, it sends out chemical signals to recruit blood vessels to gain its nourishment. When blood vessels form to bring it nutrients, the tumor grows much faster. Environmental estrogens may help it to do this. Soy, green tea, turmeric, quercetin (in onions) and zinc help to prevent the formation of this blood supply, known as 'angiogenesis', as well as stall the growth phase.

PREVENTION
Breast calcifications should be monitored closely every few months to be sure there is no change in size or shape, which might indicate cancer. Women with calcifications should be diligent in adopting a cancer prevention diet and lifestyle, following many of the guidelines in this book.

FACT
When breast cancer occurs in a younger woman, it tends to be more aggressive than cancer occurring in a post-menopausal woman.

FACT
Breast cancer begins with changes in the DNA of the breast cell initiated by a variety of causative agents, including chemicals, radiation, free radicals, toxic metals, electromagnetic fields, genetic defects, drugs, viruses, and stress.

Metastasis

Single cancer cells can separate from the original tumor and travel through the blood or lymphatic vessels to the rest of the body. They can migrate to the liver, lungs, bone marrow, or brain and multiply to form another tumor, or metastasis, of the original deranged breast cell.

The body tries to put a halt to this process by attacking breast cancer cells in the lymph nodes, and sending out white blood cells to patrol the blood to seek and destroy any wandering cancer cells. Melatonin levels increase in an attempt to curtail the cancerous process. Unlike normal cells, cancer cells lose the signal to die after they reproduce. They are on a narcissistic mission of self-perpetuation at the expense of their host. Over time, they can interfere with processes essential to life. Many natural substances can be used to inhibit metastases, like bromelain (from pineapple), modified citrus pectin and proteolytic enzymes. For more information, see Chapter 8, 'Nutritional Supplements for Breast Health,' and Chapter 10, 'Breast Disease Treatments.'

Types of Breast Cancer

There are approximately 30 types of breast cancer and a series of grades or levels, indicating severity. Generally they are divided into two categories: lobular vs. ductal. Most breast cancers are ductal; this category includes mucinous, papillary, and combination cancers. Breast cancers that are neither lobular nor ductal include Paget's disease and inflammatory carcinoma.

The term 'in situ carcinoma' is used for the early stage of cancer, when it is limited to the immediate area where it began. Specifically in breast cancer, in situ means that the cancer remains confined to the ducts (ductal carcinoma in situ) or lobules (lobular carcinoma in situ). It has not invaded surrounding fatty tissues in the breast, nor has it spread to other organs in the body. If the cancer moves from the site of origin, it is called 'invasive'.

Most breast cancers begin in glandular tissue, such as the ducts or lobules of the breast and are called adenocarcinomas when this is the case. 'Adeno' means 'related to a gland'. About 86% of breast cancers start in the ducts, while 12% originate in the lobules at the end of the ducts.

Ductal Carcinoma in Situ

Ductal carcinoma in situ (also known as intraductal carcinoma) is the most common type of noninvasive breast cancer. Noninvasive means that the cancer cells are inside the ducts but have not spread through the walls of the ducts into the fatty tissue of the breast. One-fifth of all new breast cancer patients are found to have DCIS.

At this early stage, mammograms will detect DCIS before the tumor is palpable. It rarely is felt as a discrete lump, but may feel like a soft thickening, as the ducts plug up with cancer cells. If left untreated, about 20-25% of women with low grade DCIS would develop invasive cancer up to 25 years after the initial biopsy.[17] The cancer tends to spread throughout the involved duct, which may traverse a large area of the breast and can become invasive over time.

FACT
Before mammography became popular, 'in situ' cancers accounted for only about 5% of all new breast cancer cases. Now because of screening mammography, they account for about 20% of cases. The other 80% are 'invasive' cancers.

FACT
Nearly all women diagnosed in the early stage of ductal carcinoma in situ can be cured, with five-year survival rates being over 99%.

There are several types of DCIS, but the most important difference between them is whether or not there is an area of dead or degenerating cancer cells, known as 'tumor necrosis'. If necrosis is present, the tumor is considered more aggressive. The term 'comedocarcinoma' is often used to describe a type of DCIS with necrosis.

Lobular Carcinoma in Situ (LCIS)
Although it is not a true cancer, LCIS (also called lobular neoplasia) is sometimes classified as a type of noninvasive breast cancer. It is uncommon, occurring in about 2% of all breast biopsies. The atypical cells begin in the otherwise hollow milk-producing glands and can fill them up, but do not penetrate through the wall of the lobules. Usually LCIS does not become an invasive cancer, so removing the LCIS is not the answer, but women with this condition do have an increased risk of 16-27 % in developing cancer in either breast over 30 years.[18,19] If a cancer does occur, it isn't confined to where the original LCIS was discovered, but can arise in any place in either breast. This suggests that whatever is causing the LCIS also puts these women at risk of future cancer. Five-year survival with LCIS is over 99%.

Infiltrating (or Invasive) Ductal Carcinoma (IDC)
This cancer starts in a milk duct of the breast, breaks through the wall of the duct, and invades the fatty tissue of the breast. It usually feels like a hard, firm lump or an irregular-shaped mass of varying density and mobility, with fibrous extensions into the surrounding breast tissue that can create a 'crab-like' appearance. The scar tissue that forms around ductal cancer cells creates the feeling of hardness.

There is about a 15% chance of this cancer occurring in the other breast. Invasive ductal carcinoma may metastasize, or spread to other parts of the body, such as the liver, brain, bones or lungs, through the lymphatic system and bloodstream.

Medullary Carcinoma
This special type of infiltrating breast cancer has a rather well-defined, distinct boundary between tumor tissue and normal tissue. It has some other special features, including the large size of the cancer cells and the presence of immune system cells at the edges of the tumor. Medullary carcinoma accounts for about 5% of breast cancers. Because of its less aggressive nature, medullary carcinoma rarely metastasizes to distant sites, and five-year survival is 82%. Other special types of breast cancer that are less likely to spread include mucinous or colloid carcinoma (five-year survival 95%) and papillary carcinoma (five-year survival 96%).[20]

Tubular Carcinoma
Tubular carcinomas are a special type of infiltrating breast carcinoma where the cancer cells look like small tubes. They account for less than 2% of all breast cancers and are usually less aggressive than other infiltrating ductal or lobular carcinomas. Five-year survival is 96%.

PREVENTION
Women with lobular carcinoma in situ should have a physical exam 2-3 times a year to monitor for an early breast cancer, and an annual thermogram or mammogram.

FACT
About 65-80% of invasive breast cancers are infiltrating ductal carcinomas. Seventy-nine percent of women diagnosed with this type of breast cancer will be alive 5 years after being diagnosed.

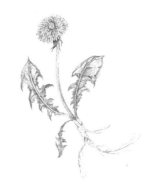

MEASURABLE FACTORS IN BREAST CANCER PROGNOSIS

Many measurable factors can be used to predict the likelihood of surviving breast cancer, but many more immeasurable factors like diet, nutritional status, immune strength, support systems, lifestyle, prayer, hope, grit, purpose, and love have profound effects on life expectancy and can alter the course of any disease. These are not taken into account with these predictions. I have seen women live 10 years or more with liver metastases and others die within a year after a stage II cancer diagnosis. Nevertheless, science uses several quantifiable parameters to predict disease outcomes.

Tumor Size: The larger the tumor at the time of diagnosis, the less favorable the prognosis. If the tumor is larger than 5 cm, it is very likely that there are microscopic cancer clusters elsewhere, while if it is smaller than 1 cm, there is not likely to be further spread.

Number of Axillary Lymph Nodes Positive for Cancer: The fewer lymph nodes that are positive for breast cancer the better the prognosis. However, about 30% of the time a woman with positive nodes doesn't have cancer elsewhere, and about 25% of the time a woman with negative nodes does have cancer somewhere else.[22]

Number of Blood Vessels Surrounding the Tumor (Angiogenesis): When tumors reach a size of 2 mm, they need a blood supply to continue to grow. Cancer cells secrete proteins that stimulate new blood vessels to form around it, bringing more nutrients for growth. Therefore the greater number of blood vessels surrounding a tumor, the faster it will grow.

Plasma Viscosity, Fibrinogen, and Plasma Fibrin D-dimers: Plasma viscosity ('stickiness of the blood') is higher in breast cancer patients in comparison to women with benign breast tumors and is an independent marker for overall survival.[23] A value higher than 1.4 mPa is associated with a poorer outcome. Higher viscosity causes a decrease in oxygen to the area of the tumor, which favors metastases. Blood levels of fibrinogen and plasma fibrin D-dimers are associated with blood coagulation, decreased movement of the blood, and lower oxygen levels in the tissues and are increased in 89% of patients with progressive metastatic disease.[24] Fibrinogen serves as a kind of scaffolding in the extracellular fluid that supports angiogenesis, tumor cell growth and spread.[25] Levels of plasma fibrin D-dimers correlates with tumor load, number of metastatic sites, angiogenesis, and rate of progression of cancer.

Whether the Cancer Has Spread Elsewhere in the Body: If it has already spread to another location, it will be more difficult to keep further growth in check.

Infiltrating (or Invasive) Lobular Carcinoma (ILC)

Infiltrating lobular carcinoma starts in the milk-producing glands, or lobules. This type of cancer can also spread to other parts of the body. About 10% of invasive cancers are ILCs. Invasive lobular carcinoma may be harder to detect by mammography than invasive ductal carcinoma. Five-year survival is 84%.

Inflammatory Breast Cancer

This rare type of invasive breast cancer accounts for about 1% of all breast cancers. It makes the skin of the breast look red and feel warm and gives the skin a thick, pitted appearance. These changes are not caused by inflammation or infection, but by cancer cells blocking lymph vessels or channels in the skin. This type of breast cancer has a poorer prognosis, with five-year survival being 18%.

If the Cancer is 'Fixed' to Adjacent Structures: The extent of the cancer is likely to be greater, and the prognosis worse.

Tumor Type: The type of cancer cells present in the tumor help to determine its aggressiveness.

Mitotic Count: This relates to how many of the cancer cells are dividing and how quickly this is occurring. The faster they divide, the more aggressive the cancer. Less aggressive cancers have very few dividing cells.

Nuclear Grade: The nucleus of the cell is the part that initiates cell division, and the grade relates to the growth rate and how unusual the nuclei look. For instance, are they small, medium or large, are they uniform in size and shape, is their outline irregular or regular? A pathologist will grade the nuclei on a scale of 1-3 or 1-4, with the highest number being the worst.

Tubule Formation: The cancer is less malignant when more of the tumor as a whole is composed of tubular structures. When over 75% of the cancer has a tubular formation, it gets a grade of 1, while when there is less than 10% tubule formation, the tubular score would be 3.

Tumor Necrosis: This means that there are dead cancer cells within the tumor, usually a sign that it is growing rapidly and has outgrown its blood supply.

Estrogen and Progesterone Receptor Status: If these receptors are present, the prognosis is improved. All healthy breast cells have receptors for estrogen, progesterone, and other hormones. Hormones attach to the receptors in order to achieve their action on the cell. As the breast cell becomes more unusual looking, it can lose its receptors for estrogen and/or progesterone. At that point, neither of these hormones will have any influence on the cell. When the receptors are present, the cancer can be influenced by substances that can bind to the receptors to block estrogen – such as Tamoxifen, soy and ground flaxseeds.

Age: Often the younger the person at the time of diagnosis, the more aggressive the cancer is likely to be.

The Bloom Richardson Grading System

This system is used to classify tumors utilizing the prgnostic factors of mitotic count, nuclear grade, and tubule formation described above. Each of these is scored on a scale of 1 to 3 and then the total is added.

A total score of 3, 4, or 5, is grade 1; a score of 6 or 7 is grade 2; and a score of 8 or 9 is grade 3, the most aggressive. The lower the grade, the better the prognosis. Generally a grade of 1 is associated with 95% survival over 5 years, a grade 2 with 75% survival, and a grade 3 with 50% survival over the same time period.[26]

Paget's Disease of the Nipple

This type of breast cancer begins in the breast ducts and spreads to the nipple and then to the areola, the dark circle around the nipple. It is rare, accounting for only 1-5% of all cases of breast cancer. The skin of the nipple and areola often appears crusted, scaly, and red, with areas of bleeding, ulceration, and oozing, similar to eczema. Symptoms may also include burning or itching of the skin around the nipple. Paget's disease may be associated with in situ (non-invasive) or with invasive breast cancer. About half the time, a painless mass can be felt underneath the reddened area, which is usually indicative of invasive cancer. If no lump can be felt in the breast tissue, and the biopsy shows DCIS but no invasive cancer, the prognosis is excellent. Five-year survival for Paget's Disease is 79%.

STAGES OF BREAST CANCER

The stages of breast cancer are ranked to reflect the severity of the disease or threat to life. They are labeled Stage 0, I, II, III, or IV.

Stage 0: Stage 0 is carcinoma in situ, which 75-80% of the time does not progress to invasive cancer. Five-year survival with a ductal cancer is 99%.

Stage I: Stage I is when the tumor is less than 2 cm and there is no lymph node involvement. Five-year survival with a ductal cancer is 96%.

Stage II: Stage II occurs when the tumor is less than 2 cm with lymph node involvement, or when the tumor is between 2-5 cm with positive or negative lymph nodes, or when it is larger than 5 cm with no lymph node involvement. Five-year survival with a ductal cancer is 81%.

Stage III: Stage III is when the tumor is larger than 5 cm with positive lymph nodes, possible skin involvement, and/or when the tumor is fixed to the chest wall. Five-year survival with a ductal or lobular cancer is 52%.

Stage IV: Stage IV occurs when the cancer has metastasized to a distant site or the diagnosis is inflammatory carcinoma. Five-year survival is 18%.[21]

Phyllodes Tumor

This very rare type of breast cancer develops in the stroma (connective tissue) of the breast, in contrast to carcinomas, which begin in the ducts or lobules. Phyllodes tumors are usually benign but on rare occasions may be malignant.

Benign phyllodes tumors are treated by removing the mass and a narrow margin of breast tissue. A malignant phyllodes tumor is treated by taking it out along with a wider margin of normal tissue, or by mastectomy. These cancers do not respond to hormonal therapies and are not as likely to respond to chemotherapy or radiation therapy. In the past, both benign and malignant phyllodes tumors were referred to as cystosarcoma phyllodes.

Diagnostic and Predictive Tests for Breast Cancer

Medical Protocol for Diagnosing Breast Cancer

If you suspect you may have a serious breast ailment because of a lump or change in breast texture, there are a variety of diagnostic tests recommended by different medical bodies, such as the American Medical Association or the Canadian Medical Association, chiefly clinical breast exam, mammography, ultrasound, fine needle aspiration, and biopsy. Until we have safer diagnostic tools, such as laser mammography, these recommendations are very useful and should be considered. There are other tests available to complement mammography, namely the AMAS blood test, MRI and advanced forms of thermography.

Mammography

A mammogram is an x-ray of the breast that can pick up lesions as small as 0.5 cm, which you are usually not able to feel. Mammography can detect approximately 85% of all breast cancers.[28] In contrast, an experienced physician can detect 61-92% of breast cancers through a breast exam, depending upon the physician.[29] Mammograms may prolong lives with earlier detection of breast cancer, resulting in less invasive treatments.[30] However, they are not ideal diagnostic tools for several reasons.

If a woman has dense breasts, a lump may not be visible through the tissue. Mammograms will miss up to 25% of tumors in women 40-49 years old.[31] Mammograms are less accurate in picking up lesions in smaller breasts. Often mammograms provide women and their doctors with a false sense of security if nothing is found — overall, mammograms will miss cancers 9-20% of the time, especially in younger women with dense breasts.[32] Approximately 5% of all mammograms are read as positive for cancer. Of these, 97.5% will be 'false' positives — there will really be no cancer present. In other words, out of every 100 mammograms read as positive or suspicious of cancer, only two or three will actually turn out to be cancer. This is why it is so critical to have a biopsy after a 'positive' mammogram; otherwise, surgery may be performed when it is entirely unnecessary. Women experience extreme anxiety in the waiting period while other testing is done to confirm or disprove the diagnosis.

One study found that women who had their mammograms during the last two weeks of their menstrual cycle were twice as likely to have false negative results.[33] This means that the x-ray was interpreted to be fine, but cancer was actually present – tumors were missed. Mammograms are not conclusive: if the lump is there and persists but the mammogram looks fine, it is imperative to have another test to find out what kind of mass it is.[34] This test might be the AMAS blood test, an ultrasound, fine needle aspiration, or biopsy. Trust your body's signals and insist on thorough testing until you come to a conclusive diagnosis.

Mammograms expose us to doses of radiation, which are cumulative and over time can increase our risk of breast cancer.[35] It can take 40 years for cancer to show up after exposure to radiation, so for women under 50, annual mammograms increase risk. For some women, even one mammogram may be too many. This is particularly applicable to women with a family history of breast cancer who are already at risk. Using diagnostic tools that increase risk doesn't make sense.

Other studies have shown that screening mammography leads to more cancer diagnosis and aggressive treatment, but does not decrease overall mortality.

FACT
Studies have shown that screening mammography reduces the death rate by 30% in women over 50 who have annual mammograms because tumors are detected earlier. However, it can increase the death rate from cancer by 50% when performed annually in women under 50 because women accumulate radiation toxicity.

The AMAS (Antimalignin Antibody in Serum) Blood Test

This is a non-specific cancer-screening test that measures antimalignin, an antibody found elevated in the serum of people with cancer. Malignin is found in the cell membranes of all cancer cells, and some of our white blood cells make antimalignin antibody in response to its presence. The antimalignin antibody is found increased in 93-100% of cases when a person has an active, non-terminal malignancy. In other words, the test is very effective in detecting small (1mm), previously undiagnosed tumors, but will not tell you where the cancer is. It is not useful for late stage cancer. It is elevated no matter where the site of the cancer and for all cell types. The test results in very few false positives — only 5% in serum kept frozen for more than 24 hours and less than 1% in serum tested within 24 hours of blood being drawn. False negatives are found in 7% of cases.

A study published in *Cancer Letters* tested 154 volunteers and 76 patients using the AMAS test. Of the 154 volunteers, three were AMAS positive and further testing confirmed that two actually had cancer and the third had ulcerative colitis, a precancerous condition. Breast tumor biopsies from 43 women with suspicious mammograms revealed that 32 were cancerous and 11 were not. For the cancer patients, 31 out of 32 were positive for the AMAS test, while 4 out of 11 of the benign cases were AMAS positive. In this group of patients, the AMAS test was 97% sensitive in detecting breast cancer. Other tumor marker tests were much less sensitive; for example, CEA (0%), CA15-3 (10%), CA 19-5 (5%) and the CA 125 (16%).[36]

Another study of 1,175 breast cancer patients found that one month to 30 years after treatment, clinical remission of breast cancer is correlated with the return of elevated AMAS values to normal values approximately 95% of the time. This is particularly useful for women who have had a lumpectomy and are considering chemotherapy and/or radiation.[37]

It makes sense for this test to be used more frequently in breast cancer monitoring. Rather than expose ourselves to hazardous radiation from mammograms, women under 50 can use it as an annual screening test, along with thermography.[38] If the test results are positive, a mammogram can be used to follow it up. The AMAS test can also be used to monitor a cancer patient's progress and response to naturopathic treatment.[39]

It is not foolproof. There are a few false negatives and false positives. Use this test as a guide rather than as a certainty for confirming the presence of cancer. See the 'Resources Directory' at the back of this book for laboratories handling the AMAS test.

The Immunicon Blood Test

A new blood test presently only available to clinical researchers has been developed by Immunicon Corporation that can detect one tumor cell among 20 million white blood cells. In studies on more than 60 breast cancer patients from two major American medical centers, the test was able to detect small numbers of tumor cells in the blood of women with very early stage breast tumors and greater numbers in those with advancing disease. Over a 12-month study of a group of patients, it was found that when the disease process worsened or when patients did not respond to treatment the numbers of tumor cells increased. When treatment was effective, the number of tumor cells dropped. In a few women thought to be in complete remission, tumor cells were found and further examination showed that they were indeed relapsing. The blood test will be positive when there are as few as 1,000 tumor cells in the entire circulation.[40]

Thermography

Thermography is the process of imaging a patient with a special digital infrared thermography camera that produces a highly detailed 'picture' of the heat levels and patterns from the skin. This is a passive (no energy transmitted to the patient) and non-contact process utilizing an electronic camera interfaced with a computer. Although thermography was considered inaccurate 20 years ago and lost favor due to inconsistent reporting methods, efficiency has improved and analysis of thermograms has been standardized by the American Academy of Thermology using the Marseilles Grading System.

Unlike a mammogram that detects changes in anatomy, thermography measures physiology. Often physiological changes precede anatomical changes. The blood vessels used by cancer cells respond differently to cold stimulation (immersing one's hands in ice water for 1 minute) than other blood vessels, and a comparison is made between temperature gradients of the breast surface before and after cold-water immersion. When the heat patterns from the surface of both breasts are compared in the stored computer images by someone trained to read them (thermologist qualified by the American Academy of Thermology), an anomaly is recognizable. Reputable thermologists use the objective numerical Marseilles grading system in written reports to relay results to the patient and health practitioner.

Canadian studies done at the Ville Marie Breast Center in Montreal have found that thermograms were positive for 83% of breast cancers, compared to 61% for clinical breast exam alone and 84% for mammography. The 84% sensitivity of mammography was increased to 95% when infrared thermographic imaging was added.[42]

Breast cancer patients with abnormal thermograms tend to have faster-growing tumors that are more likely to metastasize.[43] Abnormal thermograms are associated with large tumor size, high grade and positive lymph nodes.[44] This information, grim as it is, can be used to encourage a patient to do everything possible to prevent breast cancer or its recurrence. An abnormal thermogram can be investigated further with an ultrasound, mammogram, biopsy, MRI, or the AMAS blood test.

Computed Tomography Laser Mammography

X-ray mammograms may soon be a thing of the past. Computed tomography laser mammography uses state-of-the-art laser technology operating in the near infrared aspect of the electromagnetic spectrum to image the breasts. In combination with sophisticated

FACT
Women under 50 can most benefit from the use of thermography. Breast cancers tend to grow significantly faster in women under 50. The average tumor doubling time for women under 50 is 80 days; for women between 50-70, it is 157 days; and for women over age 70, it is 188 days.

FACT
Because cancerous tumors have an increased blood supply, they are slightly hotter than the surrounding areas in which they are found. The faster a tumor grows, the more infrared radiation it generates, and therefore the more likely it will be picked up with thermography.[41]

FACT
Laser mammography is painless, unlike the big squeeze used in x-ray mammography. It also poses no risk because ionizing radiation is not used. It is just as accurate when used on younger women with dense breasts as with older women, unlike x-ray mammography.

PREVENTION
If you find a lump, use ultrasound to confirm the presence of a cyst, and if a cyst is not present, choose mammography, MRI, fine needle aspiration, or biopsy to rule out breast cancer.

computer systems, 4 mm thick slice planes of the breast are reconstructed giving an almost 3D representation of the breast and its internal structures. The results are then stored on a CD-Rom, accessible to patients and their doctors.

Laser mammography can easily be used when a woman has breast implants. It can distinguish between a cyst and a solid lesion, potentially eliminating the need for fine needle aspiration or biopsy. It is expected to pick up tumors as small as 2 mm, making it more sensitive than traditional mammography.

A woman lies on a scanning bed and places a breast in a chamber. The laser rotates 360° around the breast, collecting data from the way ultra-short light pulses travel through breast tissue. Benign and malignant breast tissues have different optical properties that can be translated into images through computerized technology. Cancer cells are highlighted on the screen, usually eliminating the need for biopsies.

Clinical trials have been conducted at the Nassau County Medical Center in Long Island, New York and at the University of Virginia. FDA approval for commercial use of the machine is anticipated.[45,46]

BREAST CANCER TUMOR MARKERS

Medical practitioners sometimes use blood tests to look for tumor markers indicative of breast cancer recurrence, although their use is controversial. Tumor markers that are used in the follow-up care of invasive breast cancer include the CEA, CA27.29, CA 15-3, and the C-erbB-2 (Her2-neu).

In a study of 250 breast cancer patients who all underwent mastectomies, one of these tumor markers was the first sign of recurrence in approximately 70% of the women, detectable about four months before clinical symptoms. These particular tumor markers are more sensitive in picking up metastases to the liver or bone than they are in detecting a local recurrence.[48] Another study of 550 breast cancer patients found that the CEA and CA 15-3 were effective independent prognostic factors for relapse or survival.[49]

A fourth tumor marker is CD24, which is expressed on breast cancer cells in a particular pattern different from its expression on benign breast lesions. CD24 expression increases with the histological grade of the tumor. It may be a useful marker for tracking breast cancer and its metastasis.[50]

Ultrasound

Ultrasounds are used to distinguish cysts from solid tumors. This tool uses high-frequency sound waves that are pulsed through the breast tissue. When the sound waves meet a solid obstacle, like a tumor, they bounce back, whereas if they encounter fluid or normal tissue, they pass through the breast. Ultrasounds are best at examining one lump or area of concern that has already been detected by physical exam or mammography, but are not so useful as a whole breast screening method. They are harmless and do not expose us to radiation. Cancers and fibroadenomas are solid, while cysts are hollow and filled with fluid. If the ultrasound demonstrates that the lump is filled with fluid, a biopsy is not necessary. If it shows that the mass is solid, then a biopsy must be carried out to determine whether it is a fibroadenoma or cancer.

The ultrasound can be carried out before a mammogram when a cyst is suspected. If it is a cyst, there is no need for a mammogram, and a woman is spared radiation exposure.

Magnetic Resonance Imaging (MRI)

MRIs are most useful in imaging early breast cancers, particularly in women with a genetic susceptibility who require annual screening for breast cancer in their 20s and 30s when mammography is least accurate due to increased breast density. In these women MRIs are more accurate than mammography, ultrasound, and clinical breast exams. MRIs do not expose women to radiation, but rather use a huge magnet to image tissues after a contrast dye is injected intravenously. The dye is absorbed more easily by cancer cells than by normal tissue or benign lesions. The disadvantages of MRIs are their expense, a high level of false positive test results, and the need for more doctors and technicians trained in interpreting breast MRIs.

Fine Needle Aspiration

Fine needle aspiration is easy to perform, painless, and can be carried out in a doctor's office. A needle is inserted into the tumor and some fluid is removed. If clear fluid is removed and the tumor dissolves, it was a simple cyst. If the fluid is bloody, cancer with a cystic component may exist, and the fluid is sent for analysis. If no fluid is obtained, a biopsy must be performed. Fine needle aspiration is the least invasive, fastest, and most inexpensive way to diagnose breast cancer when a physician is skilled in the technique.

Dr William Hindle of the Breast Diagnostic Center in the Women's and Children's Hospital in Los Angeles believes that fine needle aspiration should be performed on all palpable breast masses. Ninety percent of the time a diagnosis is established with this technique.[47]

Biopsy

A biopsy will confirm or negate the presence of cancer if the above tests have not been definitive. A sample of tissue is taken in one of two ways and then analyzed.

The first method is called open surgical biopsy and is ideally performed as a lumpectomy, as though the diagnosis of cancer had already been made. This reduces the need for a second surgery should the first demonstrate breast cancer, and reduces scarring. The whole mass should be removed with a margin of normal tissue so that a pathologist can be sure that all the edges of the cancer have been taken out, and nothing remains.

The second method is called a core biopsy. For a large palpable mass, one to six slender cores of tissue are taken from different sites within it. It is most accurate for lesions over 2.5 cm in diameter and is much less invasive than an open surgical biopsy.

Other Predictive Tests

Along with standard blood tests (chem screen, CBC), hormone, toxicity, and metabolic tests may be useful in assessing overall health and breast cancer risk (though not in diagnosing breast

---

Hormone Tests

1) Salivary estradiol, estrone, estriol and the estrogen quotient.
2) Ratio of C-2 to C-16 estrogen in urine.
3) Salivary progesterone, taken between days 20-23 of one's menstrual cycle.
4) Salivary melatonin at 3:00 a.m.
5) Blood TSH, free T4, free T3, reverse T3, antimicrosomal and antithyroglobulin antibodies.
6) Saliva IGF-1, IGFBP-3 and IGF-2 .
7) Cortisol levels in blood or saliva, morning and evening.
8) Fasting insulin levels in the blood, and fasting glucose.
9) Salivary testosterone.
10) Blood prolactin.

Toxicity Tests

1) Hair mineral analysis.
2) Urine toxic metals analysis.
3) Blood or fat analysis of chemical body burden.
4) Toxin clearance capacity (TCC) and chemical burden — assesses liver's ability to detoxify.
5) Cavatat (sophisticated ultrasound) or panoramic x-ray to evaluate dental toxicity.

Metabolic Tests

1) Darkfield microscopy of 'live blood'.
2) Biological terrain analysis (BTA).
3) Plasma viscosity, plasma fibrinogen and plasma fibrin D-dimer levels.
4) Stool and blood glucuronidation rate.
5) T-lymphocyte, B-lymphocyte and natural killer cell immune panel.
6) Natural killer cell activity test.
7) Complete digestive stool analysis to determine digestive strength, presence of pathogens.
8) Gastro-test (string test) to determine hydrochloric acid levels in the stomach.
9) Zinc taste test to determine zinc deficiency.
10) Immunoglobulin G food allergy panel (ELIZA test) to reduce immune system stress.
11) Oxidata test for a measure of free radical activity.
12) Ntx urine test for osteoporosis risk.

cancer) and can guide us in using intervention strategies. See the 'Resources Directory' at the back of the book for more information about the laboratories offering these tests. Consult with healthcare professionals in ordering and administering these tests.

Summary

After reviewing the anatomy and physiology of our breasts, breast conditions including cancer, prognostic factors and staging of breast cancer, as well as diagnostic tools and predictive tests, we are ready to explore the complexities of our endocrine system and the many hormones that interact in affecting breast health. Practice these guidelines for prevention of breast disease:

1) Get to know your breasts better by touching them regularly — in the shower, in bed, before or after getting dressed. Make breast self-exams a monthly habit, practicing them in a relaxed and loving way, and re-map your breast topography whenever you detect a change.
2) Take any unusual findings or concerns to your medical doctor, and follow through with diagnostic testing until you have a confirmed diagnosis.
3) Remember that if you are under 50, have a mammogram only as needed for diagnosis of a suspected lump, and then schedule it within the first 14 days of your menstrual cycle, counting day 1 as the first day of your period. If you are over 50, consider a mammogram every 2-3 years.
4) Consider the other choices for annual screening — clinical breast exams, ultrasound, thermography, MRI, the AMAS test — and decide which you feel most comfortable with, keeping in mind your age and risk factors, and then follow through by finding practitioners or clinics that can help you.
5) Assemble a team of healthcare practitioners who can assist you with carrying out, interpreting, and recommending therapies to correct any findings from the predictive tests.

CHAPTER THREE

Understanding the
Hormone Puzzle

CONTENTS

EXERCISES, CHARTS, CHECK LISTS & WORKSHEETS

*I*N ORDER TO understand the causes of breast cancer and ways to prevent this disease, we need to familiarize ourselves with the hormone so linked to breast cancer — estrogen — and its interaction with other hormones of the endocrine system. When we understand hormones and their interactions, we recognize that there is much we can do to prevent breast cancer.

What Is a Hormone?

A hormone is a chemical messenger that moves through the bloodstream, potentially affecting every cell of the body that has receptors for that hormone. Different hormones are produced by different glands. Hormones help to maintain a constant environment inside the body, despite outside changes. Hormonal secretions can be rhythmic, tied to the solar and lunar cycles, instantaneous, or active over very long periods of time, such as the action of growth hormone throughout childhood. Hormones are able to act by binding to particular receptors in or on the cells of their target tissues. Receptors usually have a strong affinity for one particular hormone. The hormone then affects the cell nucleus to create a specific protein, which usually acts as an enzyme with a characteristic action. The action causes a shift in the body's metabolism.

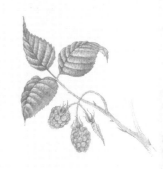

The collective actions of glands and hormones is termed the endocrine system. The function of the endocrine system is profoundly affected by what we feel and think, as well as by the environment around us and by what we put into our bodies as food and drink. Today more than ever before, environmental chemicals, radiation, electromagnetic fields, and contaminants in food are disrupting our hormones.

Components and Functions of the Endocrine System

There are nine main endocrine glands in our bodies. Other organs such as the liver, stomach, intestines, kidneys, and heart also manufacture hormones. This chart summarizes the name, location, and function of each of the main endocrine glands. In direct and indirect ways, they can be involved in the development of breast cancer.

Gland	Location	What Its Hormones Do
Hypothalamus	in the brain behind the eyes	Controls the secretions of the pituitary gland, body temperature, hunger, thirst and sexual drive.
Pineal Gland	in the center of the brain	Responds to light, dark and electromagnetic energy. Affects cell division, sleep. Inhibits cancer, slows down the aging process, protects the thymus gland, may decrease anxiety.
Pituitary Gland	in the brain behind the eyes	Controls bone growth and regulates the other glands. Often called the "master" gland.
Thyroid Gland	at the front of the throat	Controls the rate of fuel use in the body, sensitivity to heat and cold, supports immune function.
Parathyroid Glands	behind the thyroid	Control the level of calcium in the blood.
Thymus Gland	in the upper part of the sternum	Co-ordinates white blood cells and the immune system. Shrinks with age.
Liver	beneath the ribs on the right	Regulates growth, blood sugar metabolism, detoxification.
Adrenal Glands	on top of the kidneys	Controls salt and water balance in the body and our reactions to stress, glucose metabolism.
Pancreas	near the stomach	Controls the level of sugar in the blood.
Ovaries (women)	on either side of the groin	Control sexual development and egg production.
Testes (men)	behind the penis	Control sexual development and sperm production.

Hormones work in concert. Like musicians in an orchestra, they are dependent upon one another, constantly adjusting their expression to produce the music that sings through the body. Any imbalance in one hormone is likely to make the whole symphony sound out of tune.

Estrogen Balance

Estrogen stimulates breast cells to multiply. An imbalance of estrogen is a precipitating cause of breast cancer. Maintaining and restoring balance to this class of hormones is essential to our health. There are many factors affecting the balance of estrogen, including the function of our ovaries in producing estrogen, the impact of 'phytoestrogens' and 'xenoestrogens' in our food and environment, the onset of menses and menopause, the use of birth control pills and hormone replacement therapy, and the influence of other hormones – progesterone, thyroid hormone, IGF-1, insulin, cortisol, growth hormone, and melatonin.

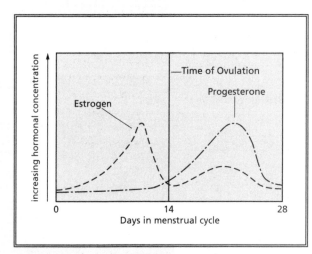

Estrogen Production

The ovaries begin to produce estrogen during puberty — when a girl is anywhere between 10-14 years of age. The pituitary hormone, FSH, signals the ovaries to produce estrogen from puberty onwards. During a single menstrual cycle, the ovaries produce increasing amounts of estrogen from the first day of the period leading up to the day of ovulation in an effort to prepare the uterus for a possible pregnancy. Estrogen levels peak just before ovulation. After ovulation, estrogen levels drop for a few days and then increase less dramatically between days 18-23, followed by a gentle decline until the end of the menstrual cycle. The monthly rise in estrogen levels is the link that puts some women at higher risk for breast cancer. Women with ovarian failure who produce little or no estrogen or whose ovaries have been removed reduce their breast cancer risk by 70-90%. Men also have very little breast cancer because their estrogen levels are low.

Kinds of Estrogen

The body produces three main types of estrogen: estrone (E1), estradiol (E2), and estriol (E3). These are categorized as either 'strong' estrogens (estrone and estradiol) or 'weak' estrogens (estriol).[1,2]

Strong Estrogens: Estradiol and Estrone
Over 50% of the body's estrogen is a form of estrone, produced in the ovaries and fat cells. Estrone is made in turn into a storage form called estrone sulphate. Breast cancer cells tend to accumulate large amounts of estrone sulphate, which can convert back to

estrone or estradiol as required. Drugs or supplements that block the conversion of estrone sulphate to estrone may become promising breast cancer treatments.[3]

Estradiol, produced in the ovaries, is the strongest of the three estrogens, being 12 times more active than estrone and 1,000 times more potent in its effects on breast tissue than estriol.

The ovaries shut down production of estradiol and estrone during menopause. After menopause, the adrenal glands produce the hormones testosterone and androstenedione in higher amounts, which can be converted to estradiol and estrone in fat cells (and in breast, skin, bone, and other tissues) through the action of the enzyme, aromatase. If we block the aromatase enzyme, we can decrease the production of estradiol and estrone after menopause. We can block the aromatase enzyme by using chrysin (a flavonoid from passion flower), ground flaxseed, genistein in soy, the mineral zinc, and natural progesterone.[4,5,6,7]

Weak Estrogens: Estriol

Estriol, a short-acting weak estrogen, is produced by the placenta during pregnancy and is otherwise a breakdown product of estrone, synthesized in the liver. Estriol matures breast cells during pregnancy, making them less vulnerable to damage from radiation and chemicals. The liver can convert estradiol and estrone to estriol. Women who excrete more estriol in their urine may have a lower risk of breast cancer.[8] Cancer remission in patients receiving endocrine therapy occurs when estriol levels increase.[9] Estriol may protect the breasts from the tumor-producing effects of estradiol and estrone.[10]

In pregnancy, estriol is produced in large quantities and becomes the dominant estrogen as ovarian production of estradiol and estrone decreases. Estriol is produced in milligram quantities, while estrone and estradiol are made only in microgram amounts. Nature may have engineered this to protect the fetus from overstimulation via estradiol and estrone. All estrogens compete for the same receptor sites, so estriol exerts its protective effect when it binds to breast cell receptors, preventing the attachment and action of estradiol and estrone. Few women are diagnosed with breast cancer while pregnant.

After menopause estrone continues to be made when a hormone from the adrenal glands called androstenedione is converted in body fat and muscle cells to estrone with the help of the aromatase enzyme. The more fat cells we have after menopause, the more estrogen we are exposed to 'in house'. Some obese women produce more estrogen after menopause than thin women make before menopause. Paradoxically, the better a woman's bone density, the greater her risk of breast cancer.

The types of food we eat can facilitate or block the conversion of estradiol and estrone to estriol. Improving liver function with specific nutrients, like indole-3-carbinol (or DIM), assists this conversion.[11] The use of iodine compounds or sea vegetables may increase estriol levels in pre- and post-menopausal women. There is, however, a risk in too much estriol. If we were to take high

ESTRADIOL

ESTRONE

FACT

Of the three forms of estrogen, estradiol and estrone are linked with increased breast cancer risk, particularly in post-menopausal women. Estriol is associated with decreased risk except when given at very high concentrations.

ESTRIOL

amounts (5-15 mg daily) from external sources, it can act like or convert to estradiol, causing increased division of breast cells, possibly promoting cancer.[12,13]

Estrogen's Role in the Cancer Process

Estrogens have particular physiological effects that influence the development of cancerous cells, for better or for worse. Estrogen promotes cell division, especially in tissues that have a high number of estrogen receptors, such as the breasts and uterus. The other

---

Estrogen Sources

Estrogen comes into our bodies from four possible sources:

1) **Ovaries, Placenta, Adrenal Glands, Fat Cells:** Three types of estrogen are made primarily by the ovaries. Estrogen is also made by the placenta during pregnancy (estriol) and the fat cells after menopause (estrone) from the adrenal hormone precursor, androstenedione.

2) **Food and Herbs:** We get estrogen from a class of foods and herbs called phytoestrogens. Certain plants, such as soy, flaxseeds, legumes, mung bean and clover sprouts, pumpkin seeds, wild indigo, licorice root, mandrake, bloodroot, thyme, yucca, hops, verbena, turmeric, yellow dock, and sheep sorrel, contain components that act like weak estrogens. Phytoestrogens generally protect us from breast cancer by displacing the body's estrogens from their receptor sites. Phytoestrogens are discussed further in Chapter 7, 'Eating Right for Breast Health.'

3) **Environment:** Some environmental chemicals, known as xenoestrogens, are able to mimic estrogen in our bodies and lead to an estrogen excess. Because we have inefficient mechanisms for breaking them down, they tend to persist in our bodies for life. Their cumulative and synergistic effect promotes breast cancer. These chemicals are present in some pesticides, plastics, petrochemicals, detergents, cosmetics, solvents, chlorinated water, fire retardants, lice shampoos and other sources discussed in Chapter 4, 'Environmental Impact on Breast Health.' We also consume estrogen when we eat animal products such as meat, poultry, dairy, and fish. These animals may naturally contain estrogen, may have been injected or fed estrogen to increase fat or milk production, or have accumulated xenoestrogens in their fat from environmental sources or pesticide residues over their lifespan. A meat and dairy based diet promotes breast cancer. Although fish oils protect us from breast cancer, contaminants present in many sources of fish may promote it.

4) **Synthetic Estrogens:** We are exposed to these when we take the birth control pill, fertility drugs, and/or hormone replacement therapy during menopause. Their effects also promote breast cancer.

---

growth-promoting hormones — insulin, IGF-1, growth hormone, and prolactin — also increase cell division in breast cells. The action of a carcinogen or a chance mistake in DNA replication, combined with hormonally driven increases in cell division, creates breast cancer. If the terrain in the body supports the growth of cancer, and our immune systems are unable to reverse it, the cancer acquires a life of its own, on a different track from the rest of the breast tissue.

Cancer requires several sequential events to occur before it can manifest in a body. Estrogen and other hormones can influence these events:

1) Inside a human cell nucleus are approximately 80,000 genes situated on 23 pairs of ribbon-like strands called chromosomes. Each gene is composed of smaller bits of DNA, the same way words are composed of letters. (Think of the chromosome as being the sen-

tence). A dividing cell must faithfully reproduce approximately one billion bits of genetic information. Mistakes can be made when pieces of DNA are inserted in the wrong spot, are duplicated incorrectly, or are missed altogether. The likelihood of a mistake being made is higher if the cell has been exposed to a carcinogen capable of damaging the DNA. Carcinogens include intense sunlight, toxic chemicals, radiation exposure, cooked or rancid fats and oils, and toxic minerals such as arsenic, cadmium, and lead. Mistakes in DNA replication also occur by chance and increase with age.

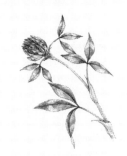

2) When genetic mistakes occur, the cell may fix them with repair mechanisms, or it may die shortly after being reproduced. Both of these processes are overseen by tumor suppressor genes, which are responsible for either activating repair mechanisms, calling a halt to cell replication when mistakes have been made, or ordering cell death. Occasionally the tumor suppressor gene itself has a mutation that makes it incompetent at its task and the aberrant cell survives, reproducing itself. We have many tumor suppressor genes but our primary one is called 'p53' and is the most commonly mutated gene in human cancer, playing a role in about 60% of tumors. Typically, cancer cells divide too frequently and lack mechanisms for controlled, programmed cell death.

3) In a good scenario, if the mutated cell survives, components of our immune system would recognize it as 'non-self' and destroy it before it became a larger tumor. When the immune system is weakened because of stressors, pollutants, glandular imbalances, poor nutrition, or emotional and spiritual factors, the renegade cell will continue to divide and reproduce, forming a cancerous tumor. Some cancer cells are particularly aggressive, reproducing quickly and requiring a very strong immune system to counteract them. Immune enhancers include many vitamins, minerals, and herbs.

4) The doubling time for breast cancer cells can range between 21-188 days. This means that during this span of time the cells will double in number. A mass of 100 billion cells is about the size of a golf ball and can take from 3-10 years or more to form. If cancer cells have a short doubling time and are particularly aggressive, pharmacological doses of melatonin administered before bed can slow down the doubling time and help to stabilize the cancer.[14]

5) When a cancerous tumor attains the size of a pinhead, it sends out chemical signals that cause small blood vessels to encircle it, providing it with nutrients. This increased blood supply encourages the tumor to grow to a large size.

6) As the tumor grows it can release clumps of cancer cells into the blood stream or into the lymphatic system from where they can colonize other bodily organs or tissues. This process is called metastasis. The most common sites for breast cancer metastases include the liver, bones, brain, and lungs.

Estrogen Dominance

Breast cancer is caused in part by the action of a carcinogen in the presence of too many strong estrogens and other growth-promoting hormones. The other ovarian hormone, progesterone, would help to protect the breasts from excess estrogen, as would thyroid hormones, melatonin and the weak estrogen, estriol, but in many of us these hormones are deficient or blocked. Estrogen dominates these other 'balancing' hormones.

Sex Hormone Binding Globulin (SHBG)

Some of the body's circulating estrogen hooks onto SHGB, a carrier molecule that shuttles estrogen (and some testosterone) through the bloodstream to its target organs. When estrogen is bound to SHBG, it is inactive. If we increase SHBG levels, we can tie up a little more estrogen so that there is less 'free' estrogen available. Adequate thyroid hormones help protect us from estrogen excess by increasing the liver's production of SHBG.

Target Sites and Effects of Estrogen

Estrogen acts only when it is able to bind to one of at least two specific receptor sites in the cells of target organs or tissues. The target sites for estrogen include the breasts, uterus, ovaries, vagina, skin, bone, brain, fat cells, liver, and blood vessels, but most of the estrogen goes to the breasts and uterus.

Target Sites	Effects of Estrogen
Breasts	Stimulates duct development in puberty and pregnancy, causes breast cells to multiply. Increases risk of breast cancer. Ensures adequate milk production.
Uterus	Causes uterine growth at puberty. Causes increased cell production and thickening of the uterine lining so that it can support a pregnancy. Increases risk of endometrial cancer.
Ovaries	Causes release of an egg each month during ovulation.
Vagina	Causes vaginal growth at puberty. Retains vaginal thickness and lubrication.
Skin	Encourages formation of collagen, which gives structural support to the skin. Causes growth of underarm and pubic hair. Causes pigmentation of the nipples and areolae.
Bone	Increases bone density by inhibiting breakdown of bone.
Brain	Affects sexual desire. Natural antidepressant.
Fat	Causes fat to be deposited on thighs, hips, and breasts; increases body fat generally.
Liver	Site of estrogen breakdown.
Blood Vessels	Encourages formation of HDL ('good' cholesterol) and keeps arteries free of plaquing. Acts as a vasodilator. May increase blood clotting when too much oral estrogen is used.
Rest of Body	Causes salt and fluid retention; depression and headaches; impairs blood sugar control. Causes loss of zinc and retention of copper; can interfere with thyroid hormone. Reduces oxygen levels in all cells; increases risk of gallbladder disease; increases risk of auto-immune diseases.

Other hormones decrease the amount of sex hormone binding globulin when their levels are too high, freeing up estrogen. These are the players we have to keep under control – insulin, IGF-1 and testosterone. High levels of cortisol, the stress hormone, can increase the production of all three of these hormones, so we need to keep it (and our stress) under control as well. If the thyroid is underactive with not enough circulating thyroid hormones, there will be less SHBG.

Estrogen Receptors

Estrogen is not active until it binds to a receptor. Estrogen fits into its receptor sites much as a key might fit into a lock. There are at least two separate receptors for estrogen, known as alpha and beta receptors, which differ in their distribution in the body, binding affinity, and physiological function. Target cells for estrogen may respond differently to the same estrogenic stimulus depending upon the numbers of each receptor present and the ratio between them. This explains why phytoestrogens and pharmaceuticals like Tamoxifen can exert different effects on different tissues, at different times.[16]

At any given time, most 'strong' estradiol is bound to SHBG, so that only a portion of it can bind to an estrogen receptor in a breast cell. 'Weak' estriol has a lower affinity for binding to SHBG and a greater percentage is available for other biological activity that exerts protection.[17]

Estrogen's Impostors

Estrogen receptors are 'promiscuous' — they attract not only the real estrogen but also its impostors. Some impostors are strong enough to activate the DNA as estrogen does, while others occupy the receptor sites so that estradiol can't attach – they just occupy the seats.

Plant estrogens, or phytoestrogens, are able to occupy estrogen's receptor sites and exert a variety of positive effects. For example, soy foods decrease a woman's risk of breast cancer by filling the breast cell receptor sites so that the body's estradiol cannot bind. The soy estrogen is too weak to exert a harmful estrogenic effect on the breast cell but acts as a weak estrogen on bone tissue, protecting us from osteoporosis by preventing bone loss. It protects the heart and blood vessels by causing more HDL or 'good' cholesterol to be made. Soy seems to exert selective activity depending on the target organ, the type of estrogen receptor it binds to, and the body's need. The plant estrogens are rapidly broken down in the body, and do not accumulate in our tissues over time. The phytoestrogens decrease the harmful effects of both the body's

PREVENTION
Decrease estrogen's activity by increasing SHBG with improved thyroid function, a low fat vegetarian diet, and the phytoestrogens ground flaxseed, soy, and red clover sprouts.[15] Keep insulin, IGF-1, testosterone, and cortisol in check to prevent a lowering of SHBG, which would make more estrogen available.

FACT
The greater the number of estrogen receptors we have in our breast cells, the more vulnerable we are to breast cancer. The hormone melatonin, produced by the pineal gland, decreases the production of estrogen receptors in breast cells.

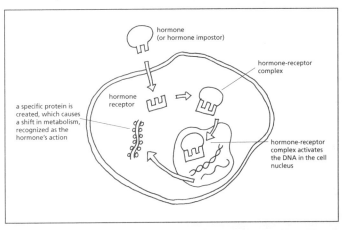

hormone (or hormone impostor)

hormone-receptor complex

hormone receptor

a specific protein is created, which causes a shift in metabolism, recognized as the hormone's action

hormone-receptor complex activates the DNA in the cell nucleus

strong estrogens and of the chemical estrogens. The plant chemicals quercetin and indole-3-carbinol are also able to attach to estrogen receptors, decreasing estrogen's effect.

Xenoestrogens, or environmental estrogens, exert a quite different influence. These imposters are also called 'hormone disruptors' because they affect not only estrogen but other hormones, particularly thyroid hormone, testosterone, and progesterone. The environmental estrogens include many pesticides, plastics, commercial detergents, fire retardants, drugs, fuels, and chlorine-based chemicals called 'organochlorines'.

Environmental estrogens bind to the 'promiscuous' estrogen receptor sites in the target cells and affect the DNA in the same way that estrogen does. When only two environmental estrogens are present in a breast cell, they can exert an effect 1000 times stronger than a single xenoestrogen.[18] It is estimated that an average North American has at least 86 hormone disrupting chemicals present in their fat cells. We have no idea what the combined effect of these is on breast tissue.[19] They may either cause mutations in the genes that regulate cell division or cause abnormal cell growth; in either case, the breast cell multiplies out of control and its DNA is altered in the process.

Xenoestrogens can stimulate breast cells to produce new blood vessels needed for tumor growth and spread.[20] Unlike the plant estrogens, environmental estrogens tend to accumulate to high levels in our bodies because they resist breakdown by our detoxification pathways. We store them in our fat cells — and breast cells are nestled among fat cells. Most of the environmental estrogens are foreign chemicals unknown to biological systems before the 1940s. Because we have inefficient mechanisms for breaking down and eliminating them, they can persist in our bodies for decades.

Breakdown of Estrogen

Estrogen is broken down or 'metabolized' by enzymes in the liver, where it is eventually bound to another substance called glucuronic acid through a process called glucuronidation. The glucuronide complex passes from the liver into the bile, then into the intestines and out through the stool. Ellagic acid, found in red raspberries (especially Meeker raspberries), can increase glucuronidation by 75%. This reaction is also assisted by high fiber, probiotics, vitamin B6, fish oil, and calcium-D-glucarate, naturally present in oranges and apples.

During the breakdown of estradiol and estrone in the liver several products or metabolites are formed. Among these metabolites, those called 'C2' estrogens are harmless. However, 'C16' and especially the 'C4' estrogen metabolites can be harmful and carcinogenic. The C4 estrogen accumulates in breast cells and can attach to DNA to cause mutations, specifically damaging the p53 tumor suppressor gene, whose job is to stop cancer cells from dividing. The C4 estrogen pathway is activated by pollutants like pesticides and other xenoestrogens. Fortunately, once made, the C4 estrogens can be inactivated in the liver through detoxification pathways called Phase 2 methylation and glutathione conjugation, assisted by specific nutrients.

The ratios between these estrogen metabolites may be a useful way to assess the activity of estrogen in our bodies. It seems that breast cancer patients have significantly lower ratios of the C2 estrogen metabolite to C16 metabolite, in contrast to women without breast cancer, who have higher ratios.[21] Women with breast cancer and women with a family history of breast cancer tend to have nearly five times as much of the C16 metabolite as other women.[22,23,24] Studies haven't been done yet on the C2 and C4 ratio in women, but it may prove to be more significant than the C2:C16 ratio in assessing risk.

Other dietary and nutritional substances that help with the conversion of estrogen to the 'good' C2 metabolite are a low fat diet, ground flaxseeds, fiber, EPA fish oil, vitamin B complex, D-limonene, magnesium, zinc, N-acetyl cysteine, rosemary, schizandra, milk thistle, curcumin (from turmeric), soy, and red clover.[25,26]

Substances which interfere with this conversion and promote the C16 metabolite are environmental estrogens, dioxin, car exhaust, paint fumes, alcohol, caffeine, pharmaceutical drugs, sugar, a high fat diet, fried or rancid fats, and inadequate protein.

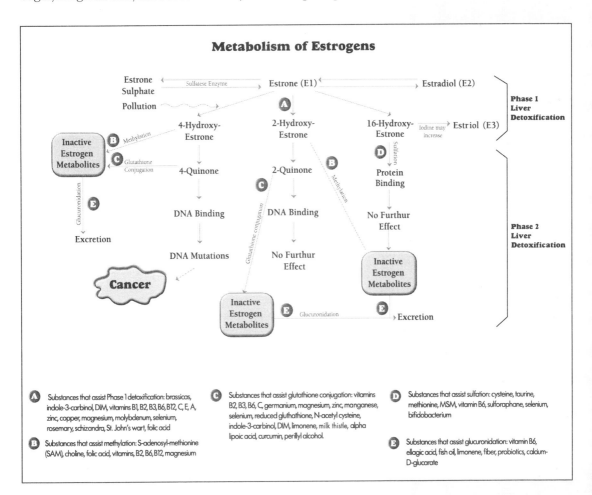

Metabolism of Estrogens

Ⓐ Substances that assist Phase 1 detoxification: brassicas, indole-3-carbinol, DIM, vitamins B1, B2, B3, B6, B12, C, E, A, zinc, copper, magnesium, molybdenum, selenium, rosemary, schizandra, St. John's wort, folic acid

Ⓑ Substances that assist methylation: S-adenosyl-methionine (SAM), choline, folic acid, vitamins, B2, B6, B12, magnesium

Ⓒ Substances that assist glutathione conjugation: vitamins B2, B3, B6, C, germanium, magnesium, zinc, manganese, selenium, reduced gluthathione, N-acetyl cysteine, indole-3-carbinol, DIM, limonene, milk thistle, alpha lipoic acid, curcumin, perillyl alcohol.

Ⓓ Substances that assist sulfation: cysteine, taurine, methionine, MSM, vitamin B6, sulforaphane, selenium, bifidobacterium

Ⓔ Substances that assist glucuronidation: vitamin B6, ellagic acid, fish oil, limonene, fiber, probiotics, calcium-D-glucarate

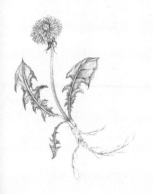

Elimination of Estrogen

Estrogen by-products are excreted through our urine and stools. While urinary estrogen is eliminated completely, the estrogen journeying down the intestines can be recycled to be used again, adding to our cumulative estrogen exposure. High levels of an enzyme present in the intestines called beta glucuronidase (made by certain intestinal bacteria) can separate the estrogen from the glucuronide complex made by the liver. The more beta-glucuronidase that is present, the more free estrogen will be reabsorbed back into the bloodstream through the intestinal wall.[27,28]

A diet high in saturated fat and meat increases specific bacteria that produce beta-glucuronidase. It is possible to measure the amount of harmful beta-glucuronidase activity in women through a stool test. Vegetarians excrete two to three times more estrogen in their stools than non-vegetarians.[29] Circulating estradiol and estrone levels are 50% higher in meat-eaters than in vegetarians.[30] One study with rats found that equal amounts of wheat bran and psyllium provided maximum protection against breast cancer tumors, rather than either fiber alone. Beta-glucuronidase activity was especially lowered by the psyllium.[31]

In studies on rats, a natural, non-toxic substance called calcium D-glucarate was able to prevent the separation of estrogen from the glucuronide conjugate so that the estrogen was eliminated and not reabsorbed into the bloodstream. When rats were fed calcium D-glucarate after treatment with a carcinogen that would stimulate breast cancer, tumor development was inhibited by over 70%.[32] Although there is no confirmation from human studies that this actually works in women, calcium D-glucarate is present in oranges and apples, so have at least one a day of each.

Estrogen Quotient

Some research has demonstrated that a mathematical formula, called the 'estrogen quotient', is also a valuable index for predicting breast and endometrial cancer. The estrogen quotient is determined by:

$$\text{Estrogen quotient} = \frac{\text{Estriol}}{\text{Estrone} + \text{Estradiol}}$$

The functional ability of the liver and bowel elimination influences these estrogen ratios; accordingly, improving liver and bowel function will increase both the amount of C-2 estrogen and estriol, thus decreasing risk.

Six epidemiological studies of estrogen quotients found higher estrogen quotients (more 'weak' estriol in relation to 'strong' estradiol and estrone) in populations with a lower risk of breast cancer.[33,34] In one study, 34 pre- and post-menopausal women without breast cancer showed an estrogen quotient of 1.2 to 1.3, respectively, as determined from urine, while 26 pre- and post-menopausal women with breast cancer had an estrogen quotient of 0.5 to 0.8, respectively. The estrogen quotient of the women with breast can-

The Hormone Puzzle

cer was about half of that of the women free of cancer.[35] A few studies do not support this link.[36]

In my own practice using repeated saliva testing on individual patients, I have been able to manipulate the estrogen quotient favorably with supplements like curcumin, ground flax, DIM, methionine, cysteine, liver herbs, and fiber. Estriol levels can be increased naturally with the inclusion of sea vegetables (for iodine), flaxseeds, soy products, and other phytoestrogens in our diet to decrease breast cancer risk.

See the 'Resources Directory' at the end of this book for laboratories that do saliva and other specialized hormone tests. Either you or your doctor can order them.

Early Onset of Menstruation, Late Menopause

Higher breast cancer risk is associated with early onset of menstruation (before age 11) in women and late menopause (after age 52). The more menstrual cycles a woman has, the more estradiol her ovaries produce over her lifetime, and consequently the greater is her risk of breast cancer. The late onset of menstruation, pregnancy, breast-feeding, and early menopause will reduce the number of menstrual cycles and decrease overall estradiol.[37] If a girl begins to menstruate before the age of 11, she increases her lifetime risk of breast cancer.[38]

One of the factors associated with early onset of menstruation and late menopause is dietary fat. Young girls raised on a high-fat diet begin menstruating about four years earlier than girls eating low-fat starch-based meals — at 12 rather than 16 years.[39] Menopause begins about four years later for women consuming a high-fat diet compared to those on a low-fat diet — at 50 rather than 46 years.[40] The increased years of menstruation are caused by the extra estrogens produced as a result of high dietary fat intake.[41,42,43]

The age of onset of menstruation has become younger in the last century. In the 1800s the average age was 16-17, compared to 11-12 today. Today, many girls are entering puberty one year or more earlier from the dates recognized in current medical texts, which state that only 1% of girls show signs of breast development and pubic hair before age 8.[44,45]

Often early puberty is linked with higher estradiol levels that persist into early adult life.[46,47,48]

This seems to be a product of industrialization, due in part to electric light at night, increased dietary fat, the consumption of hormones in animal products, and exposure to environmental estrogen-mimickers. Some organochlorines have been linked to early onset of menstruation.[49] A *New Scientist* study demonstrated that the girls with the highest prenatal exposure to environmental estrogens such as PCBs and DDE entered puberty 11 months earlier than girls with lower exposures. The mothers of these girls were exposed to the chemicals through normal diet and environmental sources, not from environmental accidents or other abnormally high exposures.[50] Puerto Rico has the highest global incidence of early breast development in girls. Since 1970, there have been 4674

PREVENTION
To evaluate your balance of estrogens and risk of breast cancer, check your ratio of C2 estrogen to C16 estrogen and your sex hormone profile yearly through a saliva or urine test. This can be used as a routine annual test to assess women at risk for breast cancer, followed by work at prevention with diet changes and nutritional supplementation.

FACT
Early onset of menstruation and late menopause are each linked with roughly twice as high a risk of developing breast cancer relative to women with a shorter menstrual life.

PREVENTION
Stall puberty in your daughters by keeping lights out at night, eating organic food, eliminating or drastically reducing animal products in their diets, giving them flaxseed oil regularly while limiting other fats, and protecting them from environmental estrogens. Use less plastic. Serve and store food in glass.

reported cases of breast development in girls younger than 8, and as young as six months, which is a ratio of 8 out of every 1000 girls. It is also occurring in boys. The culprit seems to be phthalates, environmental estrogens found in soft plastics used in packaged food, children's toys, and baby bottles.[51]

With puberty, there is also an increase in the production of growth hormone and other hormone-like substances called insulin-like growth factors, or IGF-1 and IGF-2.[52] Higher levels of insulin-like growth factors are linked to higher breast cancer incidence.[53,54] This is compounded by the increased exposure to radiation, a breast carcinogen, from nuclear power plants and weapons.

Shorter Menstrual Cycles

Women who have menstrual cycles shorter than 25 days have double the risk of breast cancer. This is due to more doses of estradiol, which is produced in greatest concentrations at mid-cycle. Women whose cycles are longer than 30 days are also at twice the risk.[55] These women are exposed to more doses of estradiol because the estrogen-secreting phase of their menstrual cycle is prolonged.[56]

Menstrual cycles can usually be normalized by balancing hormones with liver-supporting herbs, acupuncture, or homeopathic remedies. See Chapter 5, 'Detoxifying Our Bodies,' for a list of these herbs.

Birth Control Pills

Birth control pills have variable effects on breast cancer. When used before the age of 20 or if used for more than 5 years before the age of 35, they can triple the likelihood of developing breast cancer.[57,58] Although birth control is a dilemma for many, natural methods that focus on an awareness of the body are safer. The Justisse method, the Luna Fertility Indicator, and barrier methods are alternatives.

The birth control pill is also an environmental hazard. When women on the Pill urinate, the urine contains estrogens that end up in the wastewater of sewage treatment plants. Fish exposed to this water show hormonal abnormalities. We may be exposed to synthetic hormones ourselves through our drinking water.

Hormone Replacement Therapy

Oral estrogens prescribed for menopausal and post-menopausal women have been linked to 8% of breast cancers, especially when used for more than 5 years.[59] Natural progesterone used alone seems to provide increased protection from breast cancer.[60] When a woman stops hormone replacement therapy, the risk is reduced and is greatly diminished after 5 years.[61]

Naturopathic therapies are successful in preventing or reversing osteoporosis, as explained by Dr Alan R. Gaby, in his book *Preventing and Reversing Osteoporosis*, and by Dr John Lee, in *What Your Doctor May Not Tell You About Menopause*.[62] Other menopausal symptoms can be treated with the use of Chinese or Western herbal formulas, nutritional supplements, homeopathy and/or natural progesterone cream.

PREVENTION
To help regulate your periods, consult a practitioner of Traditional Chinese Medicine, a naturopath, herbalist, or homeopath.

PREVENTION
Do not use the birth control pill for longer than 5 years or before the age of 20; preferably, avoid it altogether. Investigate other methods, such as the Justisse and barrier methods.

FACT
The risk of having breast cancer increases for every year a woman has been on horse estrogen/synthetic progestin therapy. There will be an extra 12 cases of breast cancer by the age of 70 for every 1000 women who start taking hormones at age 50 and continue until age 70.

Fertility Drugs

Most studies show that fertility drugs do not increase breast cancer risk. However, in one study of over 20,000 women who used fertility drugs, there was a significantly higher incidence of breast cancer within 1 year of using the drugs, even though the overall incidence of breast cancer was no greater over 5 years than in the general population.[63] What this tells us is that women should be especially vigilant in adopting many of the strategies in this book during the first year after fertility drugs. Before resorting to fertility drugs to become pregnant, consult with a natural medicine practitioner.

DES (Diethyl Stilbestrol)

DES was given to four million pregnant American women between 1940 and 1971 to prevent miscarriage. A synthetic chemical that mimicked estrogen, it was considered a wonder drug in its time, prescribed liberally by doctors. In the daughters of the women to whom it was given, there is increased incidence of clear-cell vaginal cancer, malformations of the reproductive tract, infertility, and a reduction in T-helper cells and T-killer cells, which are essential components of our immune systems in their surveillance against cancer. DES exposed women are more likely to develop autoimmune diseases as they age. In one study, women who took the drug DES (diethyl stilbestrol) had a 44% increased risk of breast cancer and their daughters were 2.5 times more likely to develop the disease after age 40 than women who were not exposed in utero.[64] All this 20 or more years after initial exposure.

The timing of the exposure to DES in utero is more important than the amount that the mother received. The fetus is most sensitive to estrogen-mimicking chemicals early on in pregnancy, between the sixth and the sixteenth week when the reproductive organs are developing. Women whose mothers took DES before the tenth week of pregnancy have a greater chance of developing vaginal or cervical cancer, while those exposed after the twentieth week of pregnancy are spared reproductive tract deformities. DES seems to sensitize the developing fetus to estrogens, making the individual more likely to develop certain cancers later in life, such as those of the breast, ovaries, uterus, and prostate.

DES also has effects on the brain and the pituitary gland. In animal studies, exposure to DES or higher than normal levels of estrogen at a sensitive time in utero caused permanent and dramatic changes in brain structure and behavior. Female rodents exposed to excess estrogen before or just after birth showed a more masculine pattern of reproductive behavior, causing them to act more like males with a decrease in feminine mating patterns.

In studies of women exposed to DES in utero, there was a higher than average rate of bisexuality and homosexuality. There are also higher rates of depression, anorexia, anxiety, and phobias in women and men exposed to DES.[65]

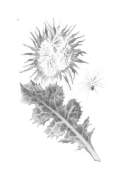

High Estrogen Levels During Pregnancy

Women born to mothers with high estrogen levels during pregnancy are at increased risk of breast cancer when they reach adulthood.[66,67] This fact indicates that we should be cautious during pregnancy to avoid exposure to xenoestrogens and to monitor our intake of phytoestrogens.

We do not know how high amounts of phytoestrogens during pregnancy or breast-feeding affect infants over their lifespan. The fetus is much more sensitive to hormonal stimulation and excess estrogen, particularly before four months of pregnancy. The blueprint for the child's sexual development and orientation are laid down in utero. The effects of excess estrogen may not visibly manifest until years later. Therefore, we should be cautious about quantities of phytoestrogens consumed during pregnancy and lactation, both for mother and child, until we know that high amounts are safe.

Some scientists are also concerned about the use of soy formulas in infants. Although they have been used for 30 years without noticeable effects, the daily exposure to infants of the plant estrogens in soy (called isoflavones) is 6-11 times higher on a body-weight basis than the dose that exhibits hormonal effects in adults. The amount of these phytoestrogens that circulate in the infant's blood are 13,000-22,000 times higher than plasma estradiol concentrations in early life. Though they are weak estrogens, soy formulas may have hormonal effects on young children that we have been unaware of so far, although one study demonstrated that 4-month-old infants did not yet have the intestinal bacteria needed to convert genistein into its active phytoestrogen, equol. Long-term follow-up studies are needed to assess the benefits or harmful effects of soy formulas in infants.[68]

In the meantime, it makes sense to vary the substitutes for breast milk, so that it is not exclusively soy-based. Alternatives are almond milk and organic goat milk. If you are trying to conceive or are pregnant, don't over-consume soy products, flaxseeds, and other phytoestrogens. They are fine in moderation but should not be the dietary mainstay. Use instead a variety of beans, grains, vegetables, fruits, nuts, and seeds.

Low Progesterone

Estrogen metabolism and breast cell proliferation are influenced strongly by the activity of many other hormones, which also need to be carefully monitored. Prime among these hormones is progesterone, estrogen's 'partner'. Like estrogen, progesterone is secreted by the ovaries. The hormone LH from the pituitary gland stimulates the ovaries to make progesterone.

Estrogen and progesterone are complementary hormones that need to be balanced. Low progesterone may lead to menstrual irregularities, PMS, uterine fibroids, ovarian cysts, breast tenderness, breast cysts, and breast cancer.[69]

This imbalance between estrogen and progesterone levels has several causes, including exposure to hormone-disrupting chemicals that affected ovary development during the embryo stage.[70] Studies have shown that environmental chemicals like phthalates, PCBs, herbicides, and hexachlorobenzene can suppress progesterone synthesis.[71,72] Low progesterone can also be the result of prolonged stress and high levels of the adrenal hormone, cortisol. Progesterone competes with cortisol inside the cell, so when progesterone levels are raised naturally or with progesterone cream, cortisol levels decline, and women experience fewer stress symptoms. Persistently high insulin levels can also prevent progesterone from being secreted by the ovary — testosterone is produced instead. Testosterone then converts to estrogen in fat cells.

FACT
High estrogen without the opposing balance of natural progesterone is linked to elevated rates of breast cancer.

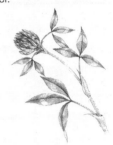

Target Sites and Effects of Progesterone

Target Sites	Effects of Progesterone
Uterus	Prepares uterus for implantation.
	Maintains the development of the placenta.
	Protects against endometrial cancer.
Breasts	Responsible for breast enlargement or 'ripening' during pregnancy.
	Develops milk-secreting cells during pregnancy.
	Protects against fibrocystic breast disease.
	Helps protect against breast cancer, in most cases.
Kidneys	Acts as a natural diuretic.
Brain	Restores libido.
	Acts as a natural tranquilizer.
Adrenal Glands	Helps to normalize blood sugar levels.
	Acts as a precursor to adrenal hormones.
Bone	Stimulates osteoblasts and may help to build bone.
Thyroid	Facilitates action of thyroid hormone, raises body temperature.
Fat cells	Helps to use fat for energy.
Rest of Body	Normalizes zinc and copper levels; normalizes oxygen levels in the cell.
	Stimulates the pancreas to release insulin. Acts as a vasodilator.

Whatever the cause, in each of these scenarios, the effect is estrogen dominance, causing uterine cells to multiply faster and stimulating breast tissue, resulting in breast swelling and tenderness. However, adequate progesterone decreases the rate at which breast cells multiply, eliminates breast tenderness, and stops uterine cells from multiplying.

Synthetic progestin does not protect from breast cancer, while natural progesterone (made from wild yam or soy) may help to prevent the disease.[73]

Breast Cell Maturation and Pregnancy

Progesterone levels are highest during pregnancy, when this hormone is produced by the placenta and causes growth and permanent maturation of breast cells. Mature breast cells are more resistant to cancer. If an abortion or miscarriage halts the pregnancy, this ripening process of breast cells stops as progesterone levels drop. The breast cells stay in a transitional state, still susceptible to cancerous changes.

Testing for Progesterone Deficiency

The most accurate test for progesterone levels is a salivary hormone test, best done in the morning between days 19-22 of your menstrual cycle when progesterone should be highest, counting from the first day of your previous period. To increase progesterone levels with oral progesterone, Dr John Lee suggests that the ideal amount is 400-500 mg of progesterone per ounce, which delivers the physiological amount that the ovaries normally produce when dosages of $1/4$ - $1/2$ teaspoon are taken daily or for a portion of one's menstrual cycle.[74] For more information on the benefits and usage of natural progesterone, consult Dr Lee's book, *What Your Doctor May Not Tell You about Breast Cancer*.

When supplementing with progesterone cream, it is important to monitor how the body responds to a particular dosage, as this will vary between individuals. If you are using progesterone cream or oral progesterone, consider follow-up testing of saliva levels of both progesterone and the three estrogens — estradiol, estrone and estriol — to ensure that all hormones and the estrogen quotient stay in a favorable range. Testing could occur two months after beginning use and then every six months thereafter. Progesterone cream is not curative — it only supplies you with progesterone for its duration of use.

Increasing Progesterone Naturally

Many products are available now that claim to contain natural progesterone but which in fact only contain diosgenin, a component in wild yam, which must be converted through a lab process to natural progesterone in order to have an effect. The body does not convert it to progesterone.[75] Other products actually do contain progesterone. While high-quality natural progesterone is readily available in the United States, in Canada, it is legally available only by prescription from a compounding pharmacist.

Other hormones, foods, herbs, and vitamins stimulate the production of progesterone. Melatonin has this effect. Some, though not all studies, have found that melatonin levels are higher during the luteal phase (latter half) of the menstrual cycle when progesterone levels are highest.[76] The thyroid hormone, T3, facilitates the action of progesterone, and the epidemic of apparent progesterone deficiency may also be related to widespread hypothyroidism, caused by radiation and environmental chemical exposure.

Herbs have been traditionally used to stimulate the production or availability of progesterone. These include chaste tree berry, yarrow, lady's mantle, mugwort, white deadnettle, elecampagne root, helonias root, wild yam root, birth root, black haw root bark, saw palmetto berry, Jamaican sarsaparilla root, Dong quai root, and marigold flowers.[79] However, David Zava and his co-workers tested over 150 various herbs, foods, and spices for progesterone bioactivity and found that none of the substances increased salivary progesterone in women, although many of them were able to bind to progesterone receptors in vitro. By far the strongest of these was bloodroot (Sanguinaria canadensis). Mistletoe, mandrake, and juniper were also all found to inhibit the proliferation of both estrogen receptor positive and estrogen receptor negative cell lines. Bloodroot and mistletoe have a long history of use in treating breast cancer.[80] Another herb called stoneseed has also been found to stimulate progesterone secretion.[83]

Vitamins and Minerals to Increase Progesterone

Vitamins that help increase progesterone include vitamin B6 and vitamin E. Vitamin B6 has been shown to reduce serum estrogen and raise progesterone levels.[84] Vitamin E enhances the absorption of progesterone. Minerals that assist in progesterone production are boron, zinc, and selenium. Increasing levels of boron in the diet will raise blood levels of both estrogen and progesterone, which is why it is an important nutrient in helping to maintain bone density. However, it may be best avoided if you are presently dealing with estrogen receptor positive breast cancer. Zinc supplementation has resulted in lowered blood levels of estrogen and higher progesterone as well.[85] Animal studies have shown that selenium supplementation can increase plasma progesterone levels.[86] Iodine levels may also have a bearing on progesterone, as the ovaries contain high amounts of iodine.

Progesterone as Treatment for Breast Cancer

If progesterone is so useful in preventing breast cancer, can we use it to treat breast cancer? The short answer is, we don't know enough yet.

One clinical trial has shown that breast cancer patients who were given progesterone had an improved disease-free and overall survival rate.[87] A 1999 study found that progesterone caused a 90% inhibition of cell growth in breast cancer cells in a laboratory setting when the cells were progesterone receptor positive. Progesterone had no effect on breast cancer cells that lacked the receptors for it.[88]

PREVENTION
Normalize progesterone and
thyroid function (see below)
to lower prolactin levels.
Increase dopamine to inhibit
prolactin by supplementing
with the amino acid, L-tyrosine,
which is also necessary to
manufacture thyroid and
adrenal hormones.

While these studies would seem to indicate that progesterone might be a powerful hormonal treatment for progesterone receptor positive breast cancer, other studies raise doubts. One study found that progesterone increased quantities of a growth factor called VEGF that stimulated the formation of a blood supply to breast cancer tumors, causing them to grow. VEGF increased 2-5 times between 3 and 6 hours after the hormone was added to breast cancer cells in a laboratory setting.[89]

In another study, Dr John Wiebe from the University of Western Ontario found that breakdown products of progesterone could act either to stimulate or to inhibit breast cancer. A particular enzyme called 5alpha-reductase is 30 times more prevalent in breast cancer cells than in healthy breast cells. When surgically removed cancerous tissue from the breasts of six women was incubated with progesterone over 8 hours, the metabolites of progesterone were recovered and identified. The enzyme 5alpha-reductase transformed progesterone into a metabolite called 5alpha-pregnane-3,20-dione (5alphaP) that stimulated breast cancer. A second enzyme known as 3alpha-HSO pushed progesterone to a metabolite called 3alphaHP that directly inhibited breast cancer cell growth.[90]

The deciding factor in this process is the quantity of 5alpha-reductase in the breast cell — if there is a lot of it (which there is in cancer cells), progesterone may be contraindicated. If there is not, as in healthy breast cells, progesterone may be protective. The long and short of it is that we have contradictory studies on the use of progesterone with breast cancer patients.

For the time being, I am being cautious and do not recommend progesterone to women with a breast cancer history. If there is an undetected tumor present, I do not want to risk feeding it. However, progesterone supplementation exerts a protective effect in the absence of breast cancer, particularly in pre-menopausal women.

High Prolactin

Prolactin, a hormone secreted by the anterior pituitary gland, normally stimulates the mammary glands to produce milk after childbirth. Prolactin levels may increase outside of childbirth when there is estrogen dominance, with either estrogen being too high or progesterone being too low, or both. Estrogen dominance also favors hypothyroidism, and serum prolactin levels are increased in about 40% of patients with hypothyroidism. Increased prolactin contributes to denser breast tissue, which may result in cystic breasts and elevate breast cancer risk.[91,92,93]

In pregnancy, prolactin levels are lower during the first trimester, which may help to protect women from breast cancer during this period.[94] Stress, suckling, sexual intercourse, and medications can raise prolactin levels, whereas the neurotransmitter dopamine can inhibit its release from the pituitary. Melatonin decreases the stimulating effects of prolactin on breast cancer cells.

Improving the breakdown and elimination of estrogen, while increasing progesterone and thyroid hormones may help to normalize prolactin. Reducing stress while increasing dopamine and melatonin may also counteract high prolactin. Prolactin levels can be assessed through a simple blood test. Screening for prolactin levels may show susceptibility to breast cancer.

Increased Growth Hormone

Growth hormone is secreted by the pituitary gland and regulates normal growth and development. Some forms of growth hormone stimulate milk production, which is why they are given to cattle in the United States. In some animal experiments, growth hormone is stronger than prolactin in stimulating breast development.[95] Girls who had a growth hormone deficiency and were given the hormone experienced accelerated development of breast tissue.[96] Growth hormone stimulates the ovaries to produce estradiol, causing puberty to occur earlier.[97]

Growth hormone is the main regulator of circulating IGF-1, and higher levels of IGF-1 increase breast cancer risk. Therefore, increased growth hormone will increase breast cancer risk through at least three mechanisms: indirectly by increasing circulating IGF-1; indirectly by stimulating estradiol production by the ovary, leading to earlier puberty and increased estradiol long-term; and directly by enhancing growth of breast tissue.

Increased Testosterone

Elevated testosterone production is a common finding in women with breast cancer.[98,99] The adrenal glands and ovaries make testosterone in women. When the ovaries shift gears during perimenopause, they decrease their production of estrogen and progesterone, and increase their production of testosterone. This drops after menopause. Women with polycystic ovary syndrome also make more testosterone and have an increased breast cancer risk.[100]

Increased testosterone levels can be triggered by chronically high levels of insulin, caused by prolonged stress, or a diet high in refined carbohydrates, sweets, soft drinks and desserts. Like estrogen, testosterone can increase cell growth. Breast tissue itself contains some of the aromatase enzyme, and so after menopause testosterone and the adrenal hormone androstenedione can be converted to estradiol and estrone directly in the breast, making it more vulnerable to cancer. Both estrogen and testosterone bind to the same carrier molecule in the blood, SHBG, although albumin is the main carrier protein for testosterone. However, increased testosterone may displace some estrogen from SHBG so that more is available to bind to receptor sites. Our goal then, is to maintain normal but not high testosterone levels.

FACT
Drinking milk or eating dairy products during pregnancy that are from growth hormone stimulated cows may cause an increased growth rate in the fetus, which is linked to a three fold higher risk of breast cancer later in life.

PREVENTION
Avoid dairy products from animals administered growth hormones. Lobby to ban the use of growth hormones in agricultural practice. For more information, see Chapter 4, 'Environmental Impact on Breast Health.'

FACT
Many American children are drinking milk from cows stimulated with growth hormone, which is likely to cause earlier onset of puberty, accelerated breast development, and increased risk of breast cancer.

PREVENTION
To block the enzyme aromatase, use ground flaxseeds daily and consider the use of chrysin as a strong aromatase inhibitor. Reduce insulin levels by following the guidelines presented in this chapter. Only use testosterone cream if your levels are low and you have been unable to raise them naturally.

Unbalanced Thyroid

The thyroid, located at the front of your throat, is regulated by a hormone from the pituitary gland, TSH, or thyroid stimulating hormone, which signals the gland to produce more or less thyroid hormones, depending on the need of the body. TSH is adjusted in turn by a hormone from the hypothalamus called TRH, or thyrotropin-releasing hormone, which reads the cues from the blood and signals the pituitary to produce TSH. The thyroid gland, when instructed by TSH, makes two hormones, thyroxine (T4) and triiodothyronine (T3), from iodine and the amino acids tyrosine and phenylalanine (which is converted to tyrosine in the liver). The job of thyroid hormones is to rev up the body's metabolic rate by increasing the number and activity of mitochondria, tiny 'furnaces' in every body cell that use oxygen to convert energy from food (glucose) into carbon dioxide, water, heat and energy. If thyroid hormones are deficient or unable to bind to their receptors, this process slows down and a person will feel fatigued and cold.

Testing Thyroid Function

There are several ways to test thyroid function. The simplest way is to take your underarm temperature in the morning before getting out of bed. A normal temperature is 97.8°F - 98.2°F or 36.6°C - 36.8°C with fluctuations that occur with your menstrual cycle. If your temperature is consistently lower than this, you may have an underactive thyroid (hypothyroid). If your temperature is often higher than 98.2°F, your thyroid gland may be overactive (hyperthyroid). Low progesterone, low cortisol and low iron may also contribute to a lowered body temperature, and often several of these imbalances are present simultaneously.

Blood tests for thyroid function should include TSH, free T3, free T4, reverse T3, thyroid microsomal antibodies (TPO Abs) and thyroglobulin antibodies (Tg Abs). If only one of these is abnormal and your temperature is low, there is likely a thyroid imbalance. If none are abnormal, there may still be a thyroid problem — go with the temperature test and symptoms and work with someone experienced with natural therapies to adjust it.

Thyroid, Estrogen, Progesterone, Prolactin, and Cortisol Interactions

When thyroid hormones are low, the liver will make less SHBG, the protein that would normally bind up estrogen in the blood, so that it is unable to attach to a receptor. Thus, low thyroid function correlates with more available estrogen, which can promote breast cancer.[103]

Conversely, when estrogen levels are higher or a woman is on hormone replacement therapy or the birth control pill, the levels of thyroxine-binding globulin, the carrier for thyroid hormone in the blood, are increased.[104] This protein attaches to thyroid hormone so that it is unavailable to bind to receptors in the cells, and a person may have hypothyroid symptoms. Only the 'free' thyroid hormones are active. A vicious cycle occurs — low thyroid results in higher available estrogen and higher estrogen levels keep thyroid hormones inactive. Naturopathic therapies can decrease estrogen and stimulate the production of thyroid hormones to break this cycle.

Progesterone, on the other hand, gives a boost to the thyroid. Dr David Zava has found that low progesterone and either high or low cortisol levels from the adrenal glands go hand in hand with a hypothyroid state. Use of natural progesterone cream can restore normal thyroid activity, in part by opposing the action of estrogen.[106] Normalizing adrenal function will also improve thyroid function.

Thyroid Function and Breast Cancer

Healthy thyroid function is critical to breast health. The thyroid gland is responsible for maintaining the body's normal temperature. Enzymes within the whole body work best at a particular temperature and pH. Their activity increases as body temperature rises. If temperature and pH are not maintained at optimal levels, there will be multiple enzyme deficiencies, and a decrease in the body's ability to detoxify and to fight cancer cells, among other things. When the thyroid hormone T3 binds to a receptor in a cell, enzyme production in the cell is increased up to six times, which facilitates optimal metabolism and keeps us warm. Depressed thyroid function will result in depressed immunity.

The basal metabolic rate, which the thyroid adjusts, is the rate of oxygen consumption in the body at rest. Cancer cells do not

FACT
When thyroid function is low, prolactin levels are sometimes elevated. Prolactin levels can normalize with an increase in thyroid hormones.[107] By decreasing prolactin levels, breast cancer risk is reduced.

Basal Body Temperature (BBT) Chart

The BBT chart can be used to screen for hypothyroidism by following these directions:

1) Take your temperature in your armpit for 10 minutes first thing in the morning before you get up.
2) Record the temperature on this chart with 'dots' for each day. Connect the dots with a line to see the trend in temperature.
3) Indicate the first day of your menstrual period by circling the temperature on that day.
4) Indicate the last day of your menstrual period by marking an 'x' through the temperature on the chart for that day. Your temperature will usually be higher the last 2 weeks of your cycle.

Note: A normal temperature falls between 36.6°C and 36.8°C or 97.8°F and 98.2°F.

If your temperature is consistently lower than this, you may have an underactive thyroid, underactive adrenals, low progesterone levels, low iron levels, or a combination of any of these. See a naturopath or other healthcare practitioner to help bring your hormones back into balance.

BBT Chart: Starting Date _____

Temperature   **Day of the Month**

°C	°F
38	100.4
37.9	100.2
37.8	100
37.7	99.86
37.6	99.68
37.5	99.5
37.4	99.32
37.3	99.14
37.2	98.96
37.1	98.78
37	98.6
36.9	96.42
36.8	98.24
36.7	98.06
36.6	97.88
36.5	97.7
36.4	97.52
36.3	97.34
36.2	97.16
36.1	96.98
36	96.8
35.9	96.62
35.8	96.44
35.7	96.26
35.6	96.08
35.5	95.9
35.4	95.72
35.3	95.54
35.2	95.36
35.1	95.18
35	95
34.9	94.82
34.8	94.64
34.7	94.46
34.6	94.28
34.5	94.1

thrive when there is an abundance of oxygen. It is plausible that women with hypothyroidism are more prone to breast cancer in part because of enzyme deficiencies and decreased tissue oxygenation.

One study has shown that plasma T3 concentrations were reduced significantly in both early and advanced breast cancer, and that TSH levels were elevated in women with advanced breast cancer — both signs of hypothyroidism.[108] Another study found that Hashimoto's thyroiditis was present in 44% of 310 Greek breast cancer patients and in only 19% of a control group.[109] A third study found that antithyroid peroxidase auto-antibodies/microsomal antibodies (TPO Abs) were twice as common in breast cancer patients than in controls.[110] A fourth study revealed a correlation between hyperthyroidism and breast cancer.[111] A fifth study of 102 consecutive breast cancer patients with ductal infiltrating carcinoma found that the overall prevalence of thyroid disease was 46% in the breast cancer patients studied, versus 14% in the control group.[112] A final study of 200 patients with breast cancer and a control group of 354 women with benign breast disease found an association between thyroid gland enlargement, as determined by ultrasound, and breast cancer.[113]

Dr Max Gerson, a pioneer in treating cancer, believed that the temperature and basal metabolic rate of cancer patients is often disturbed. He was able to normalize either of these extremes with supplemental iodine.[114]

Iodine's Link to Breast Health

Minerals that the thyroid system needs to produce its hormones are iodine, zinc, and selenium. The incidence of breast cancer is higher in areas where the soil is deficient in these minerals.[115,116] The thyroid gland absorbs 80 times more iodine than any other tissue (120 mcg per day) but contains only 20% of the body's iodine content, the rest being found in the skeletal muscles, liver, central nervous system, pituitary gland, breasts, and ovaries. Iodine is naturally absorbed into the epithelial lining of the ducts and lobules of the breast, where cancer most commonly occurs.[117] Breast cells are more sensitive to stimulation from estrogen when iodine is deficient, increasing breast cancer risk.[118]

It is probable that one of the reasons that Japanese women have low breast cancer rates is because they are the world's biggest consumers of seaweeds, averaging 11 grams per day. Liberal use of sea vegetables, such as kelp, dulse, nori, hiziki, and wakame, delivers plenty of iodine to the body, with kelp being the richest source. Our daily minimal requirement for iodine is 150 mcg or about 1 gram of seaweed.

Iodine therapy and thyroid metabolism must be monitored closely. With too much iodine, the thyroid can become either overactive or suppressed.

Dietary Sources of Tyrosine

Tyrosine is a building block for the neurotransmitter dopamine, the adrenal hormones, and thyroid hormones. It is often low in vegetarians who avoid dairy, so if you are one of those, be sure to choose foods daily that will give you an ample supply. Combine it with seaweed for iodine content. In our diet, we should aim to include at least 1500 mg daily of tyrosine for thyroid health.[105]

Food	Quantity	Mg. Tyrosine
Cooked oatmeal	¾ cup	161
Wheat bran	½ cup	101
Low fat cottage cheese	1 cup	1655
Fish	3 oz.	500
Figs	10 dried	247
Soy flour	½ cup	555
Soy nuts	½ cup	1287
Almond butter	1 tbsp	85
Almonds	12	100
Cashews	1 oz	139
Filberts	1 oz	129
Sunflower seeds	1 oz	189
Meat	3.5 oz	600-1000
Adzuki beans	1 cup boiled	890
Soy beans	1 cup	1084
Other beans	1 cup	400
Nori	3.5 oz	254
Dried spirulina	3.5 oz	2584
Miso	½ cup	500
Tofu, firm	½ cup	665

PREVENTION

Certain foods, when used without sufficient iodine in the diet, can block the thyroid's ability to use iodine. These include the raw brassica family – cabbage, broccoli, Brussels sprouts, cauliflower — and soy. Include seaweed in your diet daily to overcome the potential iodine-blocking effect of these foods, which are otherwise great for breast health.

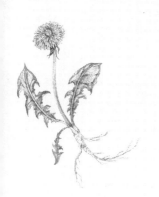

Environmental Chemicals and Toxic Metals

Even very low levels of PCBs, phthalates, and dioxins can disrupt thyroid function in the mother and fetus, causing permanent neurological damage in the developing baby that may manifest as learning disabilities, attention problems, and hyperactivity throughout childhood and adult life. It has been estimated that at least 5% of babies in the United States are exposed to quantities of environmental chemicals that would cause neurological damage.[120]

Chemicals can exert direct effects on the thyroid gland in one of several ways: they can inhibit the ability of the thyroid gland to trap iodine (thiocyanate, Tamoxifen and perchlorate do this); they can block the binding of iodine and the coupling of iodothyronines to form the thyroid hormones, thyroxine (T4) and triiodothyronine (T3) (sulfonamides, thiourea, methimazole, and aminotriazole do this); they can inhibit thyroid hormone secretion (lithium and an excess of iodine do this); they can increase the metabolism of thyroid hormones so that they are used up faster where they are needed in the body (many drugs do this — phenobarbitol, benzodiazepines, calcium channel blockers, and steroids; as do PCBs and organochlorine pesticides such as chlordane, lindane, DDT, and TCDD).[121]

Exposure to ionizing radiation disrupts thyroid function, as do many environmental chemicals. These xenoestrogens may be causing simultaneous conditions of estrogen dominance, progesterone deficiency, and thyroid dysfunction. High estrogen keeps more thyroid hormone bound to carrier proteins in the blood, so they are unavailable for use in your cells. Underactive thyroid conditions may also be related to nutritional deficiencies of iodine, zinc, selenium, or protein, resulting in a tyrosine deficiency.

Other Thyroid Conditions

A condition called Wilson's syndrome can occur when there is an excess of reverse T3 (RT3) due to the liver's inefficiency in making the conversion of T4 to T3. The enzyme required to make this conversion is dependent upon the minerals selenium and zinc, vitamin B12, and the amino acid cysteine.[122,123] The heavy metals mercury, cadmium, and lead will block this conversion in the liver.[124] Wilson's syndrome can be suspected when the underarm temperature before rising is consistently below 97.8°F, the person has symptoms of an underactive thyroid, standard blood tests for the thyroid are normal, and the ratio of T3 to reverse T3 is less than 10:1.

Hashimoto's thyroiditis is an autoimmune disease commonly resulting in a hypothyroid state. Blood tests will reveal the presence of thyroglobulin antibodies (Tg Abs) and thyroid microsomal antibodies (TPO Abs) that attack the thyroid gland, causing destruction of parts of it and/or block the production of thyroid hormone. In the early stages of the disease, the other thyroid tests — TSH, T4, and T3 — may be normal and symptoms of hypothyroidism are mild. Thus it frequently goes undiagnosed. Often the gland feels and looks enlarged and has a somewhat rubbery texture.

Grave's disease is an autoimmune hyperthyroid state that may have elevations of the same antibodies, Tg Abs and TPO Abs. Its symptoms are markedly different from hypothyroid symptoms, but like hypothyroid conditions, it is more frequently found in women with breast cancer compared to controls.

Tamoxifen and Thyroid Function

Tamoxifen, one of the drugs most commonly used in treating estrogen-driven breast cancer, interferes with thyroid function by preventing the gland from utilizing iodine and by blocking the formation of thyroid hormones.[125]

PREVENTION

If you are on Tamoxifen, use extra seaweeds in your diet or take one or more kelp tablets as well as selenium and zinc daily. Monitor thyroid function regularly and adjust any imbalances. See Chapter 10, 'Breast Disease Treatments,' for more protective natural therapies to use while on Tamoxifen.

Strategies for Improving Thyroid Function

Check your thyroid function annually with a temperature test, done for one month. If it is low, follow-up with a blood test that measures TSH, freeT4, free T3, reverse T3, thyroglobulin antibodies (Tg Abs), and microsomal antibodies (TPO Abs). If your thyroid is underactive, correct it with the help of a health practitioner using the appropriate strategies from this list:

1) Ensure adequate daily intake of selenium (200 mcg), zinc (50 mg), vitamin B12 (300 mcg), flaxseed oil (2 tbsp), and tyrosine (1500 mg).
2) Test and correct hydrochloric acid deficiency in the stomach to ensure adequate absorption of minerals.
3) Remove chemicals that may interfere with thyroid function using a sauna detoxification program. See Chapter 5, 'Detoxifying Our Bodies,' for more information on sauna programs.
4) Test for and remove heavy metals (cadmium, lead, mercury), and replace mercury fillings in the teeth with porcelain.
5) Decrease estrogen levels through improving liver detoxification (curcumin, ground flax, indole-3-carbinol or DIM, cysteine, milk thistle) and increasing bowel elimination (increase fiber, good bacteria). See Chapter 5, 'Detoxifying Our Bodies,' for information on these strategies.
6) Choose natural alternatives to the birth control pill and hormone replacement therapy.
7) Increase progesterone levels (vitamin E, B6, zinc, selenium, chaste tree, progesterone cream if appropriate).
8) Normalize the adrenal glands and cortisol levels with herbal formulas, relaxation, and nutrition.
9) If you are on Tamoxifen or Lithium, use extra iodine and selenium.
10) Exercise at least 40 minutes each day, particularly in the morning.
11) Consume small frequent meals, eating every 3 hours, with protein sources throughout the day. Avoid food sensitivities.
12) Use natural tonics for the thyroid. These include bee pollen, spirulina or chlorella algae, wheatgrass, oats, watercress, kelp, bladderwrack, saw palmetto berries, damiana leaf, guggul, and globe artichoke.[126] I have had considerable success normalizing thyroid hormones in women using a combination of L-tyrosine, zinc, selenium, guggul, spirulina, and an herbal formula containing bladderwrack, oats, skullcap, cleavers, and globe artichoke. See Chapter 7, 'Eating Right for Breast Health,' and Chapter 8, 'Nutritional Supplements for Breast Health,' for more information on these herbs. Some individuals may need bovine desiccated thyroid or combinations of T3 and/or T4 to normalize thyroid function.

High Insulin Levels

The pancreas secretes insulin in an effort to decrease blood glucose levels, particularly after eating. It helps transport glucose into muscle cells to be used for energy or into fat cells to be stored as fat. When we are overweight, we can develop 'insulin resistance', whereby the insulin less easily carries glucose to its destination, and both insulin and glucose levels rise in the blood, setting the stage for diabetes and increasing breast cancer risk.

High insulin levels can induce polycystic ovary syndrome in women, causing low progesterone and high testosterone, which both increase breast cancer risk.[127] The number of receptors for insulin on breast cancer cells is 5-10 times greater than the number on normal breast cells, making breast cancer cells very sensitive to the growth-promoting qualities of insulin.[128] Insulin is high when blood glucose is high, and we know that glucose is an energy source for the growth of breast cancer cells.[129] Dr Pamela Goodwin, a breast cancer specialist at Mount Sinai Hospital in Toronto, monitored 535 women with newly diagnosed breast cancer for up to 10 years, and found that those with higher insulin levels were about 8 times more likely to develop a recurrence and die of the disease than those with normal insulin levels.[130]

Contributing to higher insulin levels are excess sugar and sweets, soft drinks, alcohol, high glycemic carbohydrates that cause a fast rise in blood sugar, Omega 6 fatty acids (vegetable oils like sunflower, safflower), and saturated fat from animal products.[135] An Italian study of 104 postmenopausal women determined that with a radical shift to a diet that was low in refined carbohydrate and animal fat but high in low-glycemic foods, phytoestrogens, olive oil, flax, and fish oil, women could decrease insulin resistance, lose weight, and lower both testosterone and estrogen levels.[136]

Insulin and Estrogen

Insulin alters estrogen metabolism and affects breast cells in six other important ways:

1) Insulin and its cousin, insulin-like growth hormone (IGF-1), decrease the liver's ability to make SHBG, the transport truck for estrogen in the blood that keeps it from cutting loose and binding to its receptors in breast cells.[131] So the higher the insulin levels, the more 'free' estrogen is available.

2) High insulin levels triggers the adrenal glands and ovaries to produce more testosterone, which attaches to SHBG as well, and pushes estrogen out of its seat so it is free to attach to receptors in breast cells.[132]

3) Elevated insulin decreases the amount of binding protein (a different transport truck) in the blood for IGF-1, freeing more of this hormone so that it, too, can increase multiplication of breast cells when it attaches its receptors which are found in 90% of all breast cancer tumors.[133] Insulin also increases the production of IGF-1.[134]

4) Both insulin and IGF-1 stimulate the ovaries to produce more estrogen, promoting estrogen dominance.

5) Insulin resistance causes higher blood glucose levels, which eventually gets stored as fat. Increased fat storage leads to elevated estrogen levels.

6) Cancer cells depend on glucose for energy, so higher blood glucose levels feed cancer.

High Insulin-like Growth Factors-1 and -2 Levels

Insulin-like Growth Factors-1 and -2 (IGF-1 and IGF-2) are hormones produced by the liver, responsible for growth and development. Their production is stimulated by growth hormone from the pituitary gland. Our levels of IGF-1 are low at birth, rise during childhood, peak at puberty, and decline as we age. Both insulin and IGFs cause cells to hypertrophy, or enlarge. Insulin and IGFs have a similar structure, and when insulin levels fluctuate, so do the levels of IGFs. Circulating total and free IGF-1 levels are low when insulin levels are low.[137]

Women with breast cancer often have increased blood levels of IGF-1. Higher levels of IGF-1 cause a four-fold increased risk of prostate cancer and make us more prone to lung cancers.[138] It causes massive multiplication of growth when added to breast cell tissue cultures and promotes the growth and invasiveness of malignant cells. Ground flaxseed added to the diet can decrease the number of receptors for IGF-1, diminishing its effect on breast tissue.

In addition, Insulin-like Growth Factor-1 protects breast cancer cells from cell death, or apoptosis, and in so doing, interferes with the effects of chemotherapy. Receptors for IGF-1 have been found in 90% of breast cancer cell lines and in most biopsies of breast cancer tumors.[140,141] When the action of IGF-1 is blocked, breast cancer tumor growth is stalled.[142] Higher estrogen levels may make the breasts more sensitive to the growth-promoting effects of IGF-1 by increasing the number of IGF-1 receptor sites in the breasts.[143] Although we are not certain of the mechanism, it is clear that estrogen enhances the response of breast cells to the IGFs.

FACT

IGF-1 binds to its receptor sites on breast cell membranes and acts synergistically with estradiol to increase cell division, promote breast development, and increase breast density during puberty as well as breast cancer later in life.[139]

FACT

The Harvard Nurse's Study found that women whose blood contained slightly higher levels of IGF-1 had a sevenfold increase in breast cancer risk, making it one of the highest predisposing factors to the disease.

PREVENTION

Have your saliva levels of IGF-1 and serum IGFBP-3 checked annually and adopt the 'Strategies for Balancing Insulin' to reduce IGF-1 levels as well. Avoid dairy products from growth hormone treated cows. Avoid colostrum and any product that claims to increase IGF-1 or growth hormone levels.

FACT

A current health fad is to take bovine colostrum, containing growth hormone, to encourage fat loss, build muscle mass, or stimulate immunity. People who do this may simultaneously increase their cancer risk by increasing circulating IGF levels. Colostrum is meant for newborns who need rapid growth, not for adults.

PREVENTION

Have your blood or saliva levels of IGF-1 and 2 and the binding protein IGFBP-3 checked annually and reduce IGF-1 levels with a primarily vegan diet.

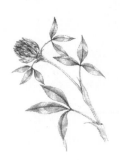

IGF-1 levels are higher in pre-menopausal breast cancer patients (compared to post-menopausal patients) and are higher in women with breast cancer recurrence. Moderate consumption of alcohol increases the liver's production of insulin-like growth factors, although IGF production declines in heavy drinkers as alcohol-related liver damage prevents their formation.[144] One of the effects of Tamoxifen is to reduce IGF-1 levels. The probability of survival is greater in breast cancer patients with plasma IGF-1 levels less than 120 ng/ml.[145] Higher serum levels of IGF-1 are associated with increased breast cancer risk in pre-menopausal women.[146]

Bovine Growth Hormones

Any substance we ingest that contains growth hormone will increase our baseline levels of IGF-1. In the United States, cows are given bovine growth hormone to increase milk production by approximately 10%. The milk of these cows contains a tenfold increase in IGF-1 beyond the milk of cows not given growth hormone. Because the IGF-1 is not protein bound, it is easily absorbed across the intestinal wall, and its digestion is blocked by casein present in the milk. This leads to higher levels of IGF-1 in the person ingesting the milk, which in turn leads to increased growth and stimulation of breast cells. IGF-1 accumulates and concentrates selectively in breast cells. We would expect that this will lead to earlier breast development and increased breast cancer risk in girls who consume milk containing bovine growth hormone.

Managing IGFs

The insulin-like growth factors are carried in the blood on one of seven binding proteins.[147] When the concentration of these binding proteins increases, the availability and activity of the IGFs decreases. Binding proteins affect the biological activity of IGFs, and can either increase or decrease their cancer-promoting activity or act independently from them. The binding protein IGFBP-3 in particular is able to inhibit breast cancer cell growth when present in high amounts.

The ratio between IGF-1 and IGFBP-3 is useful to assess the activity of IGF-1 on breast cells, and could be used as a screening tool.[148] If IGFBP-3 levels were high, it would mean that less IGF-1 would be free to attach to receptors.[149,150]

A British study compared IGF-1 levels in 92 vegan women, 99 meat eaters, and 101 vegetarians. The vegans had IGF-1 levels 13% lower than the meat-eaters or vegetarians who ate dairy.[151] If we lower plasma IGF-1 levels, we may reduce the risk of developing breast cancer; slow the progression of early stage breast cancer; lower the risk of recurrence; and increase the probability of survival. Since increased IGF-1 is the strongest hormonal risk factor for breast cancer, it makes sense to adopt a primarily vegan diet to reduce risk or assist recovery from the disease.

Unbalanced Cortisol

The adrenal glands, which sit on top of your kidneys, govern the body's ability to adapt to stress through the secretion of several hormones, including cortisol. Like insulin, cortisol affects blood glucose levels. One of its jobs is to stimulate the liver to form glucose from proteins and fats, promoting an overall increase in blood glucose levels. Cortisol levels elevate when we are under stress, and if the stress is prolonged, cortisol will promote an overall increase in blood glucose levels, insulin levels, IGF-1 levels, fat deposition in the upper body, and circulating estrogen. This is called the 'resistance phase' in the stress cycle.

Many women come in to my office with a breast cancer diagnosis after a prolonged period of stress — usually a difficult time at work, problems with a marriage, financial difficulties, or a recent loss of a loved one. High cortisol can also be caused by suppressed childhood abuse of any kind or from overexercising.[153] Hormonal imbalances will continue while the stress remains, unless we use coping mechanisms to decrease our stress response, such as relaxation breaks, meditation, counseling, or group support.

One study of 125 women with metastatic breast cancer showed that group therapy and social support was associated with lower concentrations of cortisol — signifying healthier hormonal balance.[154] Cortisol levels are usually higher in the morning to trigger wakefulness and heightened energy, and lower in the evening to induce calmness and sleep. A second study assessed salivary cortisol levels at 8:00 a.m., 12:00 a.m., 5:00 p.m., and 9:00 p.m. in 104 women with metastatic breast cancer for 3 consecutive days and found that women whose cortisol secretion pattern was 'flattened' — without the expected rise in the morning and fall in the evening —had the shortest life expectancy.[155]

FACT
Several studies demonstrate cortisol's importance to breast cancer recovery.

PREVENTION
Monitor your cortisol level through saliva testing done in the early morning, noon, late afternoon, and evening to pinpoint where you are in the stress cycle and to monitor improvement. See Chapter 9, 'Psychological and Spiritual Means for Preventing Breast Cancer,' for stress-reducing strategies.

Stress and Cancer

We know intuitively that stress plays a role in most illnesses, including cancer. High cortisol causes depressed immunity, resulting in fewer T-killer cells and less T-killer cell activity. These are the white blood cells that target cancer cells — we need lots of them and we need them to be fiercely active. Elevated cortisol levels inhibit progesterone production by the ovaries, making us more susceptible to both breast cancer and osteoporosis. The body can utilize progesterone to make cortisol if needed during periods of stress, inducing more estrogen dominance because of the lowered progesterone. Increased stress can increase the production of testosterone in the ovaries and adrenals and can increase the activity of the aromatase enzyme that converts testosterone to estrogen. High cortisol causes thyroid hormones to be less efficient in your cells, which in turn increases estrogen resistance. Finally, if cortisol levels are elevated at night, as they are for many cancer patients, less of the protective hormone, melatonin, will be produced.[152] After cortisol levels have been high for a time, the adrenals may develop exhaustion and cortisol levels can become very depressed. This is known as the "exhaustion phase" in the stress cycle. Each of the above 'stress' factors contributes to breast cancer risk.

Reducing Stress and Breast Cancer Risk

As women we must recognize when a situation is not working for us, break through our denial or desire to please, and exercise courage to change the situation. I have counseled many women newly diagnosed with breast cancer to consider leaving their relationship when it was apparent that it was the source of their inner conflict and things were unlikely to change. So, if you have been diagnosed with breast cancer, think about what you need to cut out of your life to feel whole again, and take out your sword. Find a healthcare practitioner you can talk to who can help to unravel your life and suggest coping mechanisms to guide you through it. Use the journey as a rebirth to your new self.

Decreased Melatonin

Melatonin is a hormone secreted by the pineal gland that modifies the function of the nervous system, glandular system, and immune system. The pineal gland translates changes in external light into chemical signals that impose a 'circadian rhythm' upon the body that helps orchestrate many, if not all, of the other body rhythms. In a 24-hour cycle, the highest level of melatonin production occurs during the night between 1:00 a.m. and 3:00 a.m., while we are asleep in the dark. Exposure to light or electromagnetic radiation at night reduces these levels. Electromagnetic fields from clocks, radios, electric blankets, and anything else within $2\frac{1}{2}$ feet of us while we sleep will inhibit melatonin production. Melatonin levels can be monitored through saliva testing at 3:00 a.m.

As melatonin levels decrease with aging, we are more vulnerable to disorders associated with disturbances in the body's rhythms, such as sleep disorders, hormonal imbalances, and cancer. Youthfulness and longevity are linked to high levels of melatonin secretion. Some of the health benefits ascribed to producing or taking melatonin on a regular basis are improved sleep, increased libido, resistance to viral infections, improved energy, and prevention of jet lag.

Melatonin Levels in Cancer Patients and Shift Workers

Cancer patients have melatonin levels that are 30-40% lower than people who are cancer free at similar ages.[156] Autopsies of cancer victims reveal shrinkage and decreased weight of the pineal gland.[157] Patients with aggressive breast tumors have lower levels of melatonin than women with a low rate of malignant cell growth.[158]

Melatonin levels are low in women who work night shifts, sleep in the day and don't experience regular night-time sleep periods of total darkness.[159] One study of 800 women with breast cancer found that women who were awake between 1:00 a.m. and 2:00 a.m., when melatonin levels peak, had an increased breast cancer risk compared to a control group. There were 60% more cases of breast cancer in women who worked at least one night shift per week for a minimum of 3 years in the 10-year period leading up to their diagnosis, compared to women who never worked night shifts.[160] It takes about 6 days for the pineal gland to adjust to a changing sleep schedule.[161]

Blind women, on the other hand, have a 20-50% lower rate of breast cancer, because the visual signals from light are absent in these women and melatonin levels remain constant.[162]

Actions in Inhibiting Breast Cancer

When a small breast tumor begins to form, the pineal secretes more melatonin in an attempt to control it. If it fails to control the process and breast cancer is initiated, pineal exhaustion sets in and night-time blood levels of melatonin decrease as the tumor grows in size.[163] If the breast tumor metastasizes and spreads through the body, the pineal makes a last, valiant attempt to stop the cancer from spreading by sending large amounts of melatonin into the bloodstream. Usually the prognosis is poor, but occasionally the pineal's efforts are successful and the cancer retreats. Older people may have less success because the pineal has deteriorated due to aging.

Women with late stage breast cancer achieved partial remission lasting an average of 8 months when they were given high doses of melatonin in the evening (20 mg per day). If melatonin is prescribed, all doses should be taken at bedtime, since morning administration has been found to stimulate cancer growth in animal studies.[166]

Melatonin, Prolactin, Progesterone, Estrogen, and Thymus Interactions

Melatonin also decreases the stimulating effect of the hormone prolactin (secreted by the pituitary gland) on breast cancer cells. Women with breast cancer and low melatonin levels tend to have higher secretions of prolactin around noon. It seems that melatonin is involved in the complex timed release of other hormones, including prolactin. Hypothyroidism is also often linked to higher prolactin levels.

Melatonin levels vary during a woman's menstrual cycle, and melatonin itself may stimulate progesterone secretion, though research is conflicting.[169] Some studies, though not all, show that melatonin levels are low at ovulation and increase premenstrually three to sixfold, reaching their peak at menstruation.[170]

Higher amounts of melatonin will cause a decrease in the numbers of estrogen receptors and inhibit the replication of breast cancer cells in the laboratory by regulating cell division and multiplication.[171] It's as though this pineal hormone flips a breaker switch to turn off estradiol's activity on the breast cell. It may even lower estrogen levels.[172]

There is a close relationship between the function of the pineal,

FACT
Supplementation with melatonin often results in stabilizing cancer so that it ceases to grow, or can actually cause tumors to regress.[164]

Melatonin Healing Mechanisms

Melatonin inhibits the growth of breast cancer cells through several mechanisms:

1) Melatonin can directly kill breast cancer cells.

2) Melatonin inhibits the production of tumor growth factor, thereby thwarting tumor growth.

3) Melatonin stimulates the differentiation of cancer cells, shifting them towards normal cells.

4) Melatonin improves the individual's immune system to fight against the tumor.[167]

5) Melatonin decreases the ability of cancer cells to attach to basement membranes, preventing invasive cancer.[168]

6) Melatonin helps to regulate cell division and multiplication.

7) Melatonin decreases the number of estrogen receptors in breast cells, thereby decreasing estrogen's effect on breast cells. It also competes with estrogen for the existing receptor sites.

pituitary, and thymus glands, each of them playing a role in cancer prevention and immune fitness. A hormone from the thymus gland called thymosin, which improves immune function, is regulated in part by melatonin. A 240% increase in natural killer cells has been observed after melatonin supplementation.[173] This means that the immune system has more than double the ability to annihilate cancer cells directly when melatonin levels are high. Melatonin can reverse shrinkage of the thymus gland caused by psychological and physiological stress.[174]

Contraindications

Melatonin should not be taken or used cautiously by people with autoimmune diseases like rheumatoid arthritis or Hashimoto's thyroiditis, as it may increase the activity of an already overactive immune system. It should be avoided during steroid use and may worsen depression if used by depressed individuals.

Natural Sources of Tryptophan

Melatonin is synthesized in humans from the amino acid tryptophan, which is first converted to serotonin in the pineal gland and then to melatonin. Melatonin production is dependent on vitamins B3 and B6, calcium, magnesium, and zinc. Vitamin B6 in particular is needed for the conversion of tryptophan to serotonin. Melatonin's effectiveness in the body is at least partially dependent on glutathione, an amino acid complex important for the liver's detoxifying ability and immune health.

Ultradian Breath Rhythms

In his book, *Self-Healing: Powerful Techniques*, Ranjie Singh, PhD, found that practitioners of breathing exercises were able to raise their melatonin levels from 0.5 to 10 times higher, with an average of 3 times higher than baseline levels. Cancer patients experienced an average increase in melatonin levels of 230% or over double their baseline levels.

Physiological and psychological processes influenced by ultradian rhythms include the desire to eat and drink, sleep, dreaming and wakefulness, actions of the immune system, breast-feeding, hormonal secretions, stress reactions, attention and concentration, cell replication, and mood changes. These are governed by the same 90-120 minute periods as the breath cycle.[178] As the breath cycle comes into balance through practicing breathing exercises, the other ultradian rhythms normalize as well.

Breathing Balance

When the left nostril is dominant, the right hemisphere of the brain exhibits more activity.[179] The right hemisphere is linked to creative thought, intuition, non-linear thinking, a sense of timelessness, and appreciation of art, music, and poetry. With left nostril dominance the parasympathetic nervous system is activated, causing us to feel more relaxed. Blood pressure will often decrease with left nostril breathing. When the right nostril is dominant, the left hemisphere

Food Sources of Tryptophan for Elevating Melatonin

We can promote melatonin production is by ensuring an adequate dietary supply (1000 mg) of the amino acid tryptophan. Animal studies have shown that increased amounts of dietary L-tryptophan can cause a fourfold elevation in blood melatonin levels.

Food	Serving	Tryptophan (mg)	Food	Serving	Tryptophan (mg)
Spirulina, dried	3.5 oz	929 mg	Adzuki Beans, boiled	1 cup	166 mg
Soy Flour	1 cup	683 mg	Lentils, boiled	1 cup	160 mg
Soy Nuts	½ cup	495 mg	Mung Beans, boiled	1 cup	154 mg
Soy Protein Powder	1 oz	312 mg	Chick Peas, boiled	1 cup	139 mg
Cottage Cheese	1 cup	312 mg	Pumpkin seeds	122 seeds	122 mg
Tofu, raw, firm	½ cup	310 mg	Hummus	1 cup	116 mg
Tuna	3 oz	291 mg	Wheat Germ	¼ cup	110 mg
Tempeh	½ cup	234 mg	Soy Milk	1 cup	103 mg
Salmon	3 oz	231 mg	Egg	1 medium	100 mg
Cashews	20 whole	215 mg	Collards, boiled	1 cup	100 mg
Avocado	½ medium	200 mg	Sunflower Seeds	1 oz	99 mg
Oatmeal flakes	1 cup	200 mg	Brazil Nuts	8 nuts	74 mg
Miso	½ cup	197 mg	Organic Raisins	7 tbsp	60 mg
Navy Beans, boiled	1 cup	187 mg	Sweet Potato	1 small	50 mg
Kidney Beans, boiled	1 cup	182 mg	Spinach	2 cups raw	50 mg
Black Beans, boiled	1 cup	179 mg	Yogurt	1 cup	50 mg
Great Northern Beans	1 cup	175 mg	Almond Butter	1 tbsp	43 mg

Note: Tryptophan can be purchased in capsule form as 5-HTP. Usually the dosage is 100-200 mg, 2-3 times daily. Be sure to take vitamin B6 as well. If you have breast cancer, especially if it is estrogen receptor positive, consider supplementing with 5-50 mg of melatonin one half hour before bedtime (8:00-10:00 p.m.) with medical supervision. If you are at high risk for breast cancer, use 3-9 mg of melatonin nightly as prevention.

of the brain shows more activity. The left hemisphere is related to linear thinking, assertiveness and aggressiveness, concentrated study, athletic activity, mathematical problem solving, and logic.

With right nostril dominance the sympathetic nervous system is activated, causing us to feel more alert and charged, ready for action.[180] Right nostril breathing will often elevate blood pressure slightly and prepare us for intense physical activity, study, or assertive exchanges.

The 20-minute period when both nostrils are dominant is a time of integration between the hemispheres. This is often the time when we want to daydream, fantasize, reflect, have a break from what we were doing, move around, or process emotional material. It is the time of reconciliation between mind and body, when we are more open to receive and pay attention to the messages from the body. It is the time when we are primed to receive intuitive impulses, inner guidance, and connect to our spiritual selves. During this twenty-minute break, we are more apt to acknowledge emotions we have suppressed.

When we develop and practice a slow, meditative breath, melatonin levels increase throughout the body as the pineal gland

FACT
Western society chronically neglects the body's need for a 20- minute break every 2 hours or so. We replace these times of potential integration with addictions such as coffee, cigarettes, alcohol, work, television, sugar or excess food, and recreational drugs, which compound the problem. These addictions further alienate us from the messages our bodies send us, from our emotional truths, and from our spiritual identities.

Strategies for Taking Care of Your Pineal Gland

Besides ensuring adequate consumption of foods high in tryptophan, along with vitamins B3, B6, calcium, magnesium, zinc, and NAC or foods containing cystine, melatonin levels can be increased by lifestyle changes that enhance the pineal gland:

1) Avoid shift work. It confuses your body's rhythms and will interfere with melatonin production.
2) Spend at least 20 minutes outside in natural light (without sunglasses) in the early part of the day. This may help melatonin levels to be higher at night.[175]
3) Sleep in a dark room, with no light shining in from the street. Melatonin production is lower when we are exposed to light at night. Low intensity light (50 lux) is acceptable but levels of 500 lux or higher suppress melatonin release. If need be, wear a mask over your eyes as you sleep.
4) Keep regular hours, preferably going to bed early and getting up early.
5) Avoid excessive exposure to electromagnetic radiation, which interferes with melatonin production. Do not sleep within 3 feet or I meter of an electrical outlet or device.
6) Exercise regularly. One hour daily on a stationary bicycle can double or triple melatonin levels.[176]
7) Avoid the other factors that interfere with pineal function — alcohol, caffeine, recreational drugs, nicotine, intense electromagnetic fields, bright lights and medications such as beta-blockers, diazepam, haloperidol, chlorpromazine, and ibuprofen.
8) Practice a meditative or breathing exercise one or more times daily. We can stimulate our own bodies to produce melatonin through the regular practice of meditation or breathing exercises, particularly before bed.

PREVENTION
To help prevent breast cancer, keep your melatonin levels high through an evening meditation practice.

FACT
Ignoring the psychological and physiological need to relax fosters hormonal imbalances and increased cell replication leading to cancer.

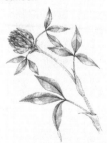

responds with renewed vigor.[181] When the pineal gland is not functioning properly, there will be increased cell division and multiplication and a greater likelihood of cancer. We know that cell division is linked with the breath cycle through ultradian rhythms, so that normalizing the breath cycle can help to normalize cell division. The complete process of cell division typically takes between $1\frac{1}{2}$ - 2 hours, with a 20-minute critical period of time when molecules called 'cyclins' accumulate in the cell to determine if and when it will divide.

Regular Relaxation

When we are chronically stressed, the breath cycle becomes derailed. Most often it speeds up, so that the nostril shift will occur within a shorter period. We may also become dominant in one nostril, rarely breathing through the other. This can lead to over dominance in one hemisphere of the brain, problems occurring particularly on one side of the body and dominance of either the parasympathetic or sympathetic nervous system. We lose our pre-programmed equilibrium. It is no wonder that breast cancer often occurs after a period of chronic stress.

Many of us live very busy lives with little time for genuine relaxation, self-reflection, meditation, prayer, or solitude. Relaxation is a necessary component of any healing process. When we relax, we activate the parasympathetic branch of the autonomic nervous system, which promotes healing. One of the most important things you can do in your healing journey is to adopt a daily practice of relaxation, visualization, or meditation.

The Hormone Puzzle

Hormone Balancing Strategies for Breast Cancer Prevention

This quick reference chart should assist you and your healthcare team to develop strategies for balancing your hormone levels to promote your good health and to prevent cancer.

Increases Risk	Protection Strategy

ESTROGEN

Increases Risk	Protection Strategy
Excessive Strong Estrogens (Estrone and Estradiol) *due to:* Lack of exercise High intake of meat High fat diet Obesity Constipation Early puberty, late menopause Birth control pill, hormone replacement therapy Light at night	Increase Estriol (Weak Estrogen) *with:* Cabbage, brassica family Indole-3-carbinol or DIM Sea vegetables Iodine Decrease Estradiol and Estrone by: Daily exercise Vegetarian, low fat diet Improve liver detoxification and elimination Stall puberty Sleep in a dark room
Increased C4 and C16 Estrogens *linked to:* Xenoestrogens, pesticides, especially lindane Dioxin, car exhaust, paint fumes Phenols, formaldehyde Mercury, lead, arsenic, thallium, tin Pharmaceutical drugs Intestinal toxins and harmful bacteria Sugar, a high fat diet, fried or rancid fats Inadequate protein	Make More C2 Estrogen, Less C4 and C16; Inactivate C4 Estrogen *with:* **1. Promote formation of C2 estrogens:** brassicas - cabbage, broccoli, brussel sprouts etc, indole-3-carbinol or DIM, rosemary, schizandra, St. John's wort **2. Assist Phase 2 methylation:** methionine, SAM, MSM, choline, betaine, vitamins B6, B12, B2, folic acid, magnesium **3. Assist Phase 2 glutathione conjugation:** milk thistle, curcumin, ellagic acid, alpha lipoic acid, cysteine, NAC, goat whey, soy nuts, broccoli sprouts (sulforaphane), green tea, limonene and perillyl alcohol (essential oils of lemon, celery, sweet orange, palmarosa, lavender), zinc, selenium **4. Assist Phase 2 sulfation:** cysteine, taurine, methionine, MSM, vitamin B6, sulforaphane, selenium, Bifidobacterium. **5. Dietary:** low fat diet, EPA (fish oil), ground flax seeds, increased fiber, wheat bran, psyllium, probiotics, soy, red clover, phytoestrogens **6. Assist glucuronidation:** ellagic acid (red raspberries), Vitamin B6, psyllium, wheat bran, legumes, high fiber, Calcium-D-glucarate (oranges, apples), fish oil, probiotics **7. Normalize progesterone**

Increased Production of Strong Estrogens (Estrone and Estradiol) *due to:*
Aromatase enzyme

Inhibit Aromatase *with:*
Chrysin (strong)>1500 mg/day
Ground flaxseed (moderate)
Genistein (soy) (weak)
Zinc

Decreased SHBG (Sex Hormone Binding Globulin) *due to:*
High cortisol
High insulin
High IGF-1
High testosterone
Low thyroid

Increase SHBG *with:*
Fiber
Ground flaxseeds, soy
Red clover sprouts
Low fat vegetarian diet
Improve thyroid function
Normalize cortisol, insulin, IGF-1, testosterone

Increased Number of Estrogen Receptors *due to:*
Pesticides
Xenoestrogens
Hormone replacement therapy
High Body Mass Index

Decrease Number of Estrogen Receptors *with:*
Melatonin

Xenoestrogens Attach to Estrogen Receptors *such as:*
Pesticides, PCBs, dioxin, PVC, phthalates, Bisphenol A, brominated fire retardants, nonylphenyl ethoxylates, cadmium, mercury, lead

Block Estrogen Receptors *with:*
Phytoestrogens: flax, soy, red clover, mung bean sprouts, pumpkin seeds
Indole-3-carbinol, DIM
Quercetin

PROGESTERONE

Decreased Progesterone *due to:*
Phthalates
PCBs
Herbicides
Hexachlorobenzene
High cortisol levels
High insulin levels
Excess refined sugars and carbohydrates
Nutritional deficiencies

Increase Progesterone *with:*
Vitamins B6 and E; selenium, zinc, boron
Chaste tree berry, stoneseed
Soy, ground flaxseed
Improve liver, bowel and adrenal function
Adequate melatonin levels
Normalize cortisol levels
Normalize insulin, avoid sugar
Normalize thyroid, use zinc seaweeds, selenium to increase T3.
Use progesterone cream as a last resort

PROLACTIN

High Prolactin *due to:*
Estrogen dominance
Underactive thyroid
Stress
Suckling
Sexual intercourse
Medications

Normalize Prolactin *with:*
Normalize low progesterone
Normalize low thyroid
Improve detoxification and elimination of estrogen
Use L-tyrosine to increase dopamine
Increase melatonin; sleep in dark room
Reduce stress/ use relaxation

TESTOSTERONE

Elevated Testosterone *due to:*
High insulin levels
Chronic stress
Excess sugar and refined carbohydrates
Polycystic ovary syndrome

Normalize Testosterone *with:*
Flaxseed
Chrysin
Seaweed
Iodine
Testosterone cream (last resort)

GROWTH HORMONE

Increased Growth Hormone *due to:*
Dairy containing bovine growth hormone
Colostrum products

Normalize Growth Hormone *with:*
Avoid dairy or beef products containing bovine
growth hormone

THYROID HORMONES

Low Thyroid Function *due to:*
Ionizing radiation: x-rays, nuclear power and
weapons
Lead, cadmium, mercury
PCBs, pesticides, phthalates, dioxin
Prescription drugs: tamoxifen, steroids, etc.
Excess estrogen levels
Low progesterone levels
High or low cortisol levels

Normalize Thyroid Hormone Production *with:*
Normalize progesterone
Improve detoxification and elimination of estrogen
Normalize cortisol
Use tyrosine, iodine or kelp
Use dessicated thyroid
Use T3, T4 hormones as last resort
Improve RT3:T3 Ratio;

Increase Conversion of T4 to T3 *with:*
Detoxify mercury, cadmium, lead, chemicals
Tyrosine, cysteine, iodine
Zinc, selenium, copper
Vitamin B12
Flaxseed oil

Hyperthyroid Condition *due to:*
Excess iodine
Chronic stress/ cortisol imbalance
Radiation exposure
Liver stagnation and heat

Normalize Thyroid Hormones *with:*
Decrease stress
Daily relaxation/meditation
Chinese herbs to relax the liver
Motherwort, skullcap, bugleweed, lemon balm
Magnesium, B complex
Avoid radiation

INSULIN

High Insulin Levels *due to:*
Excess sugar, soft drinks, alcohol, refined carbohydrates
Animal fats
Omega 6 fatty acids
Obesity
High blood sugar

Normalize Insulin *with:*
Protein with each meal
Low glycemic carbohydrates, avoid sugar
Increase fiber
Daily exercise
Maintain ideal weight
Chromium, magnesium, niacin
Alpha lipoic acid
Flax or fish oil

INSULIN-LIKE GROWTH FACTOR-1 (IGF-1)

Increased IGF-1 *due to:*
Moderate alcohol consumption
High insulin levels
High growth hormone levels
Drinking milk from Growth Hormone fed cows (USA)
Bovine colostrum
Low levels of binding protein IGFBP-3

Lower IGF-1 *with:*
Tamoxifen
Vegan diet
High levels of binding protein IGFBP-3
Chromium, alpha lipoic acid, omega 3 oils

CORTISOL

High Cortisol Levels *due to:*
Stress, Overexertion, Childhood Abuse
resulting in:
High blood glucose
High insulin, Increased IGF-1
Fat deposition in torso/more estrogen in breasts
Depressed T-killer cells
Low progesterone
Increased testosterone
Decreased efficiency of thyroid hormone
Decreased melatonin production

Normalize Cortisol *with:*
Meditation
Counseling
Relaxation
Find supportive people or group
B complex, vitamin C
Magnesium, zinc, MSM
Ho shou wu, Siberian ginseng, licorice root, borage, oats, schizandra, rhodiola, ashwaganda, suma

MELATONIN

Decreased Melatonin *due to:*
Shift work
Light at night
Insomnia
Chronic exposure to strong electromagnetic fields, above 2 mG
Alcohol, caffeine, nicotine, drugs
Cortisol imbalance

Increase Melatonin *using:*
Foods high in tryptophan
Vitamins B3, B6; calcium, magnesium, zinc
Meditate/pray before bed
Sleep in a dark room
20 minutes in natural light in a.m.
Exercise daily
Normalize cortisol

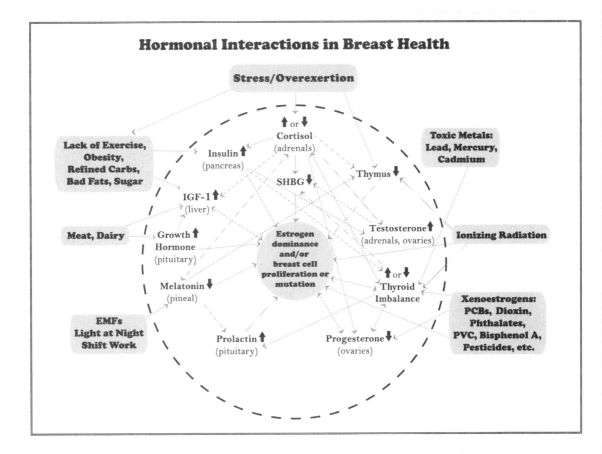

Summary

There are many interacting hormonal links to breast cancer and numerous ways that we can achieve hormonal balance to decrease risk through lifestyle and dietary changes. The need to do so is even more pressing when we consider the impact our increasingly toxic environment has on our endocrine system — and thus our breast health.

We can protect ourselves from breast cancer by managing our hormones wisely with the following practices:

1) Monitor your hormones annually with appropriate testing. See the 'Resources Directory' for a list of laboratories that can do this for you.
2) Decrease the overall production of potentially harmful estrogens by adopting a low fat, high fiber, vegetarian diet, and raise your children on such a diet. Take care to maintain a healthy weight for life. Exercise 40 minutes or more each day, doing something you enjoy.
3) Decrease the availability and activity of estrogen by increasing SHBG and filling your estrogen receptors with phytoestrogens to displace xenoestrogens and strong estrogens. Use 2 or more tbsp daily of ground flaxseeds, 30 grams or more of fiber daily, eat soy and other phytoestrogens such as clover sprouts and pumpkin seeds.

4) Balance the estrogen quotient, lower your C4 and C16 estrogens and increase the C2 estrogen with the daily intake of 150 mg DIM, 1500 mg curcumin (or 2-3 tsp turmeric), 1500 mg N-acetyl cysteine, food sources of methionine, 50 mg vitamin B complex, 300 mg magnesium, and 1 tsp fresh rosemary in your food. Use a breast oil containing palmarosa, lemon, and lavender and cleansing liver herbs which include milk thistle, dandelion, globe artichoke, bupleurum, chelidonium, and schizandra. Use 2 tbsp flaxseed oil daily in your food and 2 EPA fish oil capsules. Spend an hour a week in a sauna (avoid if you have lymphedema) to excrete xenoestrogens.

5) Decrease the reabsorption of estrogen from the bowel with regular use of a quality probiotic formula (good bacteria), 1 tbsp or more of wheat bran, 1 tbsp or more of psyllium, and the daily intake of legumes. Consider the use of calcium-D-glucarate once we know that it works in humans.

6) Optimize thyroid function with 2 tbsp or more daily of seaweeds, 50 mg zinc, 200 mcg selenium, 1500 mg daily of L-tyrosine, vitamin B12, and 2 tsp spirulina. Eat small meals frequently rather than having 3 large ones. Check for heavy metal toxicity and replace mercury amalgam fillings with porcelain.

7) To optimize insulin and cortisol levels, use at least 200 mcg chromium, 100 mg alpha lipoic acid, 2000 mg vitamin C, and consider using an herbal formula to help you adapt to stress that may contain borage, Siberian ginseng, ashwaganda, suma, licorice root, rhodiola, schizandra, and/or shou wu. Develop a daily practice of meditation, visualization, or relaxation.

8) To keep melatonin levels high and decrease the number of estrogen receptors, sleep in a dark room, avoid night shifts, meditate before bed, and make sure you have enough tryptophan in your diet or as a supplement.

CHAPTER FOUR

Environmental Impact on Breast Health

CONTENTS

Margaret Mead once stated, 'Never doubt that a small group of thoughtful citizens can change the world. Indeed, it's the only thing that ever has.' Today, we need such small groups to counteract the impact on our environment and on ourselves of radiation, electricity, petrochemicals, chlorinated chemicals, plastics, brominated fire retardants, and formaldehyde — all cancer causing agents. We absorb them, breathe them, eat them, and drink them.

We have a huge task ahead of us in decreasing the environmental links to breast cancer. How can we possibly make a difference? Start with your own body, in your own home, then reach out to your community, and keep going.

In the last five years I have witnessed committed groups of women and men creating tidal waves of change with their resolve to make this earth a safer place to live. Thanks to them, many Canadian cities and towns have recently passed bylaws restricting or banning pesticide use. The rest of North America may follow. Breast cancer action groups, like Hope Nemiroff's Mid Hudson Options Project and Benedictine Hospital in Kingston, New York, and the Breast Cancer Research and Education Fund in the Niagara region of Ontario, tirelessly educate women in breast cancer prevention, providing options and support to those newly diagnosed. Together we can change the world.

Radiation

Radiation contributes significantly to breast cancer development and thyroid dysfunction. Breast and thyroid tissue are sensitive to radiation, particularly during the childbearing years; in fact, the breasts and thyroid are the body tissues most sensitive to the cancer-causing effects of radiation.[1,2] The effects of radiation are cumulative and may manifest as cancer anytime within 40 years after exposure.

Some of these effects include:
1) damage to cell membranes caused by the formation of free radicals;
2) a decrease in white blood cell count and depressed immunity; [3]
3) irregularly shaped red blood cells, which may result in anemia, fatigue, short-term memory loss;
4) leukemia, hypothyroidism and thyroid cancer, lung cancer, bone cancer, Hodgkin's disease;[4]
5) birth defects and increased infant mortality;
6) multiple chemical sensitivities;
7) kidney damage;[5]
8) depression.

Exposure to radiation acts synergistically with environmental estrogens to increase risk significantly.[6,7,8,9]

Sources of radiation include nuclear fallout from weapons testing and from reactor failures, such as the Three Mile Island and Chernobyl accidents, fission materials from nuclear power plants, leaking radioactive disposal sites, flying at high altitudes, mammograms, and x-rays. Even the lowest level of radiation can cause cancer in susceptible individuals. There is no level that is safe.[10,11]

Nuclear Testing and Power Generation

Nuclear weapons testing by the American government in the 1950s put the population at risk. When Dr Carl Johnson compared cancer incidence in women, he found that those living in the fallout path from the Nevada nuclear test site had double the incidence of breast cancer after the testing (between 1967-1975) as compared to before the testing (1951).[12]

In the Soviet Union in the 1940s and '50s, nearly 500 nuclear tests were carried out in the area of present day Kazakstan. As many as 150 were above ground. More than 1.2 million people were adversely affected by the testing. The horror continues in the gene pool of its survivors. By 1997, nearly 500 out of every 1,000 babies born in the city of Semipalatinsk had some form of birth defect or serious health problem. Forty-seven of every 1,000 babies born, died. Ninety percent of the people living near the test site suffer from immune deficiency, many of them afflicted with tuberculosis, cancer, or blood diseases. Mental disability and suicide are common.[13] This is the legacy of nuclear testing.

After the Three Mile Island reactor leaked radiation, breast cancer rates increased in five counties adjacent to it, with the incidence seven times higher than rates in similar rural areas.[14] San Francisco area white women have one of the highest breast cancer rates in the world; breast cancer activists believe that this increased susceptibility to the

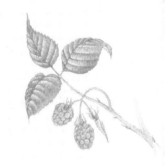

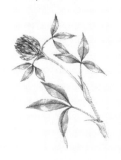

disease is linked to leakage from radioactive material at the Livermore National Laboratory nuclear site, situated close to earthquake fault lines.[15] Breast cancer rates are high in the Great Lakes region, possibly due to the combination of proximity to nuclear reactors and abundance of hormone-disrupting chemicals. Greenpeace maintains that between 1972 and 1991 more than 29 trillion picocuries (equal to the radiation released from two Three Mile Island disasters) of radioactive elements were released into the Great Lakes ecosystem.[16]

In 1991, the U.S. used depleted uranium, or DU, a toxic nuclear waste material, to coat missiles and bullets used in Operation Desert Storm during the Gulf War. Approximately 630,000 pounds of DU were fired in the Gulf in 1991. Depleted uranium bursts into flames once it hits its target and spreads radioactive dust in its wake, which remains radioactive for 4,500 million years. Since the Gulf War, Iraq has had a sixfold increase in cancers, with a particularly high increase in childhood leukemias. Depleted uranium is used in weapons manufacturing by at least 14 countries, including Britain, France, Russia, Greece, Turkey, Israel, Saudi Arabia, Kuwait, Egypt, and Pakistan.[17]

Testing for Radiation Exposure

One of the ways to assess exposure to radiation is by measuring strontium-90 in the baby teeth of children. The 'Tooth Fairy Project' has been doing that for children in the United States. Children born after 1990 show some of the highest levels of radioactive materials since the early 1960s when atomic bombs were tested in the atmosphere. Those who live downwind from nuclear power reactors in the path of their 'plumes' of radiation have more radioactive material in their teeth. Vegetables grown in these areas and dairy products also are more radioactive.[18] Some of these children are exhibiting a higher-than-normal rate of rhabdomyosarcoma, a rare form of bone cancer. The average levels of strontium-90 found in the teeth of children diagnosed with cancer are nearly twice as high as those found in the teeth of children who are cancer-free.[19]

The Tooth Fairy Project needs thousands of teeth from American children to continue this important study. For instructions on sending baby teeth to the Tooth Fairy Project, see the web site www.radiation.org.

Frequent Flying

Frequent flying is a source of excess radiation that may increase breast cancer risk. There is an observed increased incidence of breast cancer in flight attendants.[20] A jet flight of six hours exposes us to 5 millirads of radiation (a chest x-ray exposes us to 16 millirads).

X-rays and Mammograms

The radiation that women receive during mammograms may be a contributing cause of breast cancer. For some women, it will detect cancer at an earlier stage so that treatment is more effective. For others, it will be one more risk factor to already vulnerable breasts that may tip the scales towards cancer. A Canadian study of almost 90,000 women aged

40-49 at 15 hospitals across Canada found a 30-50% increase in deaths from breast cancer among women over 40 who had annual mammograms versus those who were given only physical exams. On the other hand, women between the ages of 50 and 69 benefit from regular mammograms with a 29% reduction in mortality compared to those who do not receive mammograms.[21] For more information on mammograms and alternative diagnostic tests, see Chapter 2, 'Getting To Know Our Breasts.'

Protection from Radiation

Thankfully, there are natural substances that can protect us from radiation-induced damage.

Brown seaweeds such as Kelp (Laminaria sp.), Sargassum, and Bladderwrack (Fucus vesiculosus) contain calcium and sodium alginates, gel-like substances that bind to heavy metals such as lead, mercury, cadmium, barium, radium, plutonium, strontium and cesium in the gastrointestinal tract to form insoluble salts that are excreted in the stools.[22] In laboratory studies on rats, sodium alginate reduced the uptake of radioactive particles in bone by 80% when added to the diet.[23] A combination of sodium alginate and egg-shell powder was used in Russia to prevent radiation damage in children who had been exposed to cesium-137.[24]

Seaweeds are an excellent source of minerals (particularly iodine), vitamins, and protein, and are a very alkaline food. An ounce of caution – excess quantities of kelp can cause acne, or an autoimmune thyroid condition known as Hashimoto's thyroiditis, in some individuals, and some seaweeds are contaminated with lead or arsenic.[26] Be sure to use seaweed that has been tested to be free of metal toxicity (such as kelp from the west coast of South Africa), and do not exceed 2 tbsp daily over the long term.

Electricity and Electromagnetic Fields

Electricity and electromagnetic fields are linked to a higher incidence of breast cancer.[35,36,37] We are constantly bombarded with electromagnetic fields — house wiring, phone lines, computer terminals, televisions, refrigerators, hair dryers, electric blankets, clocks, ovens, and all electrical appliances are nagging sources.

Exposure to extra low frequency electromagnetic fields disturbs the normal growth pattern of cells by interfering with their hormonal, enzymatic, and chemical signals, causing DNA damage. The deficiency in melatonin that these fields cause promotes breast cancer.

Long-term exposure to power lines has been linked to various cancers, including breast cancer, leukemia and childhood brain tumors. Computer video display monitors emit extremely low frequency magnetic fields that are probable human carcinogens. Proximity to video display monitors for prolonged periods during pregnancy has been associated with an increase in miscarriages. Frequent use of cell phones has been linked to headaches, fatigue, dizziness, and brain tumors.

FACT
The U.S. Atomic Energy Commission recommends that we consume 2-3 ounces (wet weight) of sea vegetables per week, or 2 tablespoons daily to protect from radiation toxicity. This should be increased fourfold during or after direct exposure to radiation.[27]

FACT
The Japanese population consumes more seaweed than any other population in the world, which may account for part of its low breast cancer incidence.[25]

Radiation Protection Diet Checklist

I recommend the following substances daily to protect against radiation toxicity, with dosages increased during mammography or other radiation exposure. For more information on these foods and supplements, see Chapter 7, 'Eating Right for Breast Health,' and Chapter 8, 'Nutritional Supplements for Breast Health.' Check off your use of these foods and supplements to be sure you are protected.

- ❏ Sea vegetables, 2 tbsp, or 3 kelp tablets, daily to elevate iodine and sodium alginate. Sodium alginate binds to radioactive molecules and can increase excretion by 80%.[28] Iodine protects the thyroid from radiation – we need 150 mcg to 1000 mcg daily. (575 mg of Norwegian kelp contains 359 mcg of iodine).
- ❏ Turmeric, 2 or more tsp daily, or curcumin, 500-1000 mg 3x daily, to decrease the damaging effects of radiation.[29]
- ❏ Yams, squash, carrots, Swiss chard, or spinach daily to provide beta carotene, or use a supplement containing Dunaliella algae, 25,000 - 50,000 IU daily.
- ❏ Cooked tomato sauce, 1/2 cup daily during exposure to provide lycopene content.[30]
- ❏ Whey (goat is best) or soy protein powder,1 tbsp daily, to provide cysteine.[31]
- ❏ Foods or supplements high in calcium and potassium to aid in the excretion of radioactive particles, such as cesium-137.[32]
- ❏ Antioxidant supplements containing vitamin C, E, coenzyme Q10, zinc, selenium, grape seed extract, alpha lipoic acid, and NAC to discourage free radical damage and the development of cancer. For recommended dosages, see Chapter 8, 'Nutritional Supplements for Breast Health.'
- ❏ Flax oil (unheated), 2 tbsp, or 2000 mg uncontaminated fish oil daily to protect cell membranes.
- ❏ Vitamin B3 (niacin), B12, and B complex to help to repair DNA damage.[33]
- ❏ Green tea daily to remove radioactive isotopes and protect from cancer.
- ❏ Reishi, maitake and shitake mushrooms to sustain immune health.
- ❏ Dietary fiber, 40 grams daily, to deter absorption of radiation and improve its excretion.
- ❏ Foods from the brassica family daily – kale, cabbage, broccoli, cauliflower etc. to protect the liver.
- ❏ Miso soup a few times a week to help excrete radioactive particles and deter cancer.
- ❏ Dried beans, lentils, or tofu daily in the diet to prevent the initiation of cancer.[34]

FACT
Women who work in the electrical trade have a 38% greater risk of dying from breast cancer than other working women. The risk for female electrical engineers is 73% greater. Women who install, repair, or do line work with telephones have a risk 217% times greater than average.

We need to keep a 'safe' distance from the source of the electromagnetic field because at a distance of $2\frac{1}{2}$ feet, the fields are 80% less powerful. Buy or rent a gauss meter to measure the electromagnetic field emissions in and around your home. Do not spend hours at a time in areas where the EMF readings are higher than 2 milligauss. Use less electricity, fewer electrical conveniences, and try living without a dishwasher, a clothes dryer, or a television. Turn off your electrical appliances when not in use — even use a wind-up watch rather than one with a quartz crystal or battery — these too, emit electromagnetic fields.[38]

Petrochemicals, Chlorinated Chemicals, and Formaldehyde

Petrochemicals, such as gasoline, kerosene, or those that include formaldehyde and benzene, have been linked to breast cancer in animals.[39] Chlorinated chemicals are systematically added to gasoline and will produce dioxin when burned. Germany has banned the addition of such chlorinated chemicals to fuel in recognition of this health hazard. Our countries should do the same.

Products containing formaldehyde include adhesives, air deodorizers, antiperspirants, cellophane, concrete, cleaning solutions, contraceptive creams, cosmetics, detergents, disinfectants, dry-cleaning compounds, enamels, fabric finishes, fertilizers, finger paints, gas appliances, gelatin capsules, inks, insect repellent, urea formaldehyde insulation, carpets, laminating materials, lacquers, laundry starch, mouthwashes, nail polish, tempera paint, paper towels, particle board, perfume, pesticides, pharmaceuticals, photographic chemicals, photographic film, plaster, plastics, plywood, polyester fabric, rodent poison, shampoos, shoe polish, soaps, tobacco and tobacco smoke, toilet paper, toothpaste, wood stains, and preservatives.

Organochlorines

Organochlorines are chemicals in which at least one atom of chlorine is bonded to a carbon molecule. Reacting chlorine gas with petroleum hydrocarbons produces many organochlorines. Today there are an estimated 11,000 different organochlorines being used, specifically in plastics, pesticides, solvents, dry cleaning agents, refrigerants, and other chemicals.[40]

Unfortunately, thousands more organochlorines are formed as by-products of chlorine-based industries. These include the bleaching of pulp for paper, the disinfecting of water, and the incinerating of waste containing chlorinated products. Chlorinated dioxin is one such by-product. Although chlorine is abundant in nature in its stable ionic form, the elemental chlorine that the chemical industry produces does not occur naturally. Industry first began producing organochlorines in the early 1900s; now about 40 million tons are manufactured yearly worldwide. No organochlorines are known to occur naturally in the tissues of humans, other mammals, or terrestrial vertebrates.

P.E.R.I.S.H.E.D

Organochlorines are problematic for several reasons. Use the acronym P.E.R.I.S.H.E.D to remember the first word of each of these reasons.

1) Persistent. They are stable molecules and resist breakdown in the environment for decades or centuries.
2) Environmental loading. Because they don't easily break down, organochlorines steadily accumulate in the global environment and are dispersed worldwide through air and water.
3) Remain in our tissues for life. Our bodies and the bodies of other species have not evolved ways of breaking them down and eliminating them. We do eliminate them through breast-feeding and through the intense use of saunas.
4) Increasing concentration. They concentrate in the fatty tissues of animals and humans and multiply in concentration as they move up the food chain. Meat, dairy, and fish eaters have higher body stores than vegetarians. Older animals and humans have higher concentrations than younger individuals.

PREVENTION
Avoid sources of extra low voltage electromagnetic fields by moving beds at least 2½ feet away from electrical outlets, keeping a safe distance away from computer video display terminals (2 feet from the front; 4 feet from the sides), minimizing their use while pregnant (less than 20 hours per week), moving work and sleeping areas away from the place where electricity enters the home, and limiting the use of cordless and cell phones to emergencies and brief conversations.

PREVENTION
Rid products that contain formaldehyde from your home and refrain from putting them on your body. Limit your exposure to petrochemicals, and insist that chlorine not be added to your fuel. Use your car less often, relying on public transportation, your bicycle, or your legs more often. If possible, move your residence closer to your workplace or move more of your work into your home office.

5) Subsequent generations. They are able to cross the placental barrier, affecting the very sensitive fetus, and are mobilized from the body's fat stores into the breast milk of all mammals, including humans. The infants acquire a high concentration of environmental estrogens relative to their small body mass over a short period of time. Subsequent generations pass on higher and higher concentrations from prenatal exposure, breast-feeding, and lifetime exposure.

6) Harmful. They are highly toxic, causing such things as genetic mutations, cancer, hormonal imbalances, malformations of the reproductive organs, immune suppression, birth defects, neuro-toxicity, learning disabilities and attention deficit disorders, infertility, impaired childhood development, and toxicity to the liver, kidney, skin, and brain. Natural estrogens exert their effects at low concentrations, measured in parts per trillion, which is 1000 times less than parts per billion. Organochlorines, acting as weak estrogens, are often present in breast milk, blood, and body fat in parts per billion or parts per million — 1000 or one million times more than the amount at which estrogen has an effect.

7) Effects are synergistic. A combination of only two different organochlorines together in minute doses has been found to be 1000 times more potent in affecting human estrogen receptors as either chemical alone.[41] And we have over a hundred in our systems acting synergistically, causing them to be more active than if they were present singly.

8) Death to wildlife and humans. They are harming wildlife and humans and threaten our survival. Combinations of two different PCBs at low concentrations were effective in reversing the sex of male turtle eggs to become female.[42] Eagles and gulls that consume fish from the Great Lakes (contaminated with organochlorines) have a high rate of deformities, deaths of embryos, and exhibit abnormal nesting behavior.[43] Alligators hatched in Lake Apopka, Florida have abnormally small penises and altered hormone levels due to a massive pesticide spill in 1980.[44] Panthers living in areas of south-central Florida in which soil or water contained high concentrations of heavy metals and organochlorines have a higher than normal number of males born with undescended testes.[45] Oysters taken from

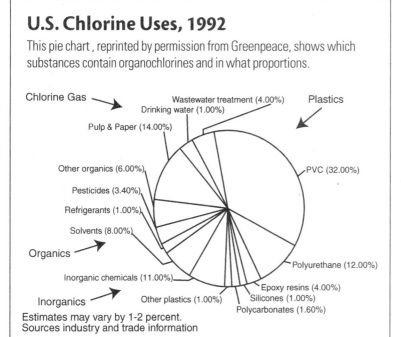

U.S. Chlorine Uses, 1992

This pie chart , reprinted by permission from Greenpeace, shows which substances contain organochlorines and in what proportions.

Chlorine Gas

Wastewater treatment (4.00%)
Drinking water (1.00%)
Plastics
Pulp & Paper (14.00%)

Other organics (6.00%)
Pesticides (3.40%)
Refrigerants (1.00%)
Solvents (8.00%)

Organics

Inorganic chemicals (11.00%)

Inorganics
Other plastics (1.00%)

PVC (32.00%)

Polyurethane (12.00%)

Epoxy resins (4.00%)
Silicones (1.00%)
Polycarbonates (1.60%)

Estimates may vary by 1-2 percent.
Sources industry and trade information

organochlorine contaminated water have shell deformities.[46] In 1994, autopsy reports on 24 stranded beluga whales in the St Lawrence River found 21 tumors in 12 specimens, including cancers of the breast, ovary, bladder, stomach, intestine, and salivary gland. The belugas are having trouble reproducing and high concentrations of PCBs, DDT, chlordane, and toxaphene were found dissolved in their fat.[47]

There has been a drop in male fertility with a 50% reduction in sperm count since 1940.[48] In Europe, some organic farmers have over double the sperm count as non-organic farmers.[49] Testicular cancer has more than tripled in the last 50 years in the United States and Europe and cases of undescended testes in infant boys has doubled.[50,51,52]

Organochlorines and Breast Cancer

At least 16 organochlorines have been found to cause breast cancer in laboratory animals.[53] Some of these have already been restricted in Canada, such as DDT, aldrin, dieldrin, and chlordane, all pesticides. Other organochlorines found to be causative agents of breast cancer have not been restricted. These include PVC, or polyvinyl chloride, used in household plumbing, and polyvinylidene chloride, familiar to us as plastic food wrap. Methylene chloride, used in paint strippers, and dichlorobenzidines, used to produce dyes, are also still being produced. There is an established relationship between the levels of certain organochlorines found in a woman's blood, fat, or breast tissue and her risk of breast cancer. Studies have found that samples taken from breast cancer biopsies showed much higher levels of DDT, DDE, and PCBs than samples from benign breast lumps or from breast tissue in women without cancer.[54] A 1990 Finnish study found that the organochlorine beta-hexachlorocyclohexane (b-HCH) was 50% higher in cancerous tissue than in healthy breast tissue. When concentrations of b-HCH were as low as 100 parts per billion, women had a 10.5 times increased risk of developing breast cancer.[55,56]

Pesticides

Approximately 90% of all chemical pesticides use chlorine in their manufacturing process. Many foods have several pesticide residues on them: for example, the average Canadian peach has 31 pesticide residues, while a strawberry may have 40. We also are exposed to pesticides through our water supply. Groundwater in Canadian and American cities was found to have residues of 39 pesticides and their breakdown products. Spraying homes, lawns, roadways, golf courses, and agricultural crops causes the pesticides to leach through the soil and enter the groundwater.[57] In 1998 world scientists were alerted to the fact that many pesticides and persistent environmental chemicals were ending up not in the areas where they were applied, but in the pristine mountainous areas of the world. When the snow melts, these chemicals are released back into the environment. They hopscotch around the world, landing on different mountains each year.[58]

FACT
The Environmental Health Committee of the Ontario College of Family Physicians warns that there is an increased risk of leukemia, brain cancer, and soft tissue sarcomas to children who have been exposed to herbicides and pesticides. Developmental problems such as poor co-ordination are occurring in children, along with smaller head size.

FACT
Women with the highest concentrations of specific organochlorine pesticides in their bodies have a risk of breast cancer 4 to 10 times higher than women with lower levels. These pesticides are one of the greatest known risk factors linked with breast cancer.

FACT
Although the amount of one pesticide residue may not be greater than the maximum allowable level, several pesticides from the same class acting at the same site in the body can have a toxic cumulative effect, particularly on children and the unborn.

Currently Used Pesticides and Breast Cancer

The following chart, adapted from the *Journal of Pesticide Reform* (Spring 1996), show the pesticides currently in use, not yet banned, and their proven impact on breast health.

Name	Use	Comments
Atrazine	A weed killer used on vegetable crops such as corn in Canada and the U.S. It is the most widely used pesticide in U.S. agriculture.	It promotes the formation of 16 alpha-hydroxyestrone that has been linked to breast cancer. Caused breast cancer and disruption of menstrual cycles in one strain of rats and inhibits the metabolism of male hormones in other animal species. In northern Italy, a link has been made between atrazine use and ovarian cancer among women farmers. Because atrazine is widely used on corn, which is the staple in animal feed, we are consuming higher amounts of it when we eat corn-fed animals, such as meat, milk, poultry and eggs. Its use has been restricted in Germany and the Netherlands.
Cyanazine	An herbicide used mostly on corn. One of the top 5 most commonly used pesticides in the U.S. Production will cease in the U.S. by Dec. 31, 1999 although its use will continue for 3 more years.	Caused significant increase in breast tumors in female rats.
1,3-dichloro-propene	Used as a soil fumigant, one of the top 10 pesticides used in the U.S.	Caused breast tumors in mice and rats.
Dichlorvos	An insecticide used in greenhouses, on fruits and vegetables and on livestock. It is used to make pet flea collars and fly strips.	Caused an increase in breast tumors in female rats.
Endosulfan	One of the most commonly used pesticides. Widely used on fruit and salad crops, found on apples, carrots, celery, cucumbers, head lettuce (not leaf lettuce), pears, peppers, plums, strawberries, and tomatoes.[59]	Causes breast cancer cells to increase in number in lab tests and promotes the formation of the C-16 "bad estrogen" linked to increased breast cancer risk.
Ethalfluralin	A herbicide used before planting soybeans, dry beans, and sunflower seeds.	Caused breast tumors in rats.
Ethylene oxide	A fumigant used on spices and to sterilize cosmetics and hospital equipment.	Increases breast tumors and several other cancers in female mice.

Name	Use	Comments
Estridiazole	A fungicide that is applied to soil and used to treat seeds.	When fed to rats there was an increase in breast tumors.
Methoxychlor	An insecticide related to DDT, used mostly on crops but also for household, garden, commercial, and industrial use.	Causes breast cancer cells to multiply in lab animals and causes changes to the ovaries in adult mice.
Oryzalin	An herbicide used on turf, almond orchards, and grape vineyards.	Caused increased breast tumors in female rats.
Prometon	An herbicide.	Causes breast tumors in rats.
Propazine	An herbicide used before planting sorghum and after planting carrots, celery and fennel.	Causes increased benign and malignant breast tumors in rats.
Simazine	An herbicide used on lawns, nut trees, corn production and fruit crops, specifically oranges, apples, plums, olives, cherries, peaches, cranberries, blueberries, strawberries, grapes, and pears.	Caused both breast and ovarian cancer in female rats.[60]
Terbuthylazine	A herbicide used to kill algae in ornamental ponds, fountains, and aquariums.	Caused increased breast tumors in female rats.
Terbutryn	A herbicide used before planting sorghum.	Increases malignant breast tumors in female rats.
Tribenuron methyl	An herbicide used in barley and wheat production.	Increases malignant breast tumors in female rats.
Lindane	Although banned from regular use in 1983, it is still allowed in lice shampoos for humans and flea dips for dogs. Some children use lice shampoos more than 20 times as well as apply insecticide sprays to the home.	Women whose breasts had the highest levels of lindane-like residues were 10 times more likely to have breast cancer than women with lower levels. Blood from women with breast cancer had 50% more of this pesticide residue than blood from women without breast cancer.[61,62,63]

Other pesticides that are known hormone disruptors include 2,4,5-T, 2,4-D, alachlor, aldicarb, amitrole, benomyl, beta-HCH, carbaryl, cypermethrin, DBCP, dicofol, esfenvalerate, ethylparathion, fenvalerate, h-epoxide, kelthane, kepone, malathion, mancozeb, maneb, methomyl, metiram, metribuzin, mirex, nitrofen, oxychlordane, permethrin, synthetic pyrethoids, transnonachlor, tributyltin oxide, trifluralin, vinclozolin, zineb, and ziram.[64]

Pesticide Residue Chart

Pesticide residue on fruits and vegetables often varies by species. Fruits and vegetables in Canada and the U.S. containing the most and least amount of pesticides are summarized here. I have this list memorized and now when I shop, I find it impossible to buy the fruits and vegetables in either 'contaminated' list unless they are organic.

Most Contaminated Foods		Least Contaminated Foods	
FRUITS	VEGETABLES	FRUITS	VEGETABLES
1. Peaches	1. Spinach	1. Avocado	1. Cauliflower
2. Apples	2. Bell peppers	2. Pineapple	2. Brussels sprouts
3. Strawberries	3. Celery	3. Plantains	3. Asparagus
4. Nectarines	4. Potatoes	4. Mangoes	4. Radishes
5. Pears	5. Hot peppers	5. Watermelon	5. Broccoli
6. Cherries	6. Green beans	6. Plums	6. Onions
7. Red raspberries	7. Head and leaf lettuce	7. Kiwi	7. Okra
8. Imported grapes	8. Cucumbers	8. Papaya	8. Cabbage
9. Blueberries	9. Carrots	9. Grapefruit	9. Eggplant

To find out more about what pesticides and herbicides are in your foods and which foods are safest, view the web site www.foodnews.org. or ewg.org.

For more information on pesticides and alternatives to pesticides, see the *Journal of Pesticide Reform*, published by the Northwest Coalition for Alternatives to Pesticides in Eugene, Oregon.

FACT

In 2002, the Windsor Regional Cancer Centre collected the work histories of its patients and compared the occupational histories of 299 women with newly diagnosed breast cancer to those of 237 women with other cancers. The breast cancer incidence in women under 55 years of age who lived on farms was 9 times higher that the average.[67]

Banning Lindane

In Israel prior to 1976, the levels of three pesticides, lindane, DDT, and alpha-BHC, were present in cow's milk at concentrations 100 times higher than those found in U.S. dairy products. Significantly, the concentration in Israeli women's breast milk was approximately 800 times more than that found in American women's breast milk. Israel had one of the highest breast cancer rates in the world.

A small consumer organization, Consumer Shield, brought the issue into the open and forced the Israeli government to ban these chemicals, despite being attacked in the media by the milk producers and even the Cancer Association. The ban resulted in a marked reduction of the chemicals in Israeli milk, and ten years later, in 1986, breast cancer mortality in Israel had fallen 8% from a decade earlier, a rare occurrence in any country.[65]

Farmers are often the unwitting victims of their own pesticide use. In Canada, I was intrigued to find that the farming community of Marquette, Manitoba had the highest death rate from breast cancer out of any Canadian community, 64.8 deaths per 100,000 women. Out of all the Canadian provinces, Manitoba has the highest breast cancer incidence.[66] In Marquette, the primary crop grown is canola, and until Canada banned its use in 2001, the canola was sprayed with lindane to exterminate flea beetles. In response to the lindane ban, an American-based chemical company is suing the Canadian government under Chapter 11 of the North American Free Trade Agreement (NAFTA), seeking lost revenue damages of $100 million.

Banned Pesticides: Aldrin and Dieldrin

Even though Dieldrin has been banned in the United States and Europe for many years, it persists in the environment and accumulates in our bodies. Aldrin was used as an insecticide on corn, citrus, cotton, and other crops. Banned in 1975, it was nevertheless allowed as a termite poison until 1987.[68]

Banned Pesticides: Chlordane and Heptachlor

Chlordane and heptachlor were used agriculturally and as termite killers until 1988 and have been linked to leukemia and childhood cancer. They cross the placenta, contaminate breast milk and act as hormone disruptors linked to decreased fertility. Even now, despite their ban, residues of chlordane are found in oysters in the Gulf of Mexico, in coastal North American whales, and in the fat of Arctic polar bears whose food source is contaminated seals. Polar bears are having trouble reproducing and are creating offspring that demonstrate both male and female reproductive organs.

Banned Pesticides: DDT

DDT reached its peak usage in the U.S. in 1959 and was banned in the U.S. in 1972. DDT was routinely sprayed over rural and residential areas as an insecticide to control mosquitoes, gypsy moths, and Dutch elm disease; was brushed on porches, window screens, and baseboards; and was added to the dry-cleaning process to mothproof woolen clothing and blankets. Its use triggered population explosions of insects that became resistant to the drug or whose natural enemies were killed by it. DDT is a persistent chemical, found in soil, hazardous waste sites, and the tissues of most life forms. It has a half-life in soil of 10-35 years, so we are still being exposed to it. Global air currents carry it worldwide from countries, such as Mexico and India, where it is still allowed for use on food crops and to combat malaria. DDT may come back to us on the food we import. We cannot convert DDT into anything excretable. DDT is converted to DDE in our bodies. DDE crosses the placenta to affect the fetus and is passed into breast milk. DDE acts to block androgens (male sex hormones) by blocking their receptor sites. The consequences for men are lowered sperm counts, smaller testes, an increased incidence of testicular cancer, and more cases of undescended testes.

PVC (Polyvinyl Chloride) Plastics

Over 20 million tons of PVC plastic or vinyl are manufactured each year and used in cars, children's toys, food containers, credit cards, raincoats, furniture, building supplies, water pipes, window frames, flooring, and even wallpaper. Dioxins and phthalates are two groups of hormone-disrupting chemicals often added to PVC. Large quantities of dioxins are formed in the production, disposal, and combustion of PVC. PVC is often present with wood furniture, with steel in cars, and with copper in cables. As these substances are recycled, dioxin is released into the environment. PVC can be identified by a number 3 in the recycling symbol. Dioxin is widely recognized as

PREVENTION

Buy organic food and/or grow your own food if possible. Establish a pesticide-free private or community garden or orchard. If you can't buy or grow all organic food, select foods that contain the least pesticide residues. Peel your fruits and vegetables, especially if they have been waxed, or wash them with a vegetable wash or diluted vinegar to remove surface pesticide residues.

Decrease or eliminate dairy consumption, particularly during pregnancy, unless it is both low fat and organic.

FACT

A 1998 study published in the *Lancet* that followed over 7,000 women for nearly 20 years found that women with the highest traces of dieldrin in their blood were twice as likely as women with the lowest levels to develop breast cancer.

FACT

DDE and PCBs have been found in higher concentrations in breast tumors than in surrounding breast tissue. This is also true of lindane, heptachlor, and dieldrin. DDT has been linked to liver and pancreatic cancer as well as tumors of the lung, liver, and thyroid.

PVC is responsible for the greatest production and use of chlorine, accounting for approximately one third of all organochlorine production.

one of the most toxic chemicals ever made. The worst of the dioxins is called TCDD or 2,3,7,8-TCDD.[69]

There is no safe way to dispose of PVC plastic. Alternatives to most, if not all PVC products exist. PVC is not a necessity — we didn't need it until the chemical industry introduced it to us. Its convenience is not a valid reason to allow our very survival and the survival of wildlife to be threatened.

Greenpeace Alternatives to PVC

Available alternatives to PVC are shown in this list prepared by Greenpeace:[71]

PVC Product	Healthy Alternative
Windows	wood (pine, larch, fir, spruce, beech), chlorine free plastics
Floorings	ceramic tiles, wood, parquetry, linoleum, rubber, stoneware tiles, cork, sisal hemp, terazzo, chlorine free plastic (polyolefine)
Walls	brickwork, pebble dash, wood, gypsum, plaster board
Wallpaper	uncoated paper (made from chlorine free recycled fibers), environmentally sound paints, paper wallpaper with protective coating on acrylate base, ceramic tiles
Facades, Curtain Walls	plaster, wood
Roll Joints, Hand Rails	wood, metal
Furniture	wood, metal, wicker
Blinds, Shutters	wood, textiles
Weather Stripping	natural rubber
Sewage Pipes	concrete, earthenware, stoneware, polyethylene (PE) and polypropylene pipes (PP)
Electrical Installations & Cables	chlorine free plastics like PE, special rubber
Packaging	minimize packaging, but when necessary, use cardboard, wood, glass, brown paper bags, waxed paper, and if plastic is necessary, use PE, PP. (We need to develop organic packaging as from hemp, straw, vegetable fibers etc. Wouldn't it be wonderful if all packaging could be composted to feed a garden or be used as mulch?)
Medical Products	switch from disposable (usually PVC) to reusable products; e.g., redden bottles, reusable scalpel handles, refillable glass bottles, and where disposable products are necessary, use chlorine free plastics such as PE for gloves, infusion bags, or use latex or natural rubber
Toys	wood, textiles

Start or join a campaign to ban the production and incineration of PVC and chlorine-based chemicals that release dioxins. Eliminate or limit your consumption of meat, fish, and dairy to reduce dioxin exposure.

Dioxins

Dioxins consist of a group of 75 chemicals that are produced during the manufacturing and combustion of other chlorine compounds. They are now widespread in our environment. The dioxin levels in the Great Lakes was zero in the 1920s but has steadily increased to be about 3200 parts per trillion today.[72] At least ten dioxins have been found in human breast milk.

TCDD, the most potent of the dioxins, blocks the male hormone testosterone. In adult males who were exposed to dioxins at work, there was a decrease in testosterone levels.[73] Dioxin exposure in men results in a higher number of female offspring from their partners. Monkeys exposed to dioxin at levels close to those found in human tissues developed an increased incidence of endometriosis.[74] Laboratory rats exposed to dioxin levels close to those encountered in our environment today gave birth to female offspring who suffered from decreased fertility and structural abnormalities of their reproductive systems.[75]

Hospital incinerators, ironically, have been a major source of dioxin release. Many medical products are made out of PVC plastic, and when these products are burned in hospital incinerators, dioxin is released into the surrounding communities. Some communities have banned the use of hospital incineration. Recent public attention has caused some hospitals to switch to using plastic that is PVC free. Municipal, industrial and sewage sludge incinerators are also significant sources of dioxin release. Accidental fires are sources of dioxin release, since so much of the building industry uses PVC in its supplies. Other sources of dioxin unrelated to PVC occur during the bleaching of pulp and paper, manufacture of chlorophenols, production of chlorine, magnesium and nickel smelting, and steel production.

We are interfering with our children's ability to learn and reproduce when we use PVC plastic and support the PVC industry.

PCBs (Polychlorinated Biphenyls)

Although most industrialized countries stopped production of PCBs over 10 years ago, their concentration in human tissues has not declined. PCBs are persistent and may not degrade for decades or centuries. PCBs can still be found in old paints, varnishes, inks, pesticides, microscope oil, and hydraulic fluids. They were used to make wood and plastic products nonflammable and stucco waterproof. However, the majority of PCBs were used in electrical transformers, where they are still subject to accidental release into the environment.

PCBs are now present in the body fat of almost all living creatures. The most contaminated waters of the Northern Hemisphere are the Baltic Sea and the St Lawrence River estuary. People who eat fish regularly from the north shore of the St Lawrence River in Quebec have a mean PCB level of 6 parts per million.[76] The Inuit, who rely on seafood as a staple, have PCB levels of 4.1 parts per million, which is 5-10 times higher than the average Canadian's. Levels this high are linked to depressed immune systems, particularly a decline in the T-cells which would ordinarily keep cancer in check.[77]

PCBs affect both thyroid and ovarian hormones. Interference with thyroid hormone during gestation may cause low birth weight, poor growth, hyperactivity, autoimmune diseases, immune suppression, and impaired learning and memory.[78]

The PCBs associated with breast cancer are PCB105, PCB118, and PCB156. In a study conducted by Dr Kristan Aronson at Queen's University in Kingston, Ontario, several PCBs were found to occur in higher amounts in the breast tumor biopsies of women with breast cancer as compared to biopsies from women with benign breast tumors. Women whose tumors had the highest amount of PCB105 were twice as likely to have breast cancer as women with lower amounts. The most consistent dietary predictor of PCB concentration in breast tissue was fish consumption.[82]

FACT

A human baby breast-fed for six months receives five times the allowable daily limit of PCBs set by international health standards for a 150-lb adult.[79] A woman passes half of her lifetime accumulation of dioxins and PCBs on to her child when she nurses for just six months.[80]

PREVENTION

Avoid eating or using animal products, particularly if you plan to breast-feed your children. Detoxify yourself and your children with regular saunas to eliminate PCBs through sweat. For instructions on how to detoxify, see Chapter 5, 'Detoxifying Our Bodies.'

PREVENTION

Take the time to wash selected clothing by hand or buy clothes that don't need dry cleaning. Find out from Environment Canada or the Environmental Protection Agency if there is a non-toxic dry cleaning or 'Green Clean' outlet in your area.

FACT

Children whose yards are treated with pesticides had a fourfold increase in soft tissue cancers over children living in homes that did not spray their lawns. Brain tumors in children have been linked to increased use of pest-repellent strips, flea collars on pets, lice shampoos containing lindane, and weed killers on lawns.

Perchloroethylene (PERC)

Perchloroethylene is used as a dry-cleaning solvent and is hazardous to workers and consumers because of its contribution to cancer and reproductive problems. It is commonly found as a contaminant in food and groundwater. Women who work in the dry cleaning industry have a greater risk of miscarriage.

2,4- dichlorophenoxyacetic acid (2,4 -D)

2,4-D was used in the Vietnam War to destroy the rain forest as a component of Agent Orange. It was introduced for agricultural use in the U.S. and Canada after that to control weeds and in the forests for shrub management. It became one of the most popular weed killers for lawns, gardens, and golf courses. It is marketed under the trade names Ded-Weed, Weedone, Plantgard, Lawn-Keep, and Demise.

It is linked to a sixfold increased incidence of non-Hodgkin's lymphoma in humans. The incidence of lymphoma doubles among pet dogs whose owners use lawn chemicals at least four times annually.[83] Pesticide residues persist for longer periods indoors than outside, where they are washed away or broken down by sunlight, rain, and soil organisms. Infants and toddlers are exposed to significant amounts of pesticides from crawling on carpets and ingesting house dust. [84,85]

Chloroform

Chloroform was used in the past as an anesthetic because of its ability to alter brain function. It is classified as a probable human carcinogen and is now used as a solvent, and fumigant, as well as an ingredient in pesticides, synthetic dyes, and refrigerants. Trace amounts of it are formed when chlorine is added to drinking water, and it is prevalent in large dump sites. Although we excrete it from our bodies within 24 hours, we are constantly exposed to it through water, food, and inhalation. According to the Commission for Environmental Cooperation, at least 4,625,354 kg of chloroform was released into the air, water, or soil in North America in 1996.[86]

Trichloroethylene (TCE)

TCE is used in industry to degrease metal parts and is one of the most common toxic substances at dump sites, from where it can trickle into groundwater. It is estimated to be in 34% of U.S. drinking water and traces are found in most processed foods.[87] It is also found in paint and spot removers, cosmetics and carpet cleaners. In the past, it was used as an obstetrical anesthetic, a grain fumigant, an ingredient in typewriter correction fluid, and as a coffee decaffeinater. Traces of it persist in the air that we breathe, especially if we live near a large dump site. In 1996, at least 10,472,026 kilograms of TCE were released into the air, water, and soil of North America.[88]

Alternatives to Chlorine Disinfectants and Bleaches

When chlorine is combined with organic matter in sewage and water, hundreds of organochlorine by-products are formed. These damage the habitat of fish and marine animals living near sewage effluent, and damage us when we drink chlorinated water. Regular consumption of chlorinated water disrupts the healthy balance of organisms in our intestines, and has been linked with colon cancer; rectal cancer, bladder cancer, birth defects, and immune related disorders. The U.S. Environmental Protection Agency has identified at least two carcinogenic chemicals that are formed when chlorine in water reacts with organic material from decayed plants. These have been detected in significant amounts in 100 municipal water systems tested in 1995.[89] Health Canada reported in its journal, *Chronic Diseases in Canada* (November 1998), that chlorinated water poses a risk to humans, particularly of bladder cancer.[90]

Disinfectants
Frequent use of chlorinated swimming pools also exposes us to chlorine toxicity. Other methods of water filtration and purification do exist, such as using ultraviolet light, ozone treatment, salination treatment for pools, and specialized filtration methods. These include reverse osmosis and charcoal or carbon filters. A public swimming pool in Vancouver uses ozonation as a purification method. The city of Montreal uses ozonation as a water purification treatment. Put pressure on your municipal governments to do the same.

Safer alternatives to using chlorine as a disinfectant are grapefruit seed extract and tea tree oil. Grapefruit seed extract has been used extensively throughout South America as an algaecide, bactericide, and fungicide rather than chlorine in hot tubs, jacuzzis, and swimming pools. The concentration of grapefruit seed extract needed to do the job of disinfecting is 10-15 drops per gallon of water. Grapefruit seed extract is a more powerful disinfectant than chlorine, tea tree oil, colloidal silver, and iodine.[91] Hospitals and clinics in the U.S. now use grapefruit seed extract in the laundry to ensure that the linen is fungi and bacteria free by adding 20-30 drops to the final rinse.[92]

To reduce the need for disinfecting chlorine products, we can install composting toilets that recycle human waste and contribute nothing to global pollution. They also avoid the water wasting of flush toilets and the many chemicals used to clean up sewage.[93]

Bleach
The pulp and paper industry releases thousands of kilograms of organochlorines into our rivers and lakes each year and is the largest North American discharger of organochlorine pollutants into water. Fish and wildlife downstream from pulp and paper mills are severely affected, with female fish taking on male characteristics, general increases in tumors, and decreased fertility. In Sweden and Finland, oxygen and hydrogen peroxide are used to bleach pulp for paper and diapers. The impetus for this transition came from the recognition and concern around organochlorine pollution in the Baltic Sea and aggressive regulations from government that forced industry to reduce and eliminate it. Pressure from the public and industry for access to chlorine-free paper will also cause the

PREVENTION
Educate your neighbors who use pesticides on their lawns about risks to their health. Minimize your use of carpeting in the home, using hardwood floors and natural fiber throw rugs instead. If you do have carpets, steam clean once or twice yearly with non-chlorinated cleansers. Insist on shoe removal in your home. Do not allow outdoor pets onto carpeted areas.

PREVENTION
Minimize your use of processed foods and stock your kitchen with what you need to cook from scratch.

FACT
People who use chlorinated water for 35 years raise their cancer risk 1.5 times. Approximately 10-13% of bladder cancers in the province of Ontario can be blamed on chlorinated water.

PREVENTION
Install a reverse osmosis or charcoal filter on your water supply to decrease chemical exposure. Insist upon safe, non-chlorine purification methods in your public and private drinking water and swimming pools, such as ozonation and the use of grapefruit seed extract.

pulp and paper industry to switch to chlorine-free processing. Totally chlorine free (TCF) paper products are available from eco stores, progressive printers, and copy shops.

Phthalates

Phthalates are not organochlorines but are used in about 50% of all PVC products to soften them and add flexibility. They are a family of over 20 different compounds used as ingredients in plastic food wraps and packaging, paints, inks, adhesives, blood bags, syringes, heart valves, medical tubing and cosmetics. Fatty foods, such as cheese and oils, are easily contaminated with phthalates and

Phthalate Sources and Health Effects

Phthalates comprise several compounds used in making a variety of goods, each with a documented effect on our breast and whole body health.[98,99,100,101]

Phthalate Compound	Where It Is Found	Known Health Effects
Di(2-ethylhexyl) phthalate (DEHP)	building products, children's toys, children's polymer clay, food packaging, medical devices, in PVC resins for teething rings, pacifiers, balls, vinyl upholstery, tablecloths, shower curtains, raincoats, adhesives, food containers, medical tubing, animal glue	probable human carcinogen, toxic to thyroid (decreases T4), liver and kidney; harmful to male reproductive tract
di-isononyl phthalate (DINP)	garden hoses, shoes and shoe soles, toys, construction materials	reproductive and developmental harm
di-isodecyl phthalate (DIDP)	car undercoating, wires and cables, shoes, carpet backing, pool liners	liver and reproductive toxicity
di-n-butyl phthalate (DBP)	latex adhesives, cellulose plastics, solvent for dyes	reproductive and developmental toxicity, skin irritation, nervous system and blood pressure impacts, disrupts estrogen
butyl benzyl phthalate (BBP)	vinyl tile, artificial leather, food conveyor belts, traffic cones, children's polymer clays	reproductive disorders, birth deformities, nerve disorders, suspected carcinogen, disrupts estrogen
di-n-octyl phthalate (DnOP)	flooring and carpet tile, canvas tarps, notebook binders, plastic food containers, medical tubing and blood bags, wire and cables, carpetback coating, floor tile, adhesives, cosmetics, pesticides	reproductive toxicity, liver and thyroid toxicity, birth deformities, genetic mutations
di-n-hexyl phthalate (DnHP)	car parts, tool handles, dishwasher baskets, flooring, tarps, flea collars	liver and thyroid toxicity, reproductive toxicity, genetic mutation

bisphenol-A when packaged in plastic. Phthalates may be present and can be absorbed from plastic baby bottles, nipples, and plastic 'soothers'. They have been linked to cancer, kidney damage, and may interfere with your children's ability to reproduce.

Phthalates are one of the most abundant environmental contaminants and are persistent, accumulating in living tissues. When male rats were exposed to phthalates before and after birth, they had lower testicular weights and a reduced sperm count. Two types of phthalates, DEHP and DINP, have been found to cause cancer in animals.[94] DEHP is implicated in the high occurrence of early breast development, in girls as young as two, in Puerto Rico.[95] Phthalates have been shown to be toxic to developing embryos, causing malformation and death. They also can lower thyroid hormone and progesterone levels, potentially contributing to PMS symptoms, breast cysts, breast cancer, and miscarriages.[96]

In 1998, some, but not all toys and soothers containing phthalates were removed from the shelves in Canadian stores. Through testing, the Danish and Dutch governments have found that these chemicals can be ingested from PVC toys during normal use; PVC toys have been taken off the shelves in Sweden, Spain, Italy, Argentina, Greece, Holland and Denmark.[97]

Bisphenol-A

Bisphenol-A is an ingredient in epoxy resins and polycarbonate plastics, which are hard plastics. Although it is not an organochlorine, it is an endocrine disruptor. It is used in formulas to seal cracks in water pipes, and in some dental materials designed to provide 'protection' against tooth decay and in the plastic fillings used to replace mercury amalgam fillings.

Bisphenol-A is a breakdown product of polycarbonate, present in the plastic coating that manufacturers use to line metal cans. These coatings were added to prevent a metallic taste in the food. Plastic linings are present in 85% of food cans in the United States, and bisphenol-A was found to have leached into about half the canned foods that were tested. When analyzed, some cans contained 80 parts per billion of bisphenol A, which is 27 times more than researchers have demonstrated is enough to make breast cancer cells proliferate in the laboratory.[102] At these levels, we would expect a physiological effect in women's breasts from regular consumption of canned food or oily food in hard plastic containers containing Bisphenol-A. Some men in the plastics industry have developed enlarged breasts after inhaling the chemical in workplace dust over long periods of time.[103]

Nonylphenol Ethoxylates

Although they are not organochlorines, nonylphenol ethoxylates (NPEs) are hormone disrupting chemicals used in 11 industrial areas and in household and industrial soaps and detergents, natural and synthetic textile processing, plastic manufacturing, pulp and paper

PREVENTION
Find alternatives to phthalate containing products. Buy goods, especially oils and fatty foods, in glass or paper rather than plastic containers. Use waxed paper or butcher paper to wrap sandwiches and other foods. Do not microwave food in plastic containers or plastic wrap. Use ceramic or glass containers instead.

PREVENTION
Explain to your children the hazards in their plastic toys and then discard them, replacing them with wood, cloth, or other natural fibers. Ask your children's teachers, care givers, relatives, and friends not to buy plastic toys for your children. Put pressure on toy manufacturing companies to stop using PVC. Use phthalate-free cosmetics. Do not use nail polish.

PREVENTION
Buy food in glass jars or cans without the liners. If you consume canned foods, call the manufacturer to determine if bisphenol-A is used to line the can. If it is, stop using the cans.

PREVENTION
If your dentist suggests a new plastic coating for your children's teeth, ensure that it contains no bisphenol-A or other hormone disrupting chemical. Ask your dentist to use ceramic fillings for your teeth.

making, petroleum refineries, pesticides and for oil extraction. They are one of the ingredients used to make plastic soft, and readily leach out into fluids at room temperature. We may find them in our water bottles, fruit juice containers, and packaging of convenience food.

The Paris Commission, an international body that sets standards for water quality, recommends that nonylphenols be phased out because of their toxicity to aquatic life and their persistence in the environment.[104,105] We should choose soaps and detergents, particularly liquid products, which the manufacturer guarantees do not contain NPEs. Usually there is a toll free number on product labels that can be used to find out this information. The following companies do not use nonylphenol ethoxylates in their detergents: Proctor and Gamble, Lever, Pond's, Tide, and Sunlight.[106]

PBDEs
(Brominated Flame Retardants)

Though not organochlorines, PBDEs are a class of chemicals similar to PCBs. They have been found in breast milk, human blood, food, remote rural air, wild fish, and in sewage sludge. The Great Lakes is among one of the most PBDE-contaminated bodies of water in the world, with Lake Michigan being the worst. PBDEs are similar in chemical form and in many of their actions to PCBs (polychlorinated biphenyls). Within 10 to 15 years PBDEs will have surpassed PCBs as environmental hazards.

Bromine is a highly-reactive chemical element, a halogen in the same class as chlorine and iodine. Worldwide, eight chemical corporations manufacture about 300 million pounds of brominated fire retardants each year, of which about 80 million pounds are members of the class known as polybromo diphenyl ethers, or PBDEs. PBDEs leach into the environment from the plastics in appliances, TVs and computers, foam in upholstery, and the fabrics of carpets and draperies. Many hard styrene plastics and many foam padding materials are 5% to 30% PBDE by weight. Some PBDEs can cause cancer, interfere with hormones, and disrupt normal growth and development in laboratory animals. Brominated compounds interfere with thyroid hormones, which are critical for the proper development of the brain and central nervous system in animals and humans. Baby mice exposed to PBDEs show permanent behavioral and memory problems, which worsen with age. Breast milk studies indicate that the danger to infants and children is rising.[107]

Is There Any Place Safe to Live?

In North America, in 2000, almost 220,000 tonnes of known or suspected carcinogens were released – one third into the air, one third into landfill, and the rest into underground injection, water or off-site tranfers. Ohio, Indiana, Ontario, Texas and Tennessee released over one quarter of the total North American burden. There are vast differences in the concentrations of toxins released from various states and provinces. Though environmental chemicals may be produced in one area, they are circulated widely, depending on water and wind currents. We can consider this information in choosing where to live.

North American Pollution Chart, 2000

Most Pollutants	Least Pollutants
1. Ohio	1. District of Columbia
2. Texas	2. Vermont
3. Pennsylvania	3. Alaska
4. Indiana	4. Prince Edward Island
5. Ontario	5. Hawaii
6. Illinois	6. Rhode Island
7. North Carolina	7. Newfoundland
8. Louisiana	8. Saskatchewan
9. Florida	9. New Mexico
10. Michigan	10. South Dakota

The information is taken from *Taking Stock: North American Pollutant Releases and Transfers (2000)*, available from Commission for Environmental Cooperation, Montreal, Quebec, and TRI in the United States. If you would like to know which industries are contaminating your air, water, and soil, you can find it in Canada on the website www.pollutionwatch.org and in the United States at www.scorecard.org. For North American comparisons, see www.cec.org. You can then unite with others to take action.

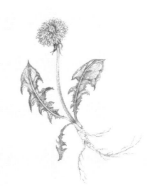

Rachel Carson Day (May 27)

Rachel Carson started the environmental movement with her book, *Silent Spring*, published in 1962. A marine biologist, ecologist, environmentalist, writer, and activist, Rachel was born on May 27, 1907 and died on April 14, 1964 from breast cancer. We can honor the spirit of Rachel and be fueled by her passion for the environment by celebrating Rachel Carson Day. Every year, on May 27, do what you can in your own corner of the world to preserve the safety and sanctity of the environment. Remove the toxins from your home. Reduce your use of plastic. Join other women and lobby against PVC, radiation, pesticides, dioxin, and chlorine. Stage a march for the environment. Create awareness for the environmental links to breast cancer every year on May 27. Be passionate, be active, be vocal, do it together. Do it for yourself; do it for your children and future generations; do it for wildlife; do it for the earth, air, and water; do it for Rachel — just do it.

Pesticide Free Municipalities

Political activism does work. About 20 towns and villages in Quebec, four in Ontario, and Halifax in Nova Scotia have passed bylaws restricting pesticide spraying on private and public green spaces. The town of Hudson, Quebec, population 5,000, takes 10 to 12 companies to court each year for illegal spraying. Its bylaw against pesticides was passed over 10 years ago.[108] We can learn from this small town and push for a moratorium on pesticide use in our own cities.

Environmental Film Festivals

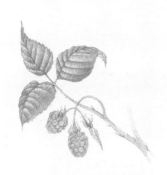

For the last three years in my small town, a group of us, calling ourselves the Rachel Carson League, have hosted a weekend environmental film festival each spring. This year we also took the films into local public schools during Earth Week and talked to the students about environmental protection. We use our film festival as our annual fundraiser, and it is genuinely a fun event.

There are three excellent films on the environmental links to breast cancer that you can show in your communities. *Exposure: Environmental Links to Breast Cancer* comes with an excellent resource guide and handbook. Another is called *Hormone Copy-Cats*. A third film is called *Rachel's Daughters*, which comes with a wonderful Community Action and Resource Guide. A fabulous new film called *The Next Industrial Revolution* offers a hopeful vision of the future presented in the work of architect William McDonough and chemist Dr Michael Braungart, two leaders in a growing movement who believe that whatever we create in industry should either be able to be used as food for something else, with no toxicity, or be recycled. Another film, *Blue Vinyl*, chronicles the humorous story of vinyl siding going on and then coming off of a family home. I encourage you to educate your communities with some of these wonderful films.

Rachel Carson Day Annual Letter Exercise

Use the occasion of Rachel Carson Day to write a letter or copy one of the samples on the following pages to your elected government officials. Send it to the mayor of your city, your provincial or state politicians, and federal government representatives. Send it every year.

May 27, Year

Minister of Agriculture	or	Secretary,
House of Commons		Agriculture, Nutrition
Ottawa, ON K1A 0A6		and Forestry
		House of Representatives
		Washington, DC 20510

Dear Minister, or Dear Secretary,

I am extremely concerned about the amount of pesticides used on the food that we eat. These pesticides end up in the groundwater and persist in the soil for many years. Many of them act as hormone disruptors linked to breast cancer and are eroding our ability to reproduce. Please tell me what steps you are making to ensure the following:

1) That the following pesticides be banned, as they are implicated in breast cancer: atrazine, cyanazine, dichlorvos, endosulfan, ethalfluralin, ethylene oxide, etridiazole, methoychlor, oryzalin, prometon, propazine, simazine, terbuthylazine, terbutyn, tribenuron methyl;

2) That organically grown food is more readily available all across the nation;

3) That the government encourage organic farmers through subsidies and educate all farmers in organic farming methods;

Sincerely,

Your address:

May 27, Year

Minister of Agriculture	or	Secretary,
House of Commons		Agriculture, Nutrition and Forestry
Ottawa, ON K1A 0A6		House of Representatives
		Washington, DC 20510

Dear Minister, or Dear Secretary,

As a woman and as a citizen of our nation, I am extremely concerned about the government's lack of resolve in enforcing environmental regulations. I insist upon immediate action in the following areas:

1) That there is an immediate ban on the production and use of organochlorines, which are causative factors in the breast cancer epidemic, and are disturbing the reproductive ability of humans, birds, fish, turtles, whales, seals, polar bears, otters, and many life forms. These chemicals are extremely toxic and extremely stable. Some do not break down for over a thousand years. The planet cannot sustain their use any longer. We must achieve zero discharge of persistent toxic substances as described by the International Joint Commission on Great Lakes Water Quality. Why has the government not acted on these recommendations?

2) That PVC plastic is speedily phased out, as it has been in Sweden, and is replaced with readily available alternatives. These alternatives should be labeled PVC free.

3) That there be a strictly enforced ban on the incineration of PVC plastic, especially by hospitals. Dioxin is one of the deadliest chemicals known, and is released through the production and burning of PVC plastic. The government must maintain a regulatory body that mandates strict enforcement of standards and severe penalties for polluters.

4) That the following pesticides be banned, as they are implicated in breast cancer: atrazine, cyanazine, dichlorvos, endosulfan, ethalfluralin, ethylene oxide, etridiazole, methoxychlor, oryzalin, prometon, propazine, simazine, terbuthylazine, terbutyn, tribenuron methyl; and that there be programs in place that encourage farmers to reduce pesticides and grow organic food.

5) That there be a ban on the production and use of alkylphenols (present in some industrial detergents) and phthalates (used in the manufacturing of plastics). Both of these chemical groups are hormone disruptors and are found throughout the environment.

6) That industry must prove its products are safe through thorough testing before they are allowed on the market or in our bodies. It has taken 40 years to realize that organochlorines are hormone disruptors, yet still they are in widespread use. Companies that make chemicals must be required to first test them thoroughly before they experiment on humans and wildlife. The testing must be done by a scientific lab without a vested interest in the industry. Industry and government must operate on the 'Precautionary Principle', which dictates that indication of harm, rather than proof of harm, is enough to restrict usage of toxic substances. We have an obligation to protect life and thousands of years of evolution. The onus must be placed on the chemical industry to prove that its products are safe rather than on us to prove that they are not.

Please let me know what specific progress you are making in each of these areas.

Sincerely,

Your address:

Non-Toxic Body and Home Care Products

There are an unprecedented number of chemicals used on the earth today We can decrease our exposure to these chemicals by using non-toxic alternatives and by encouraging others to do the same. The waters of the earth circulate in our arteries and veins; its soil becomes the nutritive base of our bodies. What we do to the earth, we do to ourselves. Please do not add toxic chemicals to this already impaired system.

Here are a few natural ways that we can support our planet as we are sustained by it.

Body Care

Baby Oil
Fill a 50 ml glass container half full with apricot kernel oil or sunflower oil, and half full with sweet almond oil. Add one capful of wheat germ oil. Add 3 drops of lavender.

Ingredients: wheat germ oil, apricot kernel oil or sunflower, sweet almond oil, lavender.

Dental Floss
Floss your teeth with 2 or 4 lb nylon monofilament fish line, available at any hardware store. Double and twist it for extra strength and rinse it in water before you begin. Cut a month's supply at a time and keep them in a small paper bag in your bathroom cabinet.

Ingredients: 2 or 4 pound monofilament fish line.

Dry Skin/Eczema Healing Oil
Pour 2 tbsp sesame oil, 1 tbsp olive oil, 2 tbsp avocado oil, and 2 tbsp almond oil in a small, dark glass jar or container. Take 10 vitamin E gelatin capsules (200 IU each) and 4 vitamin A gelatin capsules (25,000 units each) and puncture the capsules with needles or cut the ends with scissors and squeeze the contents into the bottle. Add a drop or two of your favorite essential oil to mask the aroma of the ingredients. Close the lid tightly and shake well. The best way to use this oil is at night before going to bed. After you wash your face, neck and hands take a few drops of the oil and massage into needed areas. The oil will be totally absorbed into the skin by morning.

Ingredients: sesame oil, olive oil, avocado oil, almond oil, vitamin E gelatin capsules, vitamin A capsules. This oil is based on a formula devised by Paavo Airola.

Facial Oil
Fill a 50 ml container with cold pressed almond oil and 10 drops of vitamin E. If desired, add 10 drops of lavender and 10 drops of geranium. After washing your face, apply two to three drops of oil, lightly stroking it into your face. After a few minutes the oil should be absorbed. Blot any extra with a tissue.

Ingredients: almond oil, vitamin E oil, lavender, geranium.

For an alternative to lindane-containing shampoos for lice, mix together the essential oils of:

Rosemary	20 drops
Geranium	10 drops
Lavender	20 drops
Eucalyptus	10 drops
Tea tree	20 drops

Ingredients: vegetable oil, vitamin E oil.

Ingredients: corn starch or baking soda, lavender.

Ingredients: borax liquid soap, citric acid crystals.

Ingredients: tea tree oil or citricidal, water.

Ingredients: baking soda, food grade hydrogen peroxide.

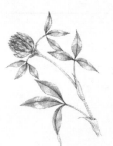

Lice Killers
Add these to ½ cup of either olive oil or mustard oil and keep the mixture in a dark glass jar. Rub the blend into the scalp and leave it overnight with a towel wrapped around the head. Wash it out in the morning. Repeat one week later. Treat the whole family at the same time and wash bedding and hair brushes. Add a small amount of the oil (5 drops) to your shampoo each time you wash your hair until the infestation is over. Buy a LiceMeister comb (other combs won't work) and comb every family member's hair daily with it to remove the nits until no more are found. Check hair weekly for nits as long as there is an outbreak in the school.

Massage Oil
Try vegetable oils like cold pressed almond, apricot kernel, sesame, sunflower, olive, or coconut oil. For 50 ml/2 oz of vegetable oil, add 5 drops of vitamin E. You can also add 5-20 drops of your favorite essential oils.

Powdered Deodorant
Stir 5 drops of lavender oil into ½ cup corn starch or baking soda and store in a glass, opaque, airtight container. Use a soft cloth, such as velvet or cotton flannel, to dust your underarms.

Shampoo
A few squirts of borax liquid soap, described above, serves as a great shampoo. The only thing you'll need to get used to is that the soap doesn't lather. After shampooing with borax liquid, use ¼ tsp citric acid crystals (not ascorbic) in a pint container of water to return your scalp to its natural acidity level.

Skin Disinfectant
For cleaning cuts and wounds add 5 drops of tea tree oil or citricidal to a small bowl of cooled, boiled water. Swab the wounded area using cotton wool or a gauze cloth.

Soap
'Soapworks' makes totally natural soaps. Some good soap choices are: evening primrose, chamomile, oatmeal, or goatmilk. These soaps are available at health food stores.

Toothbrushing
Brush your teeth with a pinch of baking soda dissolved in a glass with some water. If you have plastic, not metal, fillings dilute food grade hydrogen peroxide with equal parts water and store in a glass bottle. Brushing with this solution will help to whiten your teeth within 6 months.

Home Care

Carpet Cleaner

You can rent a machine to wash your carpet, but instead of the soap they suggest, use $\frac{1}{3}$ cup borax powder in the wash water and $\frac{1}{4}$ cup grain alcohol, 2 tsp boric acid, 20 drops citricidal, and $\frac{1}{4}$ cup white vinegar in the rinse water.

Ingredients: borax powder, grain alcohol, boric acid, citricidal, white vinegar.

Clean Air

Use 5 drops of citricidal or 10 drops of tea tree oil in 1-2 liters/quarts of water in humidifiers and air conditioners to disinfect the air and deter mold growth.

Ingredients: citricidal or tea tree oil, water.

Dish Soap

Use equal parts borax powder and washing soda to clean your dishes. For dishes that aren't greasy, just wash them with running water.

Ingredients: borax powder, washing soda.

Dishwasher Soap

Use 2 tsp borax powder pre-dissolved in water. If you use too much, it will leave a film on the dishes. You can also use vinegar in the rinse cycle.

Ingredients: borax powder, vinegar.

Disinfectant

To control bacteria, fungi and mold, add 20 drops of citricidal or up to 50 drops of tea tree oil to a bucket of water and stir well. Use this solution for mopping or wiping floors, counters, sinks, bathroom tiles, shower stalls and toilets. Put 5 drops of citricidal into a spray bottle with water and spray bathroom tiles and shower stalls to discourage mold growth.

Ingredients: citricidal or tea tree oil, water.

Drain Cleaner

First use a plunger if the sink is backed up. Push down and release a few times to dislodge debris.

Pour $\frac{1}{2}$ cup of baking soda and $\frac{1}{2}$ cup of vinegar over the drain. Let it set for one hour, then run hot water to clear. Never pour liquid grease down the drain. Always use a drain sieve.

Ingredients: plunger, baking soda, vinegar.

Dry Cleaning

Instead of dry cleaning, find a Green Clean outlet near you. They use safe water based alternatives to toxic chemicals. Ask your local dry cleaner to switch to Green Clean. The use of the organochlorine perchloroethylene ('perc') in dry cleaning impairs the health of workers and nearby residents.

Floor Cleaner

Use washing soda with a bit of borax to deter insects (except ants). Use white vinegar in your rinse water for a natural shine and to deter ants.

Ingredients: washing soda, borax powder, white vinegar.

Floor Wax

Mix beeswax and linseed oil, testing on a patch of floor to confirm desired proportions.

Ingredients: beeswax, linseed oil.

Ingredients: olive oil. ▶

Furniture Polish

Use filtered water to dampen a cloth and place a few drops of olive oil on the cloth.

Ingredients: citricidal (grapefruit seed extract). ▶

Hot Tubs, Jacuzzis, Swimming Pools

Use 10-15 drops of citricidal per gallon/ 4 liters of water to disinfect hot tubs, jacuzzis, and swimming pools.

Ingredients: boric acid. ▶

Insect Killer

Throw liberal amounts of boric acid (not borax) behind your stove, refrigerator, and under your carpets. Keep it away from food and out of children's reach.

Non-Toxic Home and Body Care Shopping Checklist

You should be able to find these natural and organic products and ingredients for the specified purposes in supermarkets, health food stores, hardware stores, and ecological supply stores. Add them to your shopping list.

Ingredient	Purpose
❑ Almond Oil, cold pressed	dry skin blend, facial oil
❑ Apricot Kernel Oil or Sunflower Oil	baby oil
❑ Avocado Oil	dry skin blend
❑ Beeswax	floor wax
❑ Borax Powder	carpet cleaner, dish soap, dishwasher soap, floor cleaner, laundry detergent, liquid soap, toilet bowl cleaner
❑ Boric Acid	carpet cleaner, insect killer
❑ Cedar Chips	moth balls
❑ Citric Acid Crystals	shampoo
❑ Citricidal Drops (Grapefruit seed extract)	disinfectant, hot tubs
❑ Essential Oils	lice killers
❑ Lavender	baby oil, facial oil
❑ Lavender Flowers and Oil	moth balls, powdered deodorant
❑ Linseed Oil	floor wax
❑ Geranium	facial oil
❑ Hydrogen Peroxide (food grade)	toothbrushing
❑ Monofilament Fish Line (2 or 4 lb)	dental floss
❑ Sesame Oil	dry skin blend
❑ 'Soapworks' Soap	body washing soap
❑ Tea Tree Oil	clean air, diaper cleaner, disinfectant, skin disinfectant
❑ Vitamin A (gelatin capsules)	dry skin blend
❑ Vitamin C (capsules)	toilet bowl cleaner
❑ Vitamin E (oil)	facial oil, massage oil
❑ Vitamin E (gelatin capsules)	dry skin blend
❑ Vegetable Oils (almond/apricot kernel/ sesame/sunflower/olive/coconut oil)	massage oil
❑ Washing Soda	diaper cleaner, dish soap, floor cleaner, laundry detergent
❑ Wheat Germ Oil	baby oil

Kitchen/Bathroom Cleanser
Use $\frac{1}{4}$ cup borax with $\frac{1}{4}$ cup of washing soda and a minimum of water to clean in the kitchen and bathroom. You can use dry washing soda to scour.

Ingredients: borax powder, washing soda.

Laundry Detergent
Use a $\frac{1}{2}$ cup of borax powder per load of laundry, or combine with washing soda for extra cleaning power. For getting out stubborn stains, try rubbing with bar soap first and/or rub with grain alcohol, vinegar, or baking soda.

Ingredients: borax powder, washing soda.

Liquid Soap
Use a funnel to put $\frac{1}{8}$ cup borax powder in a 1 gallon/ 4 liter jug. Fill the jug with cold tap water. Shake well and let it settle. After a few minutes pour off the clear liquid into dispensers for use as liquid soap. Alternatively, use vegetable oil based liquid soap.

Ingredients: borax powder, or vegetable oil-based liquid soap.

Moth Balls
Make up sachets with cedar chips sprinkled with lavender oil and flowers. Make the scent just strong enough to fill the storage area. If the closet is one you open often, you may have to refresh the oil every two months.

Ingredients: cedar chips, lavender flowers and oil.

Oven Cleaner
Scrub with baking soda on its own or mix 1 cup of pure soap, $\frac{1}{2}$ cup lemon juice with one gallon of water, and scrub. Rinse with water.

Ingredients: baking soda, pure soap, lemon juice.

Smells
Basement, pet, carpet smells… try dry herbs such as thyme, lavender, tansy, rosemary etc. strewn around the floor and swept up again after a few days. This absorbs odor and repels insects. You can also mix coarse corn meal with a few drops of essential oil, sprinkle it on the carpets, and vacuum it up after a few hours. This combination is good for upholstery, too, though not good for ingestion by children and pets.

Ingredients: dried herbs, coarse corn meal.

Toilet Bowl Cleaner
Pour 1 cup borax powder into toilet bowl and let sit overnight. Scrub with a brush and flush. For faster action, add $\frac{1}{4}$ cup lemon juice or vinegar to the borax. Wait a few hours before scrubbing. Alternatively, open two 1000 mg vitamin C capsules and drop them into the bowl, letting them sit overnight. Scrub with a brush and flush.

Ingredients: borax powder, lemon juice or vinegar, vitamin C capsules.

Window Cleaner
Mix 2 tbsp vinegar in 1 liter/ quart of water in a spray bottle. Clean your windows using newspapers.

Ingredients: vinegar, newspaper.

Summary

Once we know the sources of environmental toxins, we can set to work minimizing risk from our surroundings and cleansing our bodies from both externally and internally generated toxins. Consider these actions to decrease our collective exposure to environmental risk factors for cancer:

1) Host an environmental film festival or other event in your community each year to commemorate Rachel Carson by educating others about the links between the environment and breast cancer. Create what Margaret Mead called a "small group of thoughtful citizens."

2) Protect yourself from radiation by limiting x-rays and ingesting turmeric, sea vegetables, and foods high in beta carotene daily along with a high fiber diet.

3) Check out your home and work environment with a Gaussmeter to determine if there are any commonly used areas that consistently register higher than 2 mG. If there are, avoid them or find a way to shield yourself from the electromagnetic radiation.

4) Avoid eating the fruits and vegetables that have high amounts of pesticide residues. Choose to buy these organically grown instead. Do not use pesticides on your lawn and encourage your neighbors and community to create a pesticide ban.

5) Familiarize yourself with sources of PVC plastic, PBDEs, and phthalates. Choose non-toxic alternatives. Replace mercury fillings with ceramic (not plastic) resins and avoid the use of bisphenol A and phthalates in dentistry and food packaging.

6) If you are pregnant, take stock of your environment to learn whether there are industries, farms, toxic waste sites, plastic recycling plants, or sewage treatment plants around you that are releasing harmful chemicals. If possible, for the first four months of your pregnancy, move to a less polluted area. Filter your water using a reverse osmosis or charcoal filter.

7) Using the strategies described in the next chapter, rid your bodies of environmental chemicals through the intensive use of saunas, homeopathic or herbal cleansing formulas, and a liver and bowel detoxification program, especially before you are ready to conceive so that you do not pass on your accumulated load of environmental estrogens to the next generation.

CHAPTER FIVE

Detoxifying our Bodies

CONTENTS

EXERCISES, CHARTS, CHECK LISTS & WORKSHEETS

*T*oxins are substances that are harmful to health. They may have their origin from outside the body (exotoxins) or within the body (endotoxins). When the body is unable to break down and eliminate a toxic overload, symptoms of illness may manifest. These could include headaches, joint pain, fatigue, irritability, depression, mental confusion, digestive disturbances, cardiovascular irregularities, flu-like symptoms, or allergic reactions such as hives, runny nose, sneezing, and coughing. Toxicity may also contribute to the presence of autoimmune diseases, rheumatoid arthritis, Alzheimer's disease, Parkinson's disease, and cancer. Most bodily ailments are due in some part to toxicity.

Toxins can do their damage in several ways. They may generate free radicals, which cause cellular damage and inflammation; combine with and destroy enzymes; stagnate in tissues and interfere with circulation, causing high blood pressure; and thicken the blood, resulting in decreased oxygenation and distribution of nutrients. Toxins can block the transmission of nerve impulses, resulting in psychological disturbances. They can interact with hormones, causing imbalances in our glands. As health is impaired, there is first felt a general lowering of the body's vitality, decreased resistance to colds and flues, and irritability or depression. When our individual total toxic load surpasses our personal detoxification and eliminative capacity, disease results. We need to reduce our total toxic body burden by using regular detoxification strategies to maximize our health.

Exotoxins and Endotoxins

Exotoxins come to us from the air we breathe, food we eat, water we drink, and drugs we use. They often have an additive and cumulative effect that our bodies cannot manage.

Endotoxins are produced in the body/mind. Emotions and memories leave an imprint on organs, glands, and tissues, mediated by biochemical pathways linked to the nervous system and brain. There are real links between our emotions and our physical bodies.

Exotoxins

1) Xenobiotics (insecticides, herbicides, pesticides, food additives, plastics, drugs, solvents, etc.).
2) Toxic metals (lead, cadmium, mercury, arsenic, aluminum, nickel, etc.).
3) Organic toxins (aflatoxin, ergot toxins, fumosine, penicillium toxins, etc.).
4) Vitamin and mineral excesses (vitamin D, A, E, copper, selenium, iodine, sodium, etc.).
5) Infections (viral, fungal, bacterial, parasitic etc.).
6) Lifestyle toxins (caffeine, sugar, smoking, alcohol, recreational drugs, broiled meat, etc.).
7) Inhalants (molds, algae, pollens, etc.).
8) Food sensitivities (gluten, dairy, nightshades, individualized foods)
9) Energetic phenomena (electromagnetic fields, ionizing radiation, geopathic stress, etc.).

Endotoxins

1) By-products of intestinal bacteria and fungi, imbalanced intestinal flora (dysbiosis).
2) Intermediary metabolites (lactic acid, pyruvic acid, sulphuric acid, nitric acid, urea, homocysteine).
3) Hormonal overload (estradiol, C16, C4 estrogens, thyroxine, IGF-1, insulin, cortisol, prolactin, etc.).
4) Increased free radicals (lipid peroxides, reactive oxygen intermediates in the liver, etc.).
5) Toxic emotions (excess worry, regret, grief, fear, lust, anger, jealousy, pride, greed, attachment, etc.).
6) Toxic memories (loss, rape, embarrassment, abuse, shame, violence, abandonment, guilt, etc.).

Detoxifying Systems

Who are the selfless unpaid workers in our bodies who clean up 24 hours of the day, every day? Regardless of how well these systems work to keep us healthy, we can greatly assist them in their job of eliminating toxins and increasing our resistance to diseases, including breast cancer. In this chapter, we focus on methods for supporting and cleansing the blood, liver, kidneys, digestive organs, intestines, skin, and lungs. In Chapter 6, 'Activating the Immune and Lymphatic Systems,' we will look at ways to invigorate the lymphatic and immune systems – the white blood cells, thymus gland, spleen, and lymph vessels and nodes.

The Moving Blood

Driven by the tireless rhythmic beating of the heart muscle (70 squeezes per minute), the blood carries nutrients and oxygen to all parts of the body, and carries away carbon dioxide and cellular waste products, bringing them to the lungs, liver, and kidneys for detoxification and/or elimination. Without robust circulation, toxins accumulate as they would in a stagnant pond, creating a kind of acid sludge that deprives local tissues of oxygen. When red blood

FACT
People with cancer usually have high blood coagulability with increased 'stickiness' or blood viscosity. This interferes with circulation through the small capillaries and causes a decrease in oxygen to the area of the tumor, which can lead to tumor growth and metastases.

cells stick together or form clumps similar to a 'coin roll', less oxygen is available, viscosity increases, and this combination encourages the breaking away of single or groups of cells from a tumor site, promoting the spread of an existing cancer.[1] A plasma viscosity higher than 1.4 mPa is associated with poor disease outcome.[2]

The Liver

The liver acts as our main 'factory' for breaking down, neutralizing, detoxifying, and removing chemicals, poisons, body wastes, bacteria, antigen-antibody complexes, and unused and undigested food surpluses from our body. The liver makes bile, which it uses to carry away harmful poisons and wastes. The bile passes through the bile ducts, into the intestines, and is eliminated with its accumulated gunk.

The Kidneys

Water-soluble toxins and minerals are eliminated through the body's great filter, the kidneys. They contain about one million tiny filtration units called nephrons, which collectively cleanse 180 liters of blood in 24 hours. This means that all of our blood is filtered through the kidneys 60 times per day. The surface area that the kidneys use to do their filtering of toxins is equal to the surface area of the skin on the rest of our bodies.

The Digestive Organs and Intestines

Many of the body wastes and poisons are organic in nature — they are still much like foods. The stomach and pancreas secrete their enzymes to break these down, and change them from threatening substances into harmless ones in the same way that they digest foods. These enzymes are capable of digesting and breaking down all foreign cells, including cancer cells. The acid in the stomach, as long as we have enough of it, is a deterrent to many organisms that otherwise might gain a foothold in our intestinal tracts.

After taking the good stuff and sending it off into the blood to nourish the rest of the body, the small intestine separates 'the clean from the unclean' and drives the unclean into the large intestine with its muscular movements. The large intestine retrieves whatever water and minerals it can and eliminates the rest through bowel movements. Any excess waste will build up on the large intestine's walls, forming crusts and pockets of infection that feed hungry micro-organisms waiting for a good dinner. There are over 400 different kinds of micro-organisms in our large intestine, some beneficial and others harmful. We have more organisms in our intestines than we have cells in our bodies. One third of our stools are composed of dead bacteria.

The Skin

The skin is the envelope that protects us, opening its pores to release toxins through perspiration. The mechanism of sweating is one of the few ways we can eliminate toxins that reside in our fat cells. Stored in here are some of the environmental chemicals we have been accumulating since conception, which in sensitive persons may trigger symptoms of chronic fatigue or environmental illness.

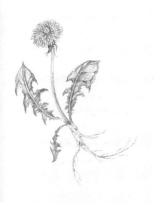

FACT
The liver handles about 40% of all the body's detoxification work, while the kidneys handle about 30% of the body's total elimination.

FACT
The skin handles about 10% of body elimination, while

The Lungs

Each time we exhale, our lungs release toxic gases and the end products of cell metabolism. When we breathe slowly and deeply we aerate a greater volume of the lungs and so improve its cleansing ability. The oxygen we take in through the breath, when delivered through the circulation, helps to deter the growth of cancer. The quality of our breathing affects so many physical and mental processes — it should be one of the first things taught in grade school.

The White Blood Cells

The function of the white blood cells is to digest and break down all foreign elements, toxins, dead cells, wastes, bacteria, and impurities in the blood stream. They congregate in the lymphatic tissue, which includes the lymph nodes, spleen, thymus gland, and specialized clean-up sites in the liver and small intestine. The white blood cells are divided into specialized troops, each equipped with remarkable defense tactics used on our behalf against toxins. Many vitamins, minerals, and herbs can activate these troops to serve us better.

The Thymus Gland

Located in the center of the chest, the thymus gland trains white blood cells in their various tasks and then sends them out to battle in the blood. Some of them take up residence in surveillance stations (lymph nodes) scattered through the body, like secret service agents. The thymus can control and turn up the volume on the elimination of wastes through the lymphatic system.

The thymus responds dramatically to our emotions and our will to live a purposeful life. It is further activated by melatonin and many vitamins, herbs, minerals, and nutritional substances. It shuts down when we are stressed and its soldiers then become fewer in number and less aggressive.

FACT

The thymus gland is the main immune organ of the body, the general of the white blood cells. The thymus develops our resistance to bacteria, cancer, viruses, toxins, and allergens of all kinds and stimulates the production of white blood cells in the bone marrow.

PREVENTION

To strengthen the function of the spleen, take herbal allies like burdock root, red clover, echinacea, and goldenseal.

The Spleen

Lying behind and slightly below the stomach, the spleen is a fist-sized organ filled with devouring macrophages — white blood cells whose destiny is to digest bacteria, foreign particles, and old decrepit red blood cells whose time is up. The spleen is a powerful filter of blood poisons and can store blood for us to be released as we need it. It is also an effective blood rebuilder.

The Lymphatic System

This is the body's 'sewage' system, comprised of drainage pipes connecting every cell and all areas of the body. The lymphatic system collects toxins from all these corners. When overloaded, a multitude of filters come into play to prevent an excessive amount of toxic debris from dumping into the bloodstream in quantities greater than the body can handle. These are the lymph nodes, small factories filled with eager, altruistic, cavalier types that defend our lives.

Promoting Blood Circulation

Decreasing Fibrinogen

Fibrinogen, a soluble protein manufactured in the liver and found in the blood plasma and extracellular fluid, is converted to fibrin, an insoluble protein, under various conditions. One of these conditions is when it comes in contact with foreign substances in the blood that may include antigen-antibody complexes, drugs, chemical toxins, heavy metals, and metabolic waste.[3] Fibrin forms an extended network of threads that impede the circulation and act as a kind of scaffolding in the extracellular fluid for tumor cell growth and spread.[4] The production of fibrin is enhanced by calcium ions, inflammation, and by increased acidity in the blood.[5] Plasma fibrinogen and plasma fibrin D-dimers, are increased in 89% of patients with progressive metastatic disease.[6] Furthermore, the cancer drugs cisplatin, doxorubicin, and cyclophosphamide cause an increase in the clumping together of red blood cells, resulting in a rise in blood viscosity.[7] Synthetic estrogens and progestin found in oral contraceptives and hormone replacement therapy also elevate plasma viscosity.[8]

Daily exercise and improved fitness decrease the production of fibrinogen while increasing the availability of oxygen.[9] Alternating hot and cold showers are another strategy to keep the heart muscle pumping strongly, allowing this river of blood to flow smoothly. Vitamin B3 (niacin) opens up the capillaries to deliver nutrients and remove waste more efficiently for us, and can decrease blood viscosity and fibrinogen levels.[10] Certain Chinese herbs, such as salvia, sparganium, ligusticum, frankincense, paeonia, and myrrh, as well as the formulas Salvia Shou Wu or Myrrh Tablets (Seven Forests), activate the blood and improve circulation.

Decreasing Plasma Viscosity

Cancer cells are by nature 'sticky', with specific cell adhesion molecules called galectins on their cell membranes that enables them to adhere to distant sites. An increased tumor load will therefore increase plasma viscosity. When taken between meals, the protein-digesting enzymes pancreatin, trypsin, chymotrypsin, papain, and bromelain, can alter these cell adhesion molecules so that they are less able to attach to distant sites.[11]

Blood viscosity increases when the red blood cells are more rigid, with less elastic cell membranes. This occurs when the pH of the blood is too acidic, when blood glucose levels are higher, and when free radicals damage cell membranes.[12] Red blood cell rigidity can be decreased by using alkalinizing minerals (magnesium and potassium or an alkaline powder), controlling blood sugar levels, and using antioxidants, along with vitamin E, fish oil, or flaxseed oil.

Assisting the Liver

Functions of the Liver

About one liter of blood passes through the liver every minute for detoxification. Found beneath the diaphragm on the right side of the body, this large organ performs many major functions vital to good health.

1) Breaks down proteins, fats, and carbohydrates, providing us with energy and nutrients.

2) Stores minerals, vitamins and sugars, to be used as needed by the body.

3) Helps to assimilate and store the fat-soluble vitamins A, E, D, and K.

4) Acts as a reservoir for blood storage, and quickly releases it when needed.

5) Helps to make blood proteins, such as albumin, which maintain fluid balance and fibrinogen, which is involved in blood coagulation.

6) Helps to maintain electrolyte and water balance.

7) Helps to regulate energy, moods, and emotions by controlling blood sugar and hormone levels.

8) Creates substances that function as part of the immune system, such as gamma globulin.

9) Filters the blood and helps to remove harmful chemicals and organisms, like bacteria and fungus.

10) Creates bile, which is stored in the gallbladder, and helps to break down fats and carry away toxins.

11) Breaks down and eliminates excess hormones as well as making its own hormones.

For breast cancer prevention, assisting the liver's detoxifying functions is vital. The liver uses a two step detoxification sequence to protect us from 'outside' chemicals (exotoxins) as well as internally generated endotoxins. This two step detoxification sequence is known simply as Phase 1 and Phase 2.

Each of these steps uses different types of enzymes for detoxification. Chemicals or hormones that are fat-soluble must first be processed through Phase 1 detoxification to be made water soluble so they can be inactivated by Phase 2 enzymes. The Phase 2 enzymes do the real clean-up.

FACT
If our liver detoxification systems are overwhelmed or inadequate, fat soluble toxins will lodge in our fatty tissues — one of their favorite resting places being our breasts.

Phase 1 Detoxification

Phase 1 detoxification uses a group of 100 different enzymes, known collectively as the 'cytochrome P450' system, each with an affinity for a different family of fat-soluble toxins. These enzymes act on toxins utilizing the biochemical reactions of oxidation (lose an electron), reduction (gain an electron), or hydrolysis (add water). Some toxic substances are inactivated completely through Phase 1, but most are not, and need Phase 2 to finish the job.

Many of the water-soluble intermediate products of Phase 1 are highly reactive and can have up to 60 times more toxic activity than their previous fat-soluble incarnations, unless they are quickly neutralized by Phase 2 enzymes. These reactive intermediate products are collectively called 'epoxides'. Some epoxides are highly carcinogenic, such as benzo[a]pyrene (BP), a polycyclic aromatic hydrocarbon found in smoked meats, and the C4 estrogen, a breakdown product of estrone. People who have a fast Phase 1 and a slow Phase 2 are at most risk of cancer because they build up epoxides during Phase 1 detoxification.

FACT
An abundance of minerals, vitamins, and amino acids is essential for liver detoxification and the prevention of cancer.

When the P450 enzymes act on a toxin, free radicals called 'superoxide radicals' are formed along with epoxides. If not quickly neutralized, both of these products have the potential to damage cell membranes, resulting in tissue injury and inflammation.

Epoxides are neutralized by Phase 2 reactions and by antioxidants like vitamins A, C, E, zinc and selenium as well as another antioxidant called glutathione. Glutathione is a protein containing the amino acids cysteine, glutamic acid, and glycine. Sugar decreases the production of glutathione.

Glutathione production and activity are dependent on healthy levels of selenium, magnesium, sulfur, manganese, vitamin B1 (thiamine), and the amino acid cysteine. The herb milk thistle can increase glutathione production by 35% in the liver, while alpha lipoic acid increases glutathione levels in red blood cells and lymphocytes by 30-70%.[13]

Speeding Up Phase 1 Liver Detoxification
Both harmful and protective substances can speed up Phase 1 detoxification. Harmful substances use up P450 enzymes faster, resulting in enzyme depletion, and a build up of other toxins. These substances are best avoided, especially if you are recovering from cancer. Protective substances place no stress on the P450 enzymes, but allow them to do their work faster, helping to eliminate toxins more quickly, so long as the Phase 2 enzymes can keep up.

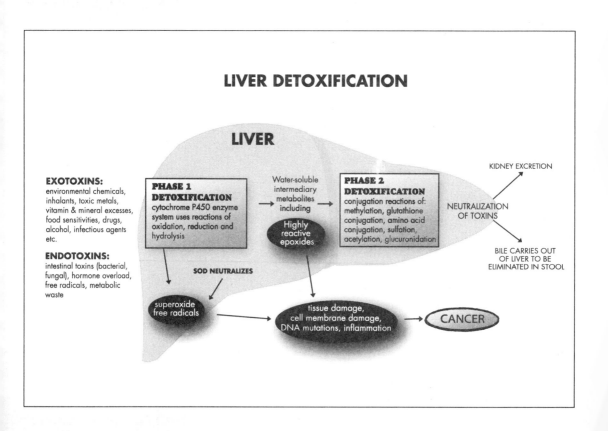

LIVER DETOXIFICATION

LIVER

KIDNEY EXCRETION

EXOTOXINS:
environmental chemicals, inhalants, toxic metals, vitamin & mineral excesses, food sensitivities, drugs, alcohol, infectious agents etc.

ENDOTOXINS:
intestinal toxins (bacterial, fungal), hormone overload, free radicals, metabolic waste

PHASE 1 DETOXIFICATION
cytochrome P450 enzyme system uses reactions of oxidation, reduction and hydrolysis

Water-soluble intermediary metabolites including

Highly reactive epoxides

PHASE 2 DETOXIFICATION
conjugation reactions of: methylation, glutathione conjugation, amino acid conjugation, sulfation, acetylation, glucuronidation

NEUTRALIZATION OF TOXINS

BILE CARRIES OUT OF LIVER TO BE ELIMINATED IN STOOL

SOD NEUTRALIZES

superoxide free radicals

tissue damage, cell membrane damage, DNA mutations, inflammation

CANCER

Harmful and Protective Substances that Speed Up Phase 1 Detoxification

Harmful Substances to Avoid	Protective Substances to Add
Dietary: alcohol, high protein, char-broiled meats, methylxanthines (found in coffee, chocolate and cola), saturated fat.	**Dietary:** brassica family (cabbage, broccoli, Brussels sprouts), oranges, tangerines, caraway seeds.
Drugs: nicotine, phenobarbitol, sulfonamides, steroids, barbiturates, valium, antihistamines. benzodiazepines, cimetidine (and other drugs used for stomach ulcers), ketoconazole, sulfaphenazole.	**Nutritional Supplements:** indole-3-carbinol or DIM, vitamin B3 (niacin), vitamin B1, vitamin C, limonene (in essential oils of lemon, orange, celery), rosemary, schizandra, St. John's wort.
Pollutants: carbon tetrachloride, exhaust and paint fumes, dioxin, pesticides.	

Note: St. John's Wort, rosemary, and schizandra all stimulate Phase 1 detoxification and can more than double the activity of some of the P450 enzymes. This is a good thing if Phase 2 enzymes can keep up, but will be harmful if they can't. These herbs can decrease the effectiveness of chemotherapy by reducing drug concentrations and should be avoided during this time and for 5 days prior. They may be useful after chemo to clear drugs out of your system, while simultaneously using substances that activate Phase 2. Tangeretin from tangerines decreases the effectiveness of Tamoxifen. Check with your pharmacist or naturopathic doctor about using these along with other medications.[14]

Phase 2 Detoxification

Phase 2 detoxification enzymes step in to bind up the water-soluble toxins and epoxides to either glutathione, methionine, glycine, glucuronic acid or sulphur compounds. These are all called conjugation reactions. Once bound, these toxins are neutralized and can no longer do damage (unless they become unbound in the large intestine). The smaller products of Phase 2 detoxification, being water soluble, are eliminated through the kidneys. The larger ones are transported in the bile to the gallbladder, then to the small intestine, and eventually are eliminated through the stools.

Overactive Phase 1 Enzymes/ Underactive Phase 2 Enzymes

If the Phase 2 enzymes can't keep up with Phase 1 detoxification, the toxic water soluble metabolites from Phase 1 may enter the bloodstream and harm any tissue, or they can be dumped into the bile and gallbladder before being inactivated, irritating the gallbladder, stomach, and small intestine.

If your Phase 2 enzymes are sluggish, you may experience food intolerances, poor cholesterol metabolism, and be hypersensitive to caffeine, perfumes, and chemicals as these persist longer in your body.

Some substances slow down the cytochrome P450 enzymes, causing the toxins they are supposed to be breaking down to circulate in the blood. This is not a good thing if your toxic burden is high, and your Phase 2 enzymes are working well and can keep up

Phase 2 Detoxification: Conjugation Reactions

During Phase 2 detoxification, six types of different biochemical interactions can occur to attach or 'conjugate' the toxic metabolites from Phase 1 to other small chemicals, which then make the original substance ready for excretion. The six types of conjugation reactions are called glutathione conjugation, amino acid conjugation, methylation, sulfation, acetylation, and glucuronidation. The chart below summarizes the substances that are detoxified, as well as the required nutrients, promoters, and inhibitors of Phase 2 detoxification reactions.[15,16] Sulfation, methylation, glutathione conjugation, and glucuronidation are important reactions in breaking down and eliminating your body's estrogen. If they are not efficient, there will be greater estrogen dominance and more of the harmful C4 and C16 estrogens.

Phase 2 System	Substances Detoxified	Assisting Nutrients	Promoters	Inhibitors
glutathione conjugation	bacterial toxins, aflatoxin, lipid peroxides, ethyl alcohol, quercetin, bilirubin, prostaglandins, acetaminophen, penicillin, tetracycline, nicotine, insecticides, styrene, benzopyrene, methylparathion, chlorobenzene, petroleum products, naphthalene, toxic metals	glutathione, vitamin B6, B2, B3, C, NAC, germanium, magnesium, manganese, selenium	brassica family, soy, whey, legumes, oatmeal, indole-3-carbinol, DIM, limonene (essential oils of lemon, celery, orange), milk thistle, alpha lipoic acid, curcumin	deficiencies of selenium, zinc, or vitamin B12, deficiency of glutathione
amino acid conjugation	bile acids, PABA, butyric acid, stearic acid, nicotinic acid, Aspirin, aliphatic amines, phenylacetic acid, solvents, benzoic acid (food preservative)	L-glycine, L-glutamine, taurine	glycine, 40 grams protein daily	inadequate dietary protein
methylation (important in estrogen metabolism)	C2 and C4 estrogens, dopamine, epinephrine, norepinephrine, L-dopa, histamine, thiouracil, morphine, paraquat,	SAM (S-adenosyl-methionine), choline, vitamin B6, B12, folic acid, B2, magnesium	soy nuts, kidney beans, black beans, org. low fat cottage cheese, methionine, choline, betaine,	deficiency of choline, folic acid, magnesium, or vitamin B12;

to Phase 1. However, there are two instances when it may be beneficial to slow down Phase 1: when someone is very toxic and you want to reduce the pace at which epoxides are generated; and when Phase 2 enzymes are sluggish and need time to catch up to Phase 1. If you spent a weekend house-painting and have a headache, you could use grapefruit juice combined with curcumin capsules to slow down Phase 1, allowing Phase 2 time to detoxify before stressing the liver with more paint fumes. Remember, it is the epoxides in the intermediate state that are most dangerous, being up to 60 times more toxic than the original substances.

Phase 2 System	Substances Detoxified	Assisting Nutrients	Promoters	Inhibitors
	mercury, lead, arsenic, thallium, tin		folic acid, B12, magnesium, MSM	excess of boron or molybdenum
sulfation (important in estrogen metabolism)	C16 estrogen, DHEA, thyroxine, testosterone, cortisol, melatonin, catecholamines, vit. D, bile acids, tyramine, coumarin, aniline dyes, amines, formaldehyde, quercetin, methyl dopa, acetaminophen, terpenes, phenols, intestinal toxins	cysteine, taurine, selenium, methionine, MSM, B6, sulforaphane (broccoli sprouts), bifidobacterium	soy, whey, cysteine, taurine, methionine, glutathione, bifidobacterium	NSAIDS, yellow food dye, excess vitamin B6, excess/def. of methionine and cysteine
sulfoxidation	garlic, sulfite food additives, preservatives, chlorpromazine, sulfite drugs (asthma)	molybdenum, legumes, whole grains	none found	deficiency of molybdenum
acetylation	serotonin, PABA, histamine, tryptamine, caffeine, choline, tyramine, clonazepam, mescaline, isoniazid, procainamide, benzidine, sulfa drugs, anilines	Acetyl-Co-A, vitamins B1, B5, C	peppers, cabbage, citrus, whole grains, green tea	deficiency of vitamins B1, B5 or C
glucuronidation (last step in estrogen metabolism)	steroid hormones, estrogen, melatonin, bilirubin, bile acids, vitamins A, E, K, D, salycilates, morphine, acetaminophen, menthol, benzodiazepine, naproxen, digoxen, valproic acid, steroids, lorazepam, propanolol, morphine, diazepam, phenols, aniline, butanol	vitamin B6, glucuronic acid, calcium-D-glucarate, fiber, probiotics	ellagic acid (red raspberries), fish oil, limonene, birth control pill, cig smoke, yellow tartrazine dye, phenobarbitol	aspirin and other NSAIDS, bowel bacteria can cause reabsorption of estrogen

Grapefruit Juice

Grapefruit, grapefruit juice, and Seville orange juice (but not sweet orange juice) contains a flavonoid called naringenin that can slow down certain cytochrome P450 enzymes by 30%.[17] Its effect can last up to 24 hours, and if we drink grapefruit juice daily, it can last up to 5 days.[18] For this reason, we should not drink grapefruit juice while taking specific medications. Grapefruit juice increases blood concentrations of oral contraceptives, many cholesterol-lowering drugs, Xanax, and numerous others. Check with your pharmacist if you are on any other medications and you consume grapefruit.

PREVENTION

Improve Phase 1 and 2 detoxification and manage your estrogens better with the following nutrients: curcumin, ellagic acid, amla, rosemary, schizandra, milk thistle, vitamins A, B complex, C, and E, choline, selenium, zinc, magnesium, manganese, coQ10, indole-3-carbinol or DIM, limonene from essential oil of lemon, flaxseed and fish oil, and foods containing cysteine and methionine (see chart in Chapter 7).

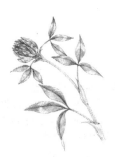

Curcumin and Ellagic Acid

Curcumin, which forms 95% of turmeric and gives it its yellow color, and ellagic acid, found in red raspberries, both slow down Phase 1 detoxification while speeding up Phase 2. They lower the formation of the toxic metabolites formed as intermediaries in Phase 1, while quickly inactivating those that have already formed, which is very helpful in preventing cancer. However, curcumin and ellagic acid should not be used during chemotherapy, as they may interfere with its effectiveness.[19]

Other dietary inhibitors of Phase 1 are quercetin, capsaicin (from red chili pepper), and eugenol from clove oil. Green tea slows down the P450 enzymes, as do blueberries, blackberries, red grapes, kiwi, watermelon, parsley, spinach, and red wine.[20,21]

Liver Protectors

We can maximize the function of these detoxification pathways and help our livers even more by including four classes of substances in our dietary and nutritional regimes: antioxidants, membrane stabilizers, choloretics, and sulphur-containing compounds.

Antioxidants

Antioxidants protect hepatic cells and all body cells from damage, neutralizing free radicals.

- Herbs: milk thistle, Chinese licorice, gingko, skullcap, Jerusalem artichoke, rosemary, bilberry, schizandra, eleuthero, chaparral, lemon balm, saffron, turmeric.
- Foods: cabbage, garlic, whole seeds, fruit, greens, red peppers, sprouts, spirulina, carrots.
- Vitamins: vitamins A, C, E.
- Minerals: zinc, selenium.
- Amino Acids: methionine, glutathione, cysteine.
- Flavonoids: catechin, quercetin, rutin, kaempferol, luteolin, pycnogenol and grape seed extract.
- Other: coenzyme Q10, alpha lipoic acid, melatonin.

Membrane Stabilizers
Membrane stabilizers protect the liver cell membranes from damage, making them less vulnerable to toxins.
- •Herbs: milk thistle.
- • Foods: cabbage, garlic, flaxseed oil, fish oil, and seeds.

Choloretics
Choloretics move the bile out of the liver with the toxins in it to be eliminated.
- • Herbs: globe artichoke, capillaris, garlic, chelidonium, burdock, barberry, blessed thistle, gentian, milk thistle, golden seal.
- • Foods: olive oil.

Sulphur-Containing Compounds
These provide the building blocks for the liver's detoxification mechanisms and glutathione.
- • Herbs: milk thistle, dandelion.
- • Foods: cabbage, cauliflower, Brussels sprouts, broccoli (brassica family), broccoli sprouts, onions, garlic, soy.

Liver Cleansers and Builders
In addition to these herbal and dietary liver 'protecting' substances, the following help to cleanse toxins from the liver.
- • Herbs: burdock, dandelion root, yellow dock, blue flag, Oregon grape root, phyllanthus, schizandra.
- • Foods: apples, other juicy fruits, apple cider vinegar, lemon juice, grapefruit juice, garlic, beets, dandelion greens, turmeric powder.
These herbs and foods help rebuild the liver and supply the nutrients it needs to operate efficiently.
- • Herbs: globe artichoke, milk thistle, butternut, oat, bupleurum, desmodium, phyllanthus.
- • Foods: seeds (flax, sesame, sunflower, pumpkin), almonds, whole grains, vitamin B rich foods (wheat germ, nutritional yeast, royal jelly, bee pollen), beets, and other foods rich in iron.

Specific Herbs for Liver Health
Certain herbs are especially effective in improving liver function and supporting other organs involved in detoxification and elimination.

Milk Thistle (Silybum marianum)
The seeds of the milk thistle plant benefit the liver, spleen, kidneys and digestion. Historically, milk thistle has been used to cure jaundice, hepatitis, and cirrhosis of the liver. Flavonoids are present in milk thistle that bind to liver cell membranes and protect them from being injured by foreign chemicals, organochlorines, hormones, radiation, heavy metals, free radicals, and endo- and exotoxins. Flavonoids protect the liver during chemotherapy and radiation and help it to regenerate after injury. Milk thistle can increase glutathione levels by 35%, promotes the flow of bile so that toxins are quickly removed from the liver, and is useful in stopping heavy menstrual bleeding. It is best taken on an empty stomach.

PREVENTION
To protect, cleanse, and rebuild the liver, choose foods and herbs from these four categories — antioxidants, membrane stabilizers, choloretics, and sulphur-containing compounds. Incorporate them into your wellness plan.

Dosage
Unstandardized liquid extract: 40 drops, 2-3 x daily. Tincture of fresh or dried seeds: 30-100 drops, 3 x daily. Powdered extract standardized to 10% silymarin: 100 mg, 2-3 x daily. Powdered extract standardized to 80% silymarin: 1-2 tablets daily.

Contraindications: None known. Can be used for nine months or more at a time, followed by a two-week break. Can be used between doses of chemotherapy to protect the liver. See Chapter 10, 'Breast Disease Treatments.'

Schizandra

Schizandra berries contain vitamin C and vitamin E. Schizandra is an adaptogenic herb, helping us to adjust to stress by increasing endurance and regulating stomach acidity. It has been used in cases of hepatitis to normalize liver enzymes; and it strongly regenerates a damaged liver. Schizandra exerts a stimulating effect on the cytochrome P450 system of the liver's Phase 1 detoxification pathway, which enhances our ability to break down toxins and estrogen. It improves energy levels and is a tonic to the eyes.

Contraindications: Should not be taken in high amounts during chemotherapy, as it will hasten the break down of medications and decrease their effectiveness. However, it is an excellent choice when the chemo has been completed, to remove toxins and regenerate the liver.

Dosage
3-9 g, or 50-100 drops 3 x daily.

Dandelion Root (Taraxicum officianalis)

Dandelion root and leaves are used to support the liver, kidneys, and breasts. Use the root in a tea, the leaves steamed, in salads or juiced with fresh vegetables. Dandelion protects, heals, and tonifies the liver, and promotes bile flow to send out toxins. It decreases breast congestion, discourages cancer, improves digestion and appetite, cleanses the kidneys, stimulates weight loss by improving metabolism, and protects the immune system by increasing interferon production and phagocyte activity. It reduces lymphatic congestion and glandular swellings. High in potassium, its leaves are a good diuretic and cellular detoxifier.

Dandelion has demonstrated estrogen-lowering properties, and both traditional use and modern research verify its ability to prevent and reverse breast cancer.

Contraindications: None known. Along with milk thistle, it would be a good choice to use between chemotherapy treatments. It can be taken long term, with 2-week breaks every 3 months.

Dosage
Cooked Greens: 1-2 cups.
Dried Root Tea: 1-5 cups (simmer the root for 20 minutes, steep for 10; can be mixed with Chinese licorice).
Tincture: 15-50 drops, 3 x daily.

Bupleurum

The root of bupleurum has been used for over 2,000 years in Traditional Chinese Medicine to remove liver congestion, improve digestion, regulate the periods, and relax tension. Bupleureum is used in formulas for hepatitis and liver cirrhosis. It increases the formation of bile, helping to digest fats and remove toxins. It is an excellent herb to restore the liver and its enzymes, harmonize its function, and protect it from chemicals. As the main ingredient in a commonly used Chinese patent herbal formula, Xiao Yao Wan, it is helpful in alleviating premenstrual breast tenderness and fibrocystic breast disease.

Contraindications: In large amounts it can cause nausea in some people; use cautiously with a persistent dry cough. Use it between chemotherapy treatments.

Dosage
Tea: add 10 g of the herb to 12 oz of water. Simmer for 45 minutes, strain off the liquid into a glass jar, add 6 oz of fresh water, simmer another 20 minutes, strain and add to the first liquid and store in the refrigerator. Drink one cup twice daily, morning and evening, starting at a lower dosage and increasing to the full dosage.
Tincture: 20-30 drops, 3 x daily.

Globe Artichoke (Cynara scolymus)

Artichoke leaf and root tonify the liver and digestion, activating bile production to help digest fats and remove toxins. The root is more stimulating to the liver than the leaf. Cynara decreases fat and cholesterol content of the blood, prevents the formation of gallstones, and encourages weight loss and removal of cellulite. It promotes urination, relieves water retention, and heals chronic constipation. The bitter taste of artichoke acts as an immune stimulant and activates the stomach to produce hydrochloric acid. A compound in this herb called cynarin enhances liver cell regeneration and protection and may slow down the aging process.

Artichoke contains very high amounts of iodine, potassium, magnesium, calcium, trace minerals and vitamins A, B1 and B2, and C. It counters hypoglycemia and hypothyroidism.

Contraindications: Use cautiously while breast-feeding, as it may clog up the milk ducts.

Dosage
Tincture: 20 drops, 3 x daily.

Celandine (Chelidonium majus)

The leaves and root of chelidonium promote bile flow and decrease liver congestion. Celandine assists the gallbladder and stimulates the pancreas to aid digestion. It improves elimination through increased bowel movements and is known to reduce tumors, benign and malignant. It stimulates the heart and circulation, with better delivery of nutrients to, and waste removal from, body cells. It decreases edema.

Contraindications: Do not use in pregnancy. If taken alone, use for 2 weeks followed by a 4-day break.

Dosage
Tincture: 12-50 drops, 3 x daily.
Fresh juice: 2 tsp.

Barberry (Berberis vulgaris)

The root of barberry helps produce and activate bile flow. Barberry's bitter taste stimulates hydrochloric acid production in the stomach, improving digestion. In combination with other herbs, it is effective against intestinal parasites such as giardia and moves out intestinal toxins. Along with acidophilus, it balances intestinal flora and is an excellent herb for chronic candidiasis. It is an immune stimulant and is useful in cases of constipation.

Contraindications: Avoid in pregnancy. If used alone, take a two week break after three months of use.

Dosage
Tincture: 20-40 drops, 2-3 x daily.
Capsules: 2 capsules, 3x daily.
Powdered Extract: 100-200 mg, 2 x daily.

Liver Loving Formula for Healthy Breasts

Many herbal formulas are available to improve liver function. Check the formulas and find one that has at least one herb from each of the above categories, or buy single tinctures of milk thistle, dandelion, and chelidonium and mix them together in equal proportions, or simply use milk thistle on its own. The potency of herbs is preserved better in tincture form rather than in capsule or tea. Always buy organic herbs.

I have designed a formula that combines organic herbs from all of the above categories. You can use the order form at the back of the book to order it, or mix it up yourself from single tinctures.

Contraindications: If you are pregnant, omit chelidonium and barberry; increase dandelion and milk thistle. Do not use this during the 5 days before or 7 days after chemotherapy treatments.

Dosage
(see recipe overleaf)
As prevention, 30-40 drops 3 x daily in a little water for 6-8 weeks at a time, 1-4 times a year. For breast cancer recovery, take it consistently, stopping for one week every 2 months.

The 10-Day Liver Flush and Cleanse

A liver flush stimulates the liver to eliminate toxins, increases bile flow, and moves liver blood. It removes impurities from the blood and lymph. Schedule a time to do a 10-day liver flush. If you can, do it within the next month. Prepare yourself physically and psychologically with relaxation and breathing exercises daily, a vegetarian diet, and consciously release negative thought patterns, old resentments, and anger. Caution: Do not use this liver flush if you know you have gallstones.

Liver Flush Directions

1) Mix together freshly-squeezed orange, lemon, and lime juices to make one cup of liquid. Do not use grapefruit unless your Phase 1 detoxification is too fast for Phase 2 and you want to slow it down. The mixture should taste sour, which activates the liver. Water it down to taste with filtered water.

2) Add 1-2 cloves of fresh garlic plus a small amount of fresh ginger juice or grated ginger. Both garlic and ginger protect the liver.

3) Mix in 1 tablespoon of high quality extra virgin olive oil from a metal or opaque glass container and blend the mixture together.

4) Drink in the morning, waiting one hour before eating. Keep your diet simple the rest of the day, either eating mainly fresh fruits and vegetables or mung beans and rice cooked with vegetables.

5) Use 2 tsp turmeric in your diet daily or take curcumin capsules to speed up Phase 2 enzymes.

Cleansing Tea Directions

1) Follow the liver flush with two cups of a cleansing tea containing a mixture of fennel, burdock, dandelion, red clover, peppermint, nettles, fenugreek, and flax. To make your own cleansing tea mix:

1 part fennel	¼ part burdock
1 part fenugreek	¼ part licorice root
1 part flax	

Using 1 oz of the herbs to 20 oz of water, simmer all the herbs for 20 minutes, then add 1 part peppermint. Let it steep for 10 more minutes. Drink two cups each morning after the liver flush.

2) Take a bowel cleansing formula which includes bentonite (or take 1 tbsp psyllium daily) and have 2-4 tablespoons of freshly ground flaxseeds daily. Drink at least 2 liters or quarts of filtered water daily.

3) Continue this regimen for 10 days. Stop for 3 days. Continue another 10 days if desired. Do it 1-4 times yearly. If you have cancer, do it under the supervision of someone experienced with detoxification regimens.

Living Loving Formula

Ingredients

25 parts milk thistle
  (Silybum marianum)
20 parts dandelion root
  (Taraxicum officianalis)
15 parts schizandra
15 parts bupleurum
10 parts globe artichoke
  (Cynara scolymus)
10 parts greater celandine
  (Chelidonium majus)
 5 parts barberry
  (Berberis vulgaris)

Castor Oil Packs

A time-honored tradition in naturopathic medicine is the use of castor oil packs, especially over the liver, although they can be used anywhere. The oil helps to draw out toxins from as deep as four inches into the body. A castor oil pack improves elimination through the bowel, kidneys, and bladder, stimulates peristalsis, and protects the mucous lining of these organs. It improves absorption and assimilation in the digestive organs, balances acid secretions in the stomach, and stimulates the liver, pancreas and gallbladder. The pack helps to regulate metabolism and stimulates the nervous system. It improves the lymphatic circulation and draws acid and infection out of the body. It can help to dissolve and remove both lesions and adhesions. The castor oil pack also increases the production of T-lymphocytes.[22]

Directions for Using a Castor Oil Pack

1) Use un-dyed cotton cloth or wool flannel and soak it in cold-pressed castor oil. Wring the cloth out so that it is wet, but not dripping. The cloth can be used several times on the same person before it is washed, and stored in a covered glass container between treatments.

2) Place the cloth on the upper right quadrant of the abdomen, over the liver area, or on any other chosen site. Cover it with a layer of plastic to prevent the oil from getting messy.

3) Place a dry towel over the plastic and a hot water bottle or heating pad on the towel. If you are using a hot water bottle, cover it with a dry towel to hold the heat. The heat should be as warm as can be tolerated.

4) Leave this on the abdomen for 1 to $1\frac{1}{2}$ hours. Use it daily or every other day for 3 weeks, and then take a break for a week before deciding if you need to repeat the procedure.

Kidney Cleansing

Our kidneys filter all of our blood 60 times a day, removing metabolic wastes and excreting them to the outside through urine. The kidneys help to control the rate of red blood cell formation, regulate blood pressure, the absorption of calcium, and the volume, composition, and pH of body fluids.

The best way to assist our kidneys with detoxification is by drinking plentiful amounts of pure water, somewhere between two to three liters or quarts daily. Unfortunately, pure water is not easy to come by. In the United States, one government report named 2,110 chemicals in drinking water.

Bottled Water

Bottled water may be an option if it is stored in glass rather than plastic containers and if it is free of bacteria. Most companies will send you laboratory reports on their water quality if you ask.

Herbs and Foods for the Kidneys

Along with plenty of clean water, we can cleanse and support our kidneys with the following herbs and foods – dandelion, uva ursi, nettle, juniper berry, sarsaparilla, horsetail, goldenrod, asparagus, parsley and watermelon. Choose 2 or 3 of these herbs and use them in a tea or tincture form for 6 weeks or longer, and use parsley in your diet almost daily to help cleanse your kidneys.

Adjusting Acid and Alkaline Balance

Different tissues of the body vary in their pH, and will become more acid or alkaline in the body's efforts to maintain the blood at a constant pH of 7.4. Whether a substance is considered acid or alkaline is determined by its pH (potential of hydrogen). A healthy person will have a urinary pH that averages between 6.4-7.2 (6.8 is ideal) and a salivary pH of 6.4-7.4 (6.8 is ideal). The pH of the blood is maintained at 7.4. The pH of the urine will fluctuate throughout the day. Usually it is more acid (lower pH) in the morning between 2:00 a.m. and

PREVENTION

Block out on your calendar 10-day periods when you will do the liver flush and cleanse, up to four times per year, perhaps combining it with a 3-week sequence of castor oil packs. Block out the 6-8 week periods when you will take a liver formula, overlapping it with the liver flush. Choose to do it one to four times yearly, or continuously if you are recovering from breast cancer.

Dates for my liver cleanse:

_____

_____

_____

PREVENTION

Drink 2-3 liters or quarts of filtered water daily, using a reverse osmosis or carbon block filter. Other choices for kidney cleansing are to add lemon juice to your water in the morning, use dandelion, uva ursi, or juniper tea or tincture regularly, drink green juices (including some parsley and watercress), and use beets, which cleanse the kidneys and liver.

Water Filters

There are several kinds of filters that can be purchased for home use to remove most water contaminants.

Type of Filter	How It Works	What It Removes
Screen Filters	A fine membrane removes bacteria from water.	bacteria
Activated Carbon Filters	Absorbs contaminants, but bacteria can proliferate in poorly functioning carbon filters. They do a good job at removing organic chemicals but do not remove toxic minerals such as aluminum, cadmium, and copper. Some of these filters contain silver to discourage bacterial growth, which can enter the water at high levels. Avoid carbon filters with silver. Use a filter with a rated capacity for 2,000 gallons. Use a filter with a carbon block rather than powdered activated charcoal.	pesticides, radon, volatile organic chemicals
Reverse Osmosis Filters	Contain a membrane that removes contaminants and some minerals. They work slowly, producing only a few gallons of water a day, discarding about 90% of incoming water. Often they are combined with an activated carbon filter in one unit. Can cost several hundred dollars.	bacteria, organic matter, inorganic matter, pesticides, PCBs, lead, aluminum, nitrates, radium, uranium, fluoride
Distillation	Water is boiled, turned to steam, and collected as water again after passing through a series of baffles. Some chemicals have lower boiling points than water and will collect in the distilled end product, unless removed by carbon. Some organisms are heat resistant and will not be killed by distillation. Minerals are removed from the water and over time mineral deficiencies may occur in the person who drinks it. The distillation process is slow and the water tastes flat.	some chemicals, most but not all organisms, minerals, fluoride
Ultraviolet Treatment	Ultraviolet rays change the molecular structure of bacteria and destroy their DNA. Some parasites and viruses are not affected, however	bacteria

In summary, the best system is a reverse osmosis system with built-in activated charcoal, if you can afford it. Otherwise, go with the activated carbon block filter without silver. Distillation does not remove the environmental chemicals. Carbon block does not remove many minerals, including aluminum and fluoride.

10:00 a.m., when the kidneys are working hard to remove acid waste, and more alkaline (higher pH) in the evening between 4:00 p.m. and 10:00 p.m. It typically becomes alkaline for two hours after eating.

If the pH of urine and saliva are characteristically outside of these ranges, certain minerals and vitamins are not absorbed. Bacteria, viruses, fungi, parasites, and cancer are more active when pH is unbalanced.[23] Enzymes and cellular metabolism work best in a precise pH range.

Acid

Acids are produced daily in the body and need to be neutralized, or they accumulate as we age. When carbohydrates, proteins, and fats are metabolized, they produce inorganic acids. The strongest acids — sulphuric acid, nitric acid, and phosphoric acid— are formed from the break down of protein, while carbohydrates produce acetic and lactic acid. High protein diets are the worst for producing a build up of acid waste that both encourages cancer growth and causes minerals to be lost from our bones, leading to osteoporosis. Our protein intake should be between 30-50 grams per day, depending on our metabolic needs.

When we exercise, our muscles produce more lactic acid. When lactic acid and carbon dioxide combine with water, carbonic acid is formed. Anyone who exercises vigorously needs to take extra care in monitoring pH levels and neutralizing acids. All of these acids are toxic and are eliminated either through the kidney, large intestine, lungs, or skin.

When the blood is burdened with excess acid, mild symptoms such as colds, headaches, sore throats, flus, aches and pains are likely to occur. The muscles and joints become stiff, energy levels drop, and we become irritable. Free radical damage occurs more readily, and antioxidants are used up faster. Vitamins and minerals from foods and supplements are less well absorbed, and enzyme function is impaired. When the extracellular fluid becomes acidic, symptoms such as excess mucus, chronic infections, fibromyalgia, arthritis, gallstones, kidney stones, cysts, and benign tumors may occur.[24] When the acids accumulate even more, they can penetrate inside the cell and cause damage to the DNA, leading to cancer.

Alkaline

The body's built-in buffer system uses minerals to protect it from being overwhelmed with toxic acids. The alkaline minerals that neutralize acids are sodium, potassium, calcium, and magnesium. A simple way to help neutralize acids is to use one or more teaspoons daily of an alkalinizing powder that contains a combination of sodium bicarbonate, calcium carbonate, potassium bicarbonate and magnesium carbonate, available through a compounding pharmacy. One of the reasons Dr Max Gerson gave potassium to all his cancer patients was to decrease acidity and encourage elimination of toxins through the kidney. See Chapter 7, 'Eating Right for Breast Health,' for a list of potassium containing foods.

The pH of most tumors is more acidic in comparison to the pH of normal tissue, and as tumors grow, they produce lactic acid, creating even more acidity.[25] There is poor removal of metabolic acids from cancer cells.[26] One strategy for healing cancer is to alkalinize the pH of the body in general and of tumors specifically. Tumor cells die at a pH of 8. Cesium and rubidium are very alkaline trace minerals that are used in treating malignant tumors by directly injecting them into the tumor site. Some women have had success using coral calcium to reverse breast cancer.

FACT
Body fluids make up roughly 70% of our body weight and maintaining the pH (acid-alkaline balance) of these fluids is essential to life. Most cancer cells thrive when there is an overproduction of acid within the cells and in the extracellular environment.

PREVENTION
In order to reduce breast cancer risk and osteoporosis, maintain a low protein (40 grams daily), vegetarian diet, with a high intake of alkaline minerals from fruits and vegetables.

PREVENTION
Deep breathing, often an integral part of yoga and Qigong, helps the lungs release more carbon dioxide, which is an acid. Breathing exercises make us more alkaline.

FACT
We can balance excess acidity through our choice of foods and through using mineral supplements if needed, particularly potassium, calcium, and magnesium. Although sodium is alkaline, it tends to cause water retention and is not advisable to use in excess, unless balanced by high potassium.

PREVENTION
Eat a diet consisting of 80%
alkaline and 20% acid-
forming foods and choose
exercises and breathing
practices to normalize pH.

Acid and Alkaline Forming Foods

When our urine has a pH that averages below 6.8, it means that fluids elsewhere in the body are too acidic and are being dumped in an effort for the body to become more alkaline. It also means that we have a shortage of alkaline minerals to neutralize the acids our bodies produce.

Foods affect our pH levels based on their mineral content. Those that have an abundance of the alkaline minerals will raise pH levels, while those that do not will lower it. (A pH above 7 is considered alkaline; below 7 is acid). Coffee, alcohol, sugar, drugs, refined foods and meat all promote acidity. Fruits and vegetables contain organic acids, which become carbon dioxide and water when oxidized in the body. Their alkaline minerals remain in the blood to neutralize acids.

Charting Your pH Balance

Urine and saliva pH can be measured easily with pH paper, also called hydrazine paper, which is usually available at drug stores and health food

Urine and Saliva Testing Directions

1) Test your saliva first thing in the morning when you get out of bed. Lick and wet the end of a strip of litmus paper, compare the color to the pH chart, and write down the number on the chart below. Do this before you brush your teeth or drink or eat anything. The pH should be 6.8. The saliva pH is a reflection of the intracellular pH and should never be below 6.8. If it is, there is no alkaline mineral reserve and the body does not have the minerals necessary to process food properly.

2) Check the pH of the first and second urine of the day. The first urine reflects the acid load from the day before that your kidneys have processed through the night. It will likely have an acid pH. The second urine should be 6.8, signifying that the acids from the day before are gone, the kidneys are no longer overwhelmed, and there are enough alkaline minerals present in the body to raise the pH. If the second urine is still acid, eat less protein and grain, drink more water, and use parsley and juniper to help the kidneys. Eat more fruits and vegetables and use alkaline minerals.

3) Check your saliva pH 5 minutes after eating something at breakfast. This number should be higher than what it was when you woke up. Ideally it should be 8.5 after breakfast. This signifies that the alkaline minerals have been utilized for digestion. The more it goes up, the more these minerals are available.

4) Check the pH of the urine between meals. It should be in the range of 7.0 to 8.5. After eating, the stomach secretes hydrochloric acid to digest the food and stimulates the pancreas to make sodium bicarbonate, which is alkaline. The urine pH 1 to 2 hours after eating should reflect the availability of sodium bicarbonate, and register as alkaline. If the urine pH is less than 7, you have too much acid waste and are more likely to have symptoms of fatigue, irritability, headaches, and tension in the neck and shoulders. You have a greater susceptibility to ulcers, diverticulitis, arthritis, osteoporosis, and sinusitis.

5) Do this testing at least once a month when you have not taken alkaline minerals for a couple of days to see that you are moving to a more alkaline state.

Note: The pH of the urine is also influenced by the time of day. It is most acid at 2 a.m. (5.0 to 6.8) and most alkaline at 10 a.m. and 2 p.m. (7.0 to 8.5), during the alkaline rise after meals. During the rest of the day, it should stay between 6.6 and 6.8.[27] The first urine of the day should be more acidic because of the removal of acid waste by the kidneys through the night. If you are taking calcium and magnesium at night, it will counteract the acid waste and the morning pH may be higher.

Acidic and Alkaline Forming Foods and Activities Chart

This chart lists in descending order the acid and alkaline-forming foods and activities that affect pH. Foods at the top of the acid group are the most acid-forming. Foods at the beginning of the alkaline group are the most alkalinizing.

Acid-Forming Foods (20 % of diet) and Activities

Animal	Grains	Beans	Other	Activities
dried squid, dried fish, egg yolk, tuna, octopus, chicken, carp, oysters, salmon, clam, scallops, pork, beef, cheese, abalone, shrimp, butter	buckwheat, rice bran, oatmeal, brown rice, pearl barley, buckwheat flour, white rice, white flour, wheat gluten, bread, cornmeal, millet	peanuts, coconut, cashews, Brazil nuts, peanuts, pecans, walnuts, black beans, chick peas, fava beans, kidney beans, pinto beans, lima beans, lentils, peas	beer, liquor, sugar, honey , maple syrup, alcohol, wine, cranberry juice, fried foods, saturated fats, pesticides, chemicals, free radical damage	vigorous exercise: jogging, rebounding, dancing, sports, hot showers or baths, shallow breathing, aging

Alkaline-Forming Foods (80% of diet) and Activities

Vegetables	Fruits	Nuts/Beans	Other	Activities
wakame, kombu, ginger, raw rhubarb, kelp, Irish moss, nori, mustard greens, shitake mushrooms, maitake mushrooms, reishi mushrooms, spinach, kale, carrots, mushrooms, potatoes, burdock root, cabbage, radish, squash, bamboo shoots, sweet potatoes, endive, celery, lettuce, broccoli, turnip, dill pickles, dulse, Swiss chard, pumpkin, zucchini,	bananas, strawberries, orange juice, grapefruit, lemon, apricots, apples, canteloupe, cherries, pineapple, all berries, persimmons, pears, grape juice, watermelon **Vegetables cont'd:** cucumbers, tomatoes, eggplant, cauliflower, asparagus, avocado, onions	soybeans, tempeh, almonds, chestnuts, adzuki beans, string beans, tofu, flaxseeds, sunflower seeds , pumpkin seeds	Greens +, Pure Synergy, Barley Green, spirulina, all sprouts, wheatgrass juice, egg white, organic milk, organic yogurt, apple cider vinegar, Celtic sea salt, antioxidants, sodium bicarbonate, stevia, good water, flaxseed oil	sea salt baths, gentle stretching, tai chi, yoga, Qigong, deep breathing, massage, meditation, walking, cold showers or baths, magnetic field therapy with negative polarity magnets, more dietary fiber, antioxidants, enzymes

stores. Purchase litmus paper with a pH range of 4.5 – 7.5. pH (potential for hydrogen) is the measurement of the hydrogen ion concentration, expressed in terms of a logarithmic expression. pH is calibrated in a scale that ranges from 0 (which would mean complete saturation of hydrogen ions) to 14 (which would mean a complete lack of hydrogen ions).

pH Balance Chart

Date	Time of Day	Urine pH	Time of Day	Saliva pH
	1ˢᵗ urine 2ⁿᵈ urine between meals		on rising 5 min. after brkfst before lunch	
	1ˢᵗ urine 2ⁿᵈ urine between meals		on rising 5 min. after brkfst before lunch	
	1ˢᵗ urine 2ⁿᵈ urine between meals		on rising 5 min. after brkfst before lunch	
	1ˢᵗ urine 2ⁿᵈ urine between meals		on rising 5 min. after brkfst before lunch	
	1ˢᵗ urine 2ⁿᵈ urine between meals		on rising 5 min. after brkfst before lunch	
	1ˢᵗ urine 2ⁿᵈ urine between meals		on rising 5 min. after brkfst before lunch	
	1ˢᵗ urine 2ⁿᵈ urine between meals		on rising 5 min. after brkfst before lunch	

PREVENTION

Monitor your urinary and salivary pH monthly until they normalize at about 6.8. You can accomplish this and discourage cancer by decreasing protein and grain, adopting an alkaline diet, drinking more water, doing deep breathing exercises, and using the minerals potassium, calcium, and magnesium.

A pH reading which falls below 7 is considered to be acidic, while a pH reading above 7 is considered alkaline, and 7 is neutral. Hormone receptor sites, enzyme activity, and cellular energy production are all pH dependent, so tracking and normalizing pH are simple yet profound practices we can use to improve health.

Eliminating Intestinal Parasites and Yeast

We may harbor parasites and yeast when our digestion is weak and when we are overly acidic and mineral deficient. A parasite is an organism that derives its food, nutrition, and shelter by living in or on another organism. It injures its host without contributing to its survival. We can free our bodies of parasites by restoring pH balance, detoxifying heavy metals and chemicals, strengthening immunity, normalizing stomach acid and candida levels, modifying

Detoxifying Our Bodies

our diet, cleansing the intestines, taking anti-parasitic formulas, healing the lining of the gut, recolonizing the gastrointestinal tract with friendly bacteria, and avoiding contact with parasites.

Increase in Parasitic Infections

Several factors have contributed to the rising incidence of parasitic infection. With increasing international travel, many organisms endemic to certain areas are spread, and with increasing immigration, parasites are hitchhiking into other countries. These include malaria, roundworm, and giardia. The growing popularity of international cuisine, with exotic foods that are prepared raw or undercooked (fish, beef, and pork), can spread parasites.

Water contaminated by raw sewage may be a source of parasites, while the increasing number of daycare centers spreads diseases through direct contact with infected feces. Parasites may come to us via our pets — there are 65 infectious diseases spread by dogs and 39 by cats. These include dog and cat roundworm, hookworm, and toxoplasmosis. Most house cats sleep with their owners.

Sexual freedom over the last 30 years has caused an increase in the number of sexual partners and practices, leading to the sexual transmission of Trichomonas vaginalis, Entamoeba histolytica, giardia, pinworms, and pork tapeworms. People who have higher chemical and persistent heavy metals in their system from dental amalgams, contaminated food, and polluted air are more susceptible to parasitic invasion. High stress lifestyles cause many people to eat quickly, without sufficient hydrochloric acid secretion from the stomach that might kill parasites.

How Parasites Harm Us

When undigested food is released into the intestine, it seeps through perforations caused by parasites into the lymphatic system, and the result is an increased allergic response and an overburdened lymphatic system. Food and environmental sensitivities and allergies are therefore often linked to the presence of parasites and can be alleviated with intestinal cleansing.

Parasites irritate the tissues in which they are present, causing an inflammatory response. This can result in pain in joints and muscles or an increased susceptibility to infection in the lungs, sinuses, vagina, bladder, or any mucous membrane. The inflammatory cascade promotes cancer growth. Parasites produce toxic substances that are poisonous to the host and difficult to get rid of. Elevated eosinophils (white blood cells that fight microscopic invaders) are a sign of parasitic infection, and eosinophils themselves can cause tissue damage, leading to pain and inflammation.

Parasites can invade the skin, causing dermatitis, itching, psoriasis, eczema, hives, swellings, and rashes. The destroyed larva or parasitic eggs can clump together forming a tumor-like mass in the colon, lungs, liver, breast, peritoneum, or uterus.

Parasites need to eat and thereby rob us of many nutrients (proteins, carbohydrates, fats, minerals, vitamins), causing anemia and fatigue. Drowsiness after meals can be a sign that parasites are present.

FACT
Over 130 types of parasites can infect the human body, including microscopic single-celled organisms (protozoa); round, pin, and hookworms (nematoda); tapeworms (cestoda); flukes (trematoda); and spirochetes. Their presence activates the immune system, and over time lowers the body's defensive energy, allowing bacterial and viral infections and cancer to take hold.

FACT
Generalized use of antibiotics kills the body's protective bacteria, upsetting the micro-ecosystem of the gastrointestinal tract and vagina. This often leads to yeast overgrowth and trichomoniasis.

PREVENTION
Two cloves of raw garlic daily help prevent roundworms, pinworms, tapeworms, and hookworms. Other foods with anti-parasitic properties are onions, carrot tops, radishes, kelp, raw cabbage, apple cider vinegar, ground almonds, pumpkin, calmyrna figs, cranberry juice, and sauerkraut. Use a variety of these foods regularly.

A combination of the following herbs and homeopathic remedies would tackle most varieties of parasites:

Wormwood
Black Walnut
Cloves
Male Fern
Goldenseal
Grapefruit seed extract
Oil of oregano (short term use)
Homeopathic Unda #39 or
Cina 4 CH

PREVENTION

Do a routine parasite cleanse twice a year, during the time of the full moon, for a minimum of six weeks each time. You may have particular sensitivities to different products, so start with a low dose.

FACT

The acid in the stomach is usually a defense against parasites, if there is enough of it. Many of us have insufficient stomach acid, particularly if we are blood type A.

PREVENTION

Once a year, check your stomach acid through use of a gastric analysis test. If your hydrochloric acid level is low, correct it with herbal or vitamin supplements or hydrochloric acid tablets.

Natural Anti-Parasitic Substances and Cleanses

Certain foods have anti-parasitic properties. Pomegranate juice (four glasses daily) is effective against tapeworm. Papaya seeds are used in Mexico to eliminate parasites and can be added to salads. Finely ground pumpkin seeds ($1/4$ cup) can be added to porridge or eaten on their own to eliminate many varieties of worms.

Herbs have long been used to eliminate parasites. Wormwood, black walnut, male fern, and cloves are an effective combination for treating roundworm, dog heartworm, hookworm, strongyloides, whipworm, pinworm, trichinella, tapeworm, and cryptosporidium. All kinds of tapeworm can also be treated with a combination of pumpkin seeds, garlic, crampbark, capsicum, and thyme, sold in a Hanna Kroeger formula called Rascal. Lung and blood flukes are eliminated with milkweed, pennyroyal, and black walnut. Liver flukes can be treated with goldenrod, goldenseal, and cloves. Spirochetes are killed with a combination of nettle, yerba santa, goldenrod, and monolaurin. Microscopic protozoa, such as amoeba and giardia, respond to grapefruit seed extract and cranberry juice. Herbs are best taken before meals and treatment is most effective if begun around the full moon when the parasites are most active. Continue for at least six weeks, then stop for two weeks, or until the next full moon. Several courses of treatment may be necessary.

Homeopathic remedies can also be used to rid the body of these unwelcome guests. Cina is best known for its effectiveness against pinworms. Chelidonium has been used for liver flukes. Unda #39 is effective against many intestinal parasites. Spigelia is an antiparasitic remedy. In the homeopathic literature, there are descriptions of cancer patients who have been given the cancer nosode scirrhinum and have responded by evacuating a clump of worms. There is a strong association between cancer and the presence of parasites.

Normalizing Stomach Acid

The pH of the stomach can be measured directly using a gastric analysis test (see the 'Resources Directory'). It should be at 1-3 if tested 15 minutes after stimulation with apple cider vinegar or coffee. Hypochlorhydria, or low stomach acid, is evident when the pH measures 4-8.

Signs and symptoms of hypochlorhydria include bloating, burning, and flatulence immediately after meals, fullness after eating, food allergies, nausea with taking supplements, anal itching, weak, peeling and cracked fingernails, iron deficiency, dilated capillaries in the cheeks, and undigested food in the stools. Stomach acid secretion decreases with age. Diseases associated with low stomach acid include asthma, diabetes, eczema, gallbladder disease, autoimmune disorders, hives, lupus, osteoporosis, psoriasis, rheumatoid arthritis, and hypo- and hyperthyroidism.

There are several ways to stimulate an increase in hydrochloric acid production. Specific herbs, such as Indian long pepper (pippali), schizandra, wormwood, gentian, and goldenseal, will do this.

Directions for Preventing Parasites

It is much easier and cheaper to prevent parasites in the first place than it is to eliminate them. Our first method of contact with them is usually through the skin and mouth. The following guidelines will help to protect you and your children:

1) Wash your hands before preparing food and eating, after going to the bathroom, after changing diapers, or handling pets.
2) Keep your fingernails short and use a nailbrush to scrub beneath them.
3) Wipe off the toilet seat before sitting on it or squat above the toilet. Wear rubber gloves while cleaning the bathroom. Clean bathrooms daily or at least twice weekly. Pinworm eggs and trichomonas can be found under toilet seats. Trichomonas can also be spread through mud and water baths and sauna benches.
4) Use sterilized lens preparations to clean contact lenses and remove them before swimming.
5) Don't walk barefoot in areas frequented by dogs, cats, raccoons, etc.
6) If you travel frequently, eat out regularly, have pets, or visit mountainous regions, have a complete parasite exam twice a year. Parasites often don't show up in stool tests, even when they are present.
7) Breast-feed your children as long as you can. Human milk has antibodies that protect against amoeba and giardia.
8) Keep away from puppies and kittens that have not been regularly dewormed. Empty kitty litter boxes daily while wearing gloves. Disinfect litter boxes frequently with boiling water and grapefruit seed extract. Keep pets and their bowls out of the kitchen.
9) Do not allow children to eat dirt or play in areas where there are animal droppings. Encourage children to keep their fingers out of their mouths and not to bite their fingernails.
10) Damp mop or vacuum bedrooms and bathrooms weekly (don't sweep) to eliminate eggs that may be in dust. Keep bedrooms well aired.
11) Try to bathe or shower daily.
12) If pinworms are present, launder bedding and personal clothing daily, wear close-fitting underwear to bed, and don't share a bed with other family members.
13) Keep toothbrushes in closed containers to avoid exposure to bathroom dust.
14) Drink filtered water. Use reverse osmosis or carbon block filters. Always boil or filter water from rivers or streams to eliminate giardia.
15) If you eat fish, use varieties that are commercially blast-frozen. Cook until it is flaky and white. Bake at 400°F, 8-10 minutes per inch of thickness. Avoid sushi.
16) If you are a meat eater, cook at 325°F or higher and use a meat thermometer to check that the internal temperature is 170°F.
17) Wash your fruits and vegetables before eating them.
18) Avoid oral-anal sex to prevent transmission of trichomonas, pinworms, ascaris, giardia, strongyloides, and Entamoeba histolytica. Use condoms when engaging in sexual intercourse unless you know that your partner is free of parasites.

So will taking one tablespoon of lemon juice or apple cider vinegar in one cup of water a half hour before meals (the vinegar is contraindicated in people with candidiasis). Chinese herbs, acupuncture, kinesiology, specific yoga exercises, and homeopathic remedies can also normalize stomach acid. Zinc, folic acid, and vitamin B6 assist in the production of stomach acid, and can be supplemented when it is deficient.

Candidiasis

The overgrowth of Candida albicans in the body interferes with hydrochloric acid secretion in the stomach and often goes hand in hand with a parasitic condition and with the presence of mercury amalgam dental filings. One of the secondary effects of candidiasis is an increase in gut permeability, which results in large molecules passing through the gut wall into the blood and lymph. The liver and the immune system are taxed in their attempts to rid the body of these substances, resulting in increased body toxicity, lowered immunity, and susceptibility to allergies.

Many herbal and nutritional products are available to decrease the levels of yeast in the body. These include grapefruit seed extract, taheebo or pau d'arco, capryllic acid, olive leaf, calcium undecylenate, oil of oregano, and garlic. Sanum isopathic formulas also neutralize fungus. Substances which help to heal the permeability of the intestinal lining include beta-carotene, glutamic acid, rice bran oil, flaxseed oil, slippery elm, comfrey, and cabbage. A probiotic supplement recolonizes the intestines with friendly bacteria.

PREVENTION
Once or twice yearly, do a candida cleanse along with a parasite, liver, and colon cleanse. Work with a healthcare practitioner to decide which supplements to use and continue for at least two months.

Cleansing the Colon

The colon, or large intestine, is our body's main route to eliminate waste. Over years of eating processed food, layers of dried mucus accumulate on the colon wall. A toxic bowel can result from using the birth control pill; steroid based medications; an overly acid condition; chlorinated drinking water; excess sugar and sweets; an overly refined diet; lack of fiber; excess meat and fat; an excess of carbohydrates; stress; eating too quickly without proper chewing; or use of antibiotics. This becomes a breeding ground for unhealthy bacteria, yeast, and parasites. We can remove this debris regularly in a gentle manner with the use of fiber supplements and/or enemas.

Fiber Supplements

Effective intestinal cleansers combine fiber to encourage bowel movements, absorbent compounds such as bentonite and pectin that attract toxins, and herbs that are soothing to the bowel lining. Intestinal cleansers may include oat bran, psyllium husks, guar gum, L-glutamine, flaxseeds, bentonite clay, apple or citrus pectin, beet root, comfrey root, agar-agar, and papaya extract. In combination, these products act like a broom to sweep out the intestinal tract. The oatbran, psyllium, flaxseeds, and agar-agar are bulking agents that expand in the colon as they absorb water and help to peel away the layers of mucus, toxins, and old fecal matter.

Occasionally, psyllium will cause abdominal bloating and discomfort to gluten-sensitive individuals. If you experience this, increase your water consumption so that you have at least two glasses with each dose of the fiber formula. If you continue to feel bloated, find a formula without psyllium or use a combination of freshly ground flaxseeds and bentonite. Apple and citrus pectin

PREVENTION
Cleanse your intestines with a fiber formula at least twice yearly for six weeks at a time, or use a fiber formula continuously, particularly if you have cancer. Use enough fiber so that you have three or more bowel movements daily. Be sure to drink sufficient water, about 2-3 liters or quarts daily, while taking a fiber supplement.

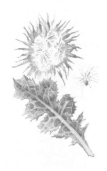

absorb toxins that can include chemicals, toxic metals, and waste produced by the body itself. Comfrey and beet root act as laxatives. These must all be taken with sufficient water for optimal effect.

Enemas

Enemas and colonics are also methods to detoxify the bowel. They are particularly useful when one must quickly remove toxins from the body, as is the case with cancer. Use them only under supervision with a naturopathic physician, herbalist, or holistic medical doctor.

There are several types of enemas. These include using distilled or spring water, herbal teas, cleansing juices, bentonite enemas, and coffee enemas.

Water Enemas

This is a basic enema, simply using water to dislodge and cleanse old fecal matter from the colon. Only distilled or spring water should be used. Avoid tap water, as the chlorine in it can combine with organic matter in the bowel to form chloroform

Herbal Tea Enemas

Many herbal teas can soothe and detoxify the bowels and improve intestinal function in general. If the intestines are spastic or irritated, then chamomile, peppermint, comfrey, or licorice can be made into a tea and used in an enema. Fenugreek is a useful herb to dissolve mucus and encrustations in the bowel lining. [28,29]

To make these teas alone or in combination, roots, barks, and stems are simmered for 20 minutes, then allowed to cool for 10 minutes before straining and using the tea. When using leaves and flowers, simmer for five minutes, turn off the heat, and let it steep for 10 minutes. Start with one part herbs to five parts of water, weight to volume. Therefore, 1 ounce of herbs would be added to 5 ounces of water to make the tea. Then approximately $\frac{1}{2}$ cup of tea is used per quart or liter of distilled or spring water to make the enema. Some people may be able to use a full cup.

Cleansing Juice Enemas

Juice enemas act as a source of nutrients to the body as well as assisting with detoxification. The nutrients are delivered through the bowel wall to the liver. Aloe vera juice can be used to soothe intestinal cramping and helps to heal the mucous membrane lining of the bowel when it is inflamed. Use one tablespoon per quart (four cups) of water. Lemon juice is cleansing and alkalinizing, useful when the body is overly acidic. Use the juice of one lemon in four cups of water. Wheat grass juice is alkalinizing and high in minerals that help to feed the liver. Use two tablespoons per quart of water. This may be the enema of choice for cases of weakness and debility, particularly when digestion and absorption are poor. The Ayurvedic herb amla can be used in a retention enema for improving energy, for detoxifying the liver, and for its anti-oxidant properties.

FACT
Enemas are simple, painless, and immediate ways to remove toxins from both the bowel and the body.

Herbal Stimulating Formula
burdock root (25%)
red clover (25%)
yellow dock (25%)
pepermint (25%)

Herbal Soothing Formula
dandelion root (35%)
chicory root (30%)
marshmallow root (25%)
licorice root (10%)

Herbal Strong Cleansing Formula
dandelion root (40%)
fennel (30%)
ginger (20%)
cascara bark (10%)

Cleanse your colon one to three times per year using either a fiber supplement or a series of enemas or colonics. Do so under the supervision of a health care practitioner familiar with detoxification regimens.

Bentonite Enemas

Bentonite is a form of volcanic ash, with no chemical action or toxic side effect. It has a negative charge, and is able to attract toxins, which are usually positively charged atoms. It can absorb and carry away 200 hundred times its own weight in toxins. Bentonite enemas are efficient at removing mucus and fecal matter attached to the colon wall. Use two tablespoons of bentonite per quart of water.

Coffee Enemas

A coffee enema helps to detoxify the liver. The caffeine acts as an herbal stimulant, which goes directly to the liver through a circulatory route from the sigmoid colon called the entero-hepatic circulation system. The caffeine is transported through the hemorrhoidal veins into the portal vein and into the liver. An integral part of the Gerson Therapy for cancer treatment, they are included here as an option to cleanse the colon and liver quickly. Dr Sherry Rogers also recommends coffee enemas in her book, *Wellness Against All Odds*.[30]

When performed properly, a coffee enema speeds up the emptying time of the bowel, removing toxins at a faster pace; empties the toxins that have accumulated in the bile ducts of the liver, allowing other bodily toxins to come in to be metabolized; stimulates the production of the enzyme glutathione-S-transferase, which assists liver detoxification; and causes an increased flow of bile. A toxic liver will dump many of its toxins into the bile and eliminate them in a few minutes. This provides quick relief to an overburdened body and may reduce symptoms of ill health and increase energy. However, the bile that is released from coffee enemas also contains valuable mineral salts that need to be replaced through the generous use of organic vegetable juices, sea vegetables and sprouted seeds, a green powder supplement, or a mineral supplement.

When coffee enemas are begun, the poisons contained in the bile produce spasms in the duodenum and the small intestines. Some of this may overflow into the stomach, causing nausea or possibly vomiting of bile. Should this occur, peppermint tea can help to wash the bile from the stomach and bring relief.

Coffee Enema Preparation

1) Add two to three tablespoons of organic, freshly ground, lightly roasted coffee beans to one quart (four cups) of distilled water. If you are particularly sensitive to coffee and become overstimulated by it, use the lesser amount. Caffeine is not detected in the blood after coffee enemas. Do not use instant, decaffeinated, or stale coffee. Store ground coffee beans in the freezer to prevent rancidity if you are not using them all right away.

2) Make the coffee fresh for each enema. Use an enamel, glass, or stainless steel pot. Do not use aluminum, teflon, or iron pots.

3) Let it boil for three minutes, then simmer for 20 minutes. Strain it and allow it to cool to the body's temperature (98.6°F), or until it feels comfortable to the touch.

4) Do not use a coffee enema if you have gallstones; if you become dizzy, nauseous, or light-headed, stop the enema process. A coffee enema should be performed only under the supervision of a naturopathic doctor or other health professional.

Directions for Giving Yourself an Enema

1) Pour the enema liquid into an enema bag connected to plastic or rubber tubing. Clamp the tube as you pour in the liquid. A fountain syringe is the best enema applicator. Lubricate the nozzle with food grade vegetable oil, such as sesame, almond, flaxseed, or olive oil. Hang the enema bag 1½ to 2 feet above the body. You can change the height to control the speed of intake into the colon. Place a large towel or mat on the floor of the washroom or in a room close by.

2) Lie on the mat or towel on your right side, with both legs drawn into the abdomen. Alternatively, you can start the enema in a knee-to-chest position with your chest on the floor and your buttocks in the air. This position allows the force of gravity to aid the flow of water into the colon. You can also lie on your back with a pillow beneath your buttocks. Breathe deeply while you begin the enema. Slowly insert the nozzle several inches into the rectum using a rotating motion. If the tube is inserted too rapidly or forcefully it can cause kinking inside of the colon, which may cause discomfort. Release the clamp and let the mixture flow in slowly.

3) If the solution comes into the colon too fast, lower the enema bag; if it comes in too slowly, raise the bag a little higher. If you experience cramping, then the solution is coming in too quickly. You can stop the flow by pinching the enema tube and then lowering the bag. Wait until the cramps have stopped before allowing the solution to flow again. It may take several minutes for the enema solution to enter the body. If it does not seem to flow freely, the enema tube may be twisted or kinked. Slowly pull it part of the way out and then insert it again until it has gone in several inches.

4) Retain the fluid for 10 to 12 minutes. Dr Gerson found that all the caffeine was absorbed from the fluid within 10 to 12 minutes. If you cannot hold all the fluid in the colon with one enema, repeat it two or more times in sequence, emptying the bowel in between.

5) While the solution is in the colon, it is helpful to change positions every few minutes. The sequence might be: 3 minutes right side, 3 minutes stomach, 3 minutes on your back, 3 minutes left side. This helps the enema solution reach all parts of the colon.

6) When the bile duct empties, you will hear or feel squirting beneath the right rib cage. This is a sign that you have succeeded in releasing toxins from the liver.

7) Sterilize the enema syringe after each use by boiling it or thoroughly cleansing it with soap and water and soaking it for 5 minutes in a solution of 2 cups water and 4 drops of tea tree oil or grapefruit seed extract.

Frequency of Enemas

The frequency of enemas is dependent upon one's symptoms. If you presently have cancer of any sort, one or two coffee enemas can be used daily until the cancer retreats, as long as you are replacing the lost minerals with several glasses of organic vegetable juices daily. The usual frequency of coffee enemas is three times a week for several weeks while you are attempting to detoxify. Consider a six-week period, twice yearly for the fiber supplement, or enemas three times a week, for several weeks at a time, one to three times per year. If you have cancer, more frequent enemas may be necessary.

Squatting

A simple way to improve elimination is by squatting when you have your bowel movements. When you use a toilet in a sitting position a portion of the large intestine is closed off, making complete elimination difficult. Over time you will have less bowel toxicity.

PREVENTION
While having a bowel movement, squat on the toilet at home or use a small 10-inch stool to place your feet on.

Bringing Back Friendly Bacteria

Functions of Intestinal Bacteria

While removing unhealthy bacteria, parasites, and yeast from our intestines, we may also remove 'good' bacteria and various nutrients necessary to maintain the health of this microscopic ecosystem. The intestinal flora is considered by some people to be a separate 'organ' in its own right because of the many functions it performs. When these good bacteria are on friendly terms, they function to synthesize certain vitamins such as vitamin K, biotin, vitamin B12, folic acid, pantothenic acid, pyridoxine, riboflavin; to make nonessential amino acids and butyric acid; to make short chain fatty acids, some of which can reduce the growth of cancer cells; to break down environmental carcinogens and other toxins; to help to reduce cholesterol levels; to break down hormones, including estrogen, to enhance absorption or elimination of estrogen; to stimulate immune function; to convert dietary flavonoids and phytoestrogens so the body can use them to protect us from cancer; to stimulate metabolic rate and help with weight loss or gain; to make 'natural' antibiotics that protect us from infections; and to maintain proper pH levels of the intestines, deterring infectious organisms.

Antibiotics

Broad spectrum use of antiobiotics is especially harmful to these 'good' bacteria. For example, a specific bacteria called *Clostridia paraputreficium* makes up only 0.4-0.8% of the intestinal flora. Clostridia has the noble task of converting the plant lignans to the weak estrogen, enterolactone, which protects us from breast cancer. When a broad spectrum antibiotic is used, this conversion is severely diminished or absent for as long as one is taking the antibiotic and can take up to 30 days to resume after stopping. In some individuals it may take as little as five days to resume — the individual variations are due to the composition of the intestinal flora.[31] This conversion happens in the beginning of the large intestine. Disturbing the ecology of organisms in the intestines can cause an overgrowth of Candida albicans in the body, which can damage the cells in the stomach that produce hydrochloric acid.

Reintroducing Good Bacteria

The reintroduction of friendly bacteria into the intestines helps to create a healthy bowel. We can promote a healthy balance of intestinal flora by supplementing with 'good' bacteria, which prevent the colonization of our intestines by unhealthy bacteria, overabundant yeast, or parasites.

The healthy bacteria are best taken in capsule form and include *Lactobacillus acidophilus*, *Lactobacillus bifidus*, *Lactobacillus bulgarus*, *Bifidobacterium bifidus*, and *Streptococcus faeceum*. The first two of these are most commonly used in probiotic formulas. They should be taken once or twice daily for a period of months.

Keep them refrigerated after opening. When taken with a plant substance called FOS, or fructo-oligosaccharides, the growth of bifidobacterium in the intestines is enhanced tenfold. FOS acts as a growth medium for these and other bacteria and is present in the following foods: asparagus, Jerusalem artichoke, onion, burdock root, honey, rye, and Chinese chive.

Dosage: Two capsules daily between meals for a total of 6-10 billion organisms per day. Food Sources: Organic yogurt, sauerkraut, kefir, olives, pickles, vinegar, tempeh, tamari, mochi.

Contraindications: None.

Assisting Digestive Enzymes

Enzymes are energized protein molecules that catalyze or initiate almost all biochemical reactions and cellular activities that occur in our bodies. Our organs, tissues, and cells are created and maintained by metabolic enzymes. Hormones, minerals, and vitamins will work only when enzymes are present. An excess of vitamins and minerals can actually deplete enzymes, as they cause more of them to be used up. Digestion is entirely dependent on enzymes. The processes of growing, living, and dying are governed by an ordered, integrated sequence of enzymatic reactions.

Enzymes are very specific in their activities. Deficiencies of single enzymes caused by a genetic defect such as occurs in muscular dystrophy can cause disease and death. Generally, enzymes transform a particular substance into a different substance by breaking or attaching molecular bonds, while they themselves remain unchanged. The names of all enzymes end with '-ase' while the first part of its name defines what it acts upon. For instance, the enzyme 'lactase' helps to break down the milk sugar, lactose.

With an abundance of enzymes we will have more energy.

FACT

The human body contains more than 2,700 different types of enzymes. Our health is dependent upon our enzyme reserve. When enzymes are depleted, we age faster and are more prone to degenerative diseases, including cancer.

FACT

We each have a limited supply of metabolic enzyme energy at birth. Enzymes are like the body's battery and must last a lifetime. The faster we use up our enzyme supply, the faster we age. The use of alcohol, drugs, stimulants, cooked food, and overeating causes us to use up enzymes. Therefore, as we age and have enzyme depletion, we have more trouble digesting foods and more chronic illness.

Enzyme Functions

There are three main groups of enzymes — metabolic, digestive, and food enzymes – all with specific functions for our health.

Type of Enzyme	What It Does
Metabolic Enzyme	Catalyzes chemical reactions within cells such as detoxification and energy production.
Digestive Enzyme	Secreted in the saliva, stomach, pancreas and small intestine to break down food so it can be absorbed into the blood.
Food Enzyme	Are naturally present in all raw foods and assist the body in breaking down the food itself. Chewing activates food enzymes, which pre-digest the food in the mouth and upper stomach, until the stomach acid inactivates them, usually 45-60 minutes later. They become active once again in the alkaline environment of the small intestine. When food is cooked above 118°F enzymes are destroyed and the assistance of food enzymes is lost, calling on more activity from the digestive enzymes.

Enzymes enhance the utilization of vitamins and minerals, and we need much less of a particular nutrient when we take enzymes along with it. There is a link between our enzyme reserve and the strength of our immune systems — the more enzymes we have, the stronger our immune systems will be. White blood cells themselves contain amylase, protease, and lipase — enzymes that help to break down carbohydrates, proteins, and fats. The white blood cells release these into the blood to act as scavengers on whatever debris needs to be digested. The same enzymes are found in the white blood cells as are found in the pancreas. After we eat cooked food, the white blood cell count increases, while when we eat raw food, it does not. This implies that cooked food results in toxicity, which the white blood cells must act upon, while raw food does not strain the white blood cells. Over time this results in immune weakness and susceptibility to cancer.

Enzymes and Cancer

Cancer cells use several self-defense mechanisms to elude detection from ever-watchful white blood cells whose job it is to seek and destroy them. They can mask their surface antigens (which the white blood cells would otherwise recognize) with a protective coat of fibrin; release their antigens into the blood to form immune complexes which act as a decoy to preoccupy and overwhelm the white blood cells; and change their appearance by turning the cell membrane inward, disguising the cell surface antigens.[32]

Systemic use of proteolytic enzymes (that digest protein) between meals works to eliminate the fibrin coat, digest the antigen-antibody complexes, and activate the immune system.[33,34] Proteolytic enzymes include pancreatin, protease, bromelain, papain, trypsin, and chymotrypsin. Wobenzyme is a quality product that contains all of these.

Studies have shown that orally ingested pancreatic proteolytic enzymes are acid stable, pass intact into the small intestine, and are absorbed into the bloodstream.[35,36,37] Animal studies on rats and mice have demonstrated inhibition of primary tumors, reduction in size of existing tumors, a decrease in metastases, and extended survival when animals inoculated with tumors were given oral proteolytic enzymes.[38,39,40,41] Human studies have demonstrated that patients given proteolytic enzymes during chemotherapy and/or radiation treatment had less deterioration, longer remission times, improved tolerance to radiation, and a decrease in mortality by 50-60%.[42,43,44]

Proteolytic enzymes can be taken every half hour between meals in extreme cases, or, alternatively, two or three times daily between meals. They should not be used if the stomach or intestinal tract is irritated or inflamed, as they may aggravate it further. Otherwise, look for an enzyme combination with high protease content (10XUSP at 500-1000 mg) or containing 600 mg of bromelain.

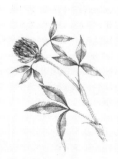

FACT

Enzymes are destroyed at temperatures above 118°F. This means that baked goods, canned food, roasted cereals, pasteurized dairy products, and cooked meat are devoid of enzymes.

PREVENTION

Use supplemental enzymes before meals to help digest your food and between meals to detoxify the blood and to break down the fibrin coat of cancer cells. If you have breast cancer, consider using proteolytic enzymes several times daily between meals. Use enzymes between meals during chemotherapy and radiation treatments to decrease side effects and improve the treatment outcome.

Conserving Enzymes

Whenever we cook our foods between 118-149°F (48-65°C) or higher, we destroy enzymes. Prolonged heat at 118°F and short heat at 149°F kills enzymes. Heating at 140-176°F (60-80°C) for one-half hour completely kills any enzymes. Boiling, baking, and microwaving destroy enzymes.

When we eat mainly cooked food, the pancreas enlarges in its efforts to produce sufficient enzymes, causing exhaustion and degeneration over time. The more digestion that can occur before the food reaches the small intestine, the fewer digestive enzymes are needed from the pancreas and small intestine. Enzyme-sparing allows metabolic enzymes to be conserved, enabling them to be used for tissue and organ repair, preserving health.

Some people suffer from abdominal pain or diarrhea with even a little raw food. In these cases, warm soups and stews cooked in a slow cooker are a good idea with supplemental enzymes taken before meals. We can soak beans and grains overnight to increase their enzyme content and decrease their cooking time.

PREVENTION

Consume at least 50%-80% of your food raw. Include fresh raw vegetable and fruit juices as part of your daily diet. Cook food on low heat or for shorter periods.

Cleansing Fast

Part of any detoxification regime is a fast. Commonly done at the change of seasons for several days, annual fasting is a good health

---

Lemon Aid Cleanse

This cleanse eliminates toxins and congestion while revitalizing the body. If continued for from 3-10 days, it usually does not cause a lack of physical energy, and is easy to follow at home, work, or while traveling. The Lemon Aid Cleanse may be done one or more times a year while fasting. Use it with medical or naturopathic supervision.

Ingredients:

2   tablespoons of the juice from freshly squeezed lemons or limes
1   teaspoon of maple syrup
$1/10$ teaspoon of cayenne pepper (more if desired)

It may be easier to make up a day's supply at one time:

2   cups of the juice from freshly squeezed organic lemons;
$3/4$-1   cup of maple syrup (B or C grade);
1   or more teaspoons of cayenne pepper.

Directions: Mix 3 tablespoons of this mixture with a glass of filtered or spring water, warm or cold.

If you are at work or traveling, you can carry enough of this in a thermos. Drink between 6-12 glasses daily (more if desired). If you also want to lose weight, keep it close to 6 glasses daily.

During the cleanse, keep your bowels moving by taking a fiber supplement containing at least some of the following: psyllium seed powder, oatbran, apple pectin, guar gum, and bentonite. If you do not have one to two bowel movements daily using the fiber formula, then consider an enema. If your energy lags, add 2-4 tablespoons of a greens supplement like Greens + to water and drink one to three times daily. You can also consider drinking fresh carrot, beet, and cabbage juice 2-3 times daily during this fast.

To end the cleanse, drink a vegetable broth soup, sipping it slowly. The following day include more food in the form of steamed vegetables, fruits, sprouts, or salads.

practice for most people. Fasting aids in recuperation by freeing the large amounts of energy used by digestion to go elsewhere, and by putting less of a burden on the liver so its enzymes can act on more internally generated toxins.

A short fast would last 1-3 days, and a longer fast than this is best done with medical supervision. Fasting can release toxins that have been stored in your fat cells, and you may feel unwell during the first two days of a fast because of this. A laxative tea or fiber supplement should be taken during a fast to eliminate the toxins that have been released. If you suffer from hypoglycemia or blood sugar irregularities, consult a health professional about the type of fast that may be appropriate for you. Do not fast if you are pregnant or breastfeeding. Do not fast if you are underweight, or if you have cancer. In these cases you will need quality nutrients from food to help rebuild your body.

Sweating It Out

The skin is a major organ of detoxification and we release toxins through it when we sweat. Perspiration carries out with it cellular and water-soluble toxins and toxic minerals. Ideally, we should sweat daily to maximize the skin's function as a detoxifying organ. Thus the importance of regular aerobic exercise, good hard physical labor, and frequent use of saunas or sweat lodges.

Saunas or sweat lodges have been used as tools for cleansing and purification by the Romans, Greeks, Turks, Russians, Japanese, and Native Americans. Used in Finland for over 1,000 years, the sauna was viewed as the 'holy place' and sauna bathing was considered the 'medicine of the poor'.[45]

L. Ron Hubbard, father of the Scientology movement, pioneered the use of saunas for people with drug dependencies in 1977, describing his method in his book *Clear Body, Clear Mind*.[46] After his success, clinical ecologists began to use sauna therapy with individuals who have chemical sensitivities, chronic fatigue, environmental illness, or who have been subjected to toxic chemical exposures. Substances that have been shown to be excreted through the skin during saunas are morphine, methadone, amphetamines, chlorinated pesticides, herbicides, and PCBs.[47]

Firemen exposed to PCBs from a transformer fire suffered memory impairment for stories, images, and numbers, attributed to the exposure. After undergoing a medically supervised diet, exercise, and sauna program, their mental function improved.[49] In his book *Diet for a Poisoned Planet*, David Steinman describes his experiences with sauna detoxification and outlines a home detoxification program that reduced his blood levels of DDT by 70%.[50] The HealthMed clinic in Los Angeles has removed over 90% of toxic chemicals from thousands of peoples' bodies through an exercise, sauna, and supplement program based on L. Ron Hubbard's work. Dr Krop, a clinical ecologist in Ontario, describes a successful protocol used for one woman overexposured to solvents.[51]

Detoxifying Our Bodies

Chemicals to Monitor During Sauna Treatments

We need studies that monitor breast cancer incidence in women who take regular saunas and compare that to incidence in those who don't, while measuring the total chemical burden of women in both groups.[52] If you were to analyze blood, or fat samples before and after a sauna detoxification program to see how successful you had been at eliminating them, you might consider testing for the following chemicals. Because these have a synergistic action together, we want to know the total body burden of chemicals that may cause breast cancer, not one or two by themselves:

1) D-ethylhexyl phthalate (DEHP), found in soft plastic, added to PVC building materials, found in household dust, linked to early puberty.

2) Di-n-butyl phthalate (DBP), found in cosmetics, nail polish, linked to earlier puberty.

3) Bisphenol A diglycidylether methacrylate (bis-GMA), found in dental materials, hard plastics, and canned food.

4) PCB 105, found in higher amounts in breast cancer tumors.

5) PCB 118.

6) PCB 156.

7) DDE, a breakdown product of DDT.

8) Dioxin, specifically TCDD or 2,3,7,8-TCDD, formed during the making of polyvinyl chloride (PVC).

9) Nonylphenol ethoxylate, found in detergents.

10) Octylphenol.

11) Butylparabens, found in cosmetics.

12) Dieldrin, a pesticide no longer used but still present in our bodies.

13) Atrazine, a pesticide on corn.

14) Endosulfan, a pesticide used on common garden vegetables.

15) Methoxychlor is related to DDT as a pesticide used on crops and vegetables.

16) Lindane, used in lice shampoos, and was used on canola, increases risk 10-fold.

17) 2,4-D, a common weed spray, somewhat linked to breast cancer.

Most of these chemicals can be tested in blood samples or fat biopsies at several labs. See the 'Resources Directory' section of this book for more details. Many naturopathic doctors now use infra red saunas in their practices as an aid to detoxification. Consult your provincial/state or national associations to locate one. We have implemented a sauna detoxification program in my office, combining saunas with a daily schedule of breathing exercises, kundalini yoga, rebounding and nature walks. For more information, see www.healthybreastprogram.on.ca. or call (519) 372-9212. You may also purchase your own portable sauna from one of several Canadian and American manufacturers. Some tips in choosing a sauna: the heat from an infra red sauna goes deeper and is more effective at releasing toxins than other types of saunas; choose a sauna with a vent to allow old air out and new air to come in; avoid the use of glues; choose poplar over cedar if you have environmental sensitivities.

Directions for a Sauna Detoxification Program

During sauna detoxification, patients are supervised for several hours daily over a 3-week period as they participate in a program as follows:

1) Before beginning sauna therapy, correct bowel function by doing a colon cleanse for several weeks. Constipation needs to be addressed and corrected.

2) Niacin should be taken as per the supplement schedule that follows before exercising. The daily dose of niacin is taken all at once. Supplemental niacin is a key ingredient in sauna therapy, as it increases peripheral circulation and mobilizes chemicals from fatty tissue. Administration of niacin will cause flushing of the skin with a burning sensation within several hours. Initially, participants are given 50-100 mg of niacin daily until they have a flushing reaction. When the reaction is not evident after the niacin, the dosage is increased incrementally in 100 mg units, usually proceeding to between 2,000 and 4,000 mg daily by the end of the third week. At 1,000 mg, most patients increase the niacin in 500 mg increments rather than 100 mg units. Any dose above 2,000 mg must be monitored with liver function tests, as niacin may injure the liver in high doses. Niacin decreases blood pressure and lowers cholesterol levels. Sauna therapy is considered complete when there is no more flushing after any amount of niacin. This usually occurs after three weeks on the program.

3) Before entering the sauna, you should not be hungry, nor have just eaten. Wait one hour after eating or two hours after a large meal before going into the sauna. Digestion requires a lot of blood, and the sauna brings the blood to the skin as a coolant. The blood cannot be effectively used for both at the same time. Alcohol and drugs are avoided during sauna detoxification.

4) Begin with 20-30 minutes of exercise in the form of rebounding, running, or using a treadmill to stimulate the circulation of blood and lymph and to move the blood deeper into the tissues, from where it can draw out toxic residues. Aerobic exercise causes the cell waste to be carried out quickly and efficiently, and should be practiced daily immediately before the sauna for 20-30 minutes.

5) After the aerobic exercise, use a dry skin brush on the legs, arms and trunk, using small circular movements and moving up the body towards the heart.

6) One liter of water or tea should be prepared and taken in to the sauna to drink over each hour of sauna time, along with 1 tsp of an alkalinizing powder containing potassium, sodium, calcium, magnesium, and some Celtic sea salt, or other electrolyte mix or tablets. Good choice of tea is a blend of burdock, cleavers, dandelion, red clover, and Chinese licorice.

7) Maintain the temperature in the sauna between 48.8°C (120°F) and 54.4°C (130°F). An infra red sauna will be the most effective, and the temperature can be slightly lower than if a dry or wet sauna is used. A dry sauna is more effective than a wet sauna.

8) Place a clean dry towel over the seat of the sauna to absorb perspiration and toxins. Use a fresh towel each time, and have each person bring her own towels and wash them daily.

9) Immediately go into the sauna after the aerobic exercise, accompanied by a partner or group. The partner is there for safety's sake, as a person undergoing sauna detoxification may experience unpleasant symptoms as chemical toxins are released. If you feel too warm or as though you are going to faint, leave the sauna and have a cool shower before returning. The sauna partner ensures that the participant does not fall asleep because salt or potassium deficiency could occur while asleep, through sweating. Symptoms of salt or potassium depletion include extreme tiredness or weakness, headache, muscle cramps, clammy skin, nausea, dizziness, vomiting, and fainting. Should any of these symptoms occur, salt tablets and potassium gluconate tablets, or alkalinizing powder are taken. Miso soup with a banana may also be on hand.

10) If suddenly your body stops sweating and your skin becomes hot and dry, this may be a sign of heat stroke. Cool off with a lukewarm or cool shower and take fluids, salt, and potassium. Drink tea with electrolytes frequently to replace what is lost through sweating while in the sauna.

11) Practice slow, long deep breathing while in the sauna to assist liver detoxification and improve lymphatic circulation.

12) Each person may be different in terms of the length of time they are able to spend in the sauna. Aim for at least four sittings of 15-20 minutes each, for five consecutive days, then off for two, for a total of 21 sauna days. Cool showers can be taken between sauna sittings to activate the circulation. Some individuals may be able to do three sittings, each an hour long, every day for three weeks. A 15-minute cool down period occurs between each of these sittings. Consider how you can do 80-100 hours of sauna time in the shortest time period, and schedule your program. David Steinman, author of *Diet for a Poisoned Planet*, recommends a home detox program that involves using saunas two to four consecutive days in a week for several months, with two or three 20-30 minute sessions in the sauna each of those days.[53]

13) Maintain a highly alkaline vegetarian diet with an ample supply of fresh fruits and vegetables, juiced or raw, while undergoing sauna detoxification. Use parsley daily to help with kidney cleansing and coriander to help with mercury removal. Use turmeric to speed up Phase 2 liver detoxification. Other vitamins, minerals, and oils should be taken along with the niacin and increased proportionately to it, as stated in the supplement schedule that follows.

14) Use calcium and magnesium in a 2:1 ratio as a drink with 1 tbsp. apple cider vinegar to improve its absorption. Vitamin C is taken at 1,000 mg daily initially and increased incrementally to 6,000 mg daily as niacin is increased. A vitamin B complex is increased incrementally with the niacin to help prevent other B vitamin deficiencies and improve liver detoxification. A multivitamin and mineral supplement is taken to provide the remaining nutrients.

15) In addition to these supplements, quality oils should be taken, varying between two tablespoons to one half cup of oil daily. For breast cancer prevention, a combination of flaxseed oil, uncontaminated fish oil, and extra virgin olive oil with added lecithin can be taken daily. Oils are cold-pressed and kept refrigerated. If your sweat becomes oily during the sauna, reduce your oil intake. Activated charcoal or 1 tbsp bentonite plus a fiber formula are used to improve excretion of toxins.

16) Sauna therapy will be more effective if liver, kidney and intestinal cleansers are taken simultaneously. These may include milk thistle, dandelion, or a formula similar to the The Liver Loving Formula. Added to this are curcumin, alpha lipoic acid, grapeseed, NAC, kelp, a fiber formula containing bentonite, guar gum, apple pectin, and citrus pectin, as well as a probiotic formula. Bowel movements should occur at least 3x daily during the sauna detox, and enemas can be used as well to achieve this.

17) Ensure you have sufficient rest while on the program, 8 hours of sleep daily. The program works best when done at the same time daily.

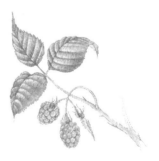

Sauna Nutritional Supplement Schedule

Nutrient	Beginning Therapy	Ending Therapy
Niacin	50-100 mg	2,000-4,000 mg
Vitamin A	5,000-10,000 IU	50,000 IU
Vitamin D	400 IU	2,000 IU
Vitamin C	1,000 mg	6,000 mg
Vitamin E	800 IU	2,400 IU
Vitamin B complex	100 mg	300 mg
Calcium	500-1,000 mg	2,500-3,000 mg
Magnesium	250-500 mg	1250-1500 mg
Iron	18-36 mg	90-108 mg
Zinc	15-30 mg	75-90 mg
Manganese	4-8 mg	20-24 mg
Copper	2-4 mg	10-12 mg
Potassium	45-90 mg	225-270 mg
Iodine	.225-.450 mg	1.125-1.350 mg
Cal-Mag Formula: mix together 1 tbsp. calcium citrate ½ tbsp. magnesium citrate 1 tbsp. apple cider vinegar ½ cup boiling water ½ cup cold water or take calcium-magnesium tablets with apple cider vinegar	1 ½ glasses	2-3 glasses

PREVENTION

Undergo a medically supervised three-week sauna detoxification program every 1-5 years, the frequency depending upon your toxin exposure, age, and general health. Develop the ritual of a weekly sauna with family or friends to release toxins regularly, not giving them time to build up to high levels.

Saunas and Cancer

Saunas must become a regular part of our lifestyle to protect ourselves and our children from breast cancer and other diseases related to chemical toxicity, including hormonal imbalances, neurological ailments such as ADD, infertility, autoimmune diseases, environmental illness, and chronic fatigue syndrome.

Many environmental chemicals are lipophilic, meaning they are attracted to fat, and so we store them in our fat cells. The skin accesses these fat stores through sweating. Better out through our sweat than into our children's mouths through breast milk.

Contraindications: Women who have lymphedema following breast cancer surgery need to be very cautious about using a sauna, as it may aggravate this condition. Don't do sauna detoxification if you are pregnant or breast-feeding. You will pass on the toxins to your child.

If you have heart, kidney, liver disease or a seizure disorder, consult with a medical doctor before beginning the program and do it with medical supervision. Do not do the program without supervision if you are anemic, or if you have sutures from a surgery.

Before getting married, consider doing the full sauna detoxification program with your partner, especially if you intend to have children in the future. At least three months before you conceive, do the full sauna detoxification program. Toxins continue to be released for several months after the therapy is completed, so do the cleansing well in advance of conception.

Detoxifying the Lungs

When we exhale, the lungs release carbon dioxide, toxic gases, and the end products of cell metabolism into the air around us. When we inhale, oxygen enters the respiratory tract to be sponged up into millions of alveoli in the lungs. Oxygen molecules diffuse across a single cell membrane to the capillaries, small blood vessels in the lungs. The oxygen then combines with hemoglobin in the red blood cells and becomes their precious cargo, delivered via the bloodstream to every nook and cranny in the body.

Deep breathing makes us more alkaline, for carbon dioxide is an acid waste. The lymphatic system depends on the pressure generated by our breathing on the thoracic duct to move the lymphatic fluid, so the deeper we breathe, the more we detoxify through the lymph. There's another bonus to deep breathing – it helps us relax and brings the glandular system and hormones back into balance. We can improve the detoxifying ability of our lungs and alkalinize the body with regular long deep breathing and some specialized yogic breathing exercises, one of which is called 'breath of fire'.[54]

FACT
Cancer cells prefer an environment with little oxygen – so the deeper we breathe to saturate our alveoli with oxygen, the more cancer may retreat.

'Breath of Fire' Lung Detoxification Exercise

This exercise will improve your energy levels, bring in more oxygen, strengthen your nerves, detoxify your lungs, and decrease susceptibility to cancer.

1) Sit cross-legged or in a chair and raise your arms up to a 60-degree angle from the horizontal, forming a 'V' above your head. Curl your fingers into the palms making a fist, but keep the thumbs pointing up straight and pull them back slightly. Close your eyes and look up between your eyebrows, holding your gaze there.

2) Begin breath of fire. Inhale as the belly comes out; exhale as you bring it in, keeping up an even rhythm with the belly pumping in and out. The inhale should equal the exhale in strength and intensity.

3) Once you have the rhythm, speed up your breathing so that you are doing 2-3 breaths per second. Continue for 1-3 minutes.

4) After a while, you can increase the time gradually to 11 minutes daily.

Summary

If we routinely detoxify each year, we can decrease our body's toxic load and improve our vitality and health. Detoxification used to be a regular part of the change of seasons in people and cultures that lived closer to nature than most of us do now. You can choose to do a cleanse at the change of seasons, in the spring and/or the fall. Continue your cleanse for 6-8 weeks or more, if needed. Write dates for your cleanse into your calendar so that you can look forward to it.

1) To enhance daily detoxification, ensure 3 or 4 bowel movements through the use of fiber, probiotics, and enemas; drink at least two liters of water to flush the kidneys; take herbs or nutritional substances to cleanse the liver and kidneys; sweat through exercising and saunas; use a skin brush to stimulate the lymphatic system and the skin; and practice breathing exercises to detoxify the lungs.

2) Invigorate the circulation of your blood with 40 minutes of exercise daily. Use flax oil, pure fish oil, niacin, and protein-digesting enzymes to decrease your blood viscosity. Evaluate plasma viscosity and fibrinogen in annual blood tests so that you can lower the possibility of breast cancer or metastases.

3) Eat foods that help your liver — beets, garlic, dandelion, cabbage and the other brassicas, turmeric, rosemary, pumpkin and sunflower seeds, lemon, grapefruit, apple cider vinegar. Use fresh organic vegetable juices regularly, such as a mixture of beet, carrot, celery, and cabbage.

4) Vitamins C and E, beta-carotene, selenium, and zinc are antioxidants, protecting the liver. Take them regularly or obtain them through diet.

5) At least two times a year, take an herbal formula for the liver, and at the same time, do a bowel-cleansing program for 6-8 weeks. If you have breast cancer, do it continuously, with short breaks every 3 months. Find a time in your calendar when you can do this. In this way, you will decrease the chemical load in the body and eliminate excess estrogen. Consider using castor oil packs to detoxify your liver over several weeks.

6) Become an expert at monitoring your urinary and saliva pH, and use the foods and minerals necessary to maintain an ideal pH range.

7) Exercise daily, and use saunas regularly, as some toxins are only eliminated through perspiration. Schedule a sauna detoxification program that will fit your needs and schedule.

8) Cleanse your body of yeast and parasites twice yearly for at least 6 weeks at a time.

CHAPTER SIX

Activating Our
Lymphatic *and*
Immune Systems

CONTENTS

EXERCISES, CHARTS, CHECKLISTS & WORKSHEETS

*T*he lymphatic system plays a vital role in detoxifying our bodies. Every 24 hours, the heart receives about 3 liters of lymph, rich in white blood cells, to fight viruses, bacteria, infection, and cancer. This system consists of a network of tubes and cleansing stations that move body fluids and debris away from the spaces between cells, and then returns the fluid to the bloodstream. The rate of flow of lymph back into the bloodstream is proportional to the depth of our inspiration and breathing rate. Powered by the squeezing action of breathing, the lymphatic fluid with its debris is drawn into a thin fabric of very small tubules that empty into larger tubes called lymphatic vessels. During exercise, the flow of lymph into the circulation can increase as much as 10 to 15 times. The fluid is cleansed by different types of white blood cells housed in lymph nodes (the cleansing stations), before being returned to the bloodstream to be recycled. This resembles our water treatment plants: ideally, the dirty water from our homes goes to a treatment plant where it is cleansed and then is returned to us as clean water. The job of lymphatic fluid is to carry proteins, foreign particles, bacteria, viruses, and wandering cancer cells away from the fluid that bathes the body's cells.

The health of our lymphatic systems is closely connected to the power of our immune system, which protects the life of the body by distinguishing 'self' from 'non-self' and recognizes what needs to be destroyed (a cancer cell, virus, bacteria, environmental toxin, internal toxin). The stronger our immune system is, the more resistant to breast cancer we will be.

Parts of the Lymphatic System

The lymphatic system comprises the lymph nodes, lymph vessels, lymphatic fluid, spleen, tonsils, and the thymus gland.

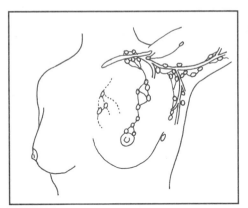

Lymph Nodes

These are small round capsules that contain well-trained armies of white blood cells. There are about 600 of them in total scattered throughout the body and they vary in size from microscopic to about an inch in diameter. The white blood cells include phagocytes which ingest and destroy bacteria, foreign particles, and worn out cells from the lymph, as well as T-Lymphocytes which co-ordinate attacks on viruses and cancer cells and B-Lymphocytes which make antibodies. The lymph nodes are like islands along the rivers of the lymphatic vessels draining all the major areas of the body. Although they exist throughout the body, lymph nodes are clustered in a few key spots such as the groin, underarm, and neck, where we easily recognize them when they are swollen and overworked.

Lymph Vessels

The lymphatic vessels are a one-way transport system that can easily get clogged up when there is an excess of debris and not enough movement through the cleansing stations. (Sort of like a long line-up of cars waiting at a car wash.) This is when you notice that you have a swollen lymph node. The debris is most often linked to a bacterial or viral infection, the presence of toxins, or cancer.

The axillary (underarm) lymph nodes are strategically placed close to our breasts. As long as our breasts and armpits move, we will circulate the lymphatic fluid around them so that effective cleansing can occur. Wearing a bra for long periods of time or wearing a tight bra restricts lymphatic circulation in the breast area and can impair our ability to cleanse the breasts, indirectly promoting breast cancer.

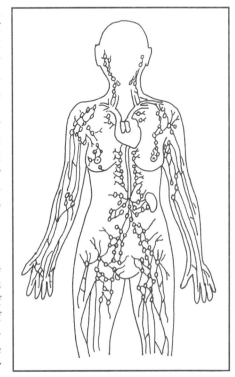

Lymphatic Fluid

Regular muscular exercise and deep breathing makes the lymphatic fluid move so that there is not a back up of debris and fluid. Lymphatic fluid is pumped by the contraction of skeletal muscle and pressure changes due to the action of breathing. The more efficiently your lymphatic fluid circulates, the less cellular debris you have, the quicker your white blood cells can get to work on bacteria, viruses, and cancer cells in the lymph nodes, and the healthier you and your breasts will be. We want the white blood cells housed in the lymph nodes to be real warriors — alert, quick, devouring, efficient, co-operative.

Spleen

Our spleen is situated beneath the diaphragm and behind the stomach, on the left side of the abdomen. The spleen has two different kinds of tissue in it, known as white pulp and red pulp. The white pulp contains large numbers of white blood cells. The red pulp contains red blood cells, white blood cells, and macrophages. Macrophages engulf and destroy bacteria and foreign particles they find in the blood as it circulates through the spleen. The spleen has the capacity to store a lot of blood, and as it does this, the macrophages can get to work gobbling up what shouldn't be in the blood, defending the body from infection. An initiate in the mysteries of blood, the spleen plays a central role in the formation of blood, the storage of blood, and the filtration of blood.

Tonsils

If you have managed to keep them, your tonsils can be seen on either side in the back of your throat. They are composed of masses of lymphatic tissue, filled with macrophages that protect you from bacteria roaming around in your eustachian tubes, mouth, and throat.

Thymus Gland

Tap the upper part of your sternum, or breast bone. The thymus gland is under here. Think of the thymus gland as a teaching station where some of the white blood cells (the T-lymphocytes) are educated and taught to cooperate in coordinated attacks against viruses and cancer cells. The warriors that the thymus breeds are there to protect our lives — hence they are fueled by our own self-love. If they don't get the message that we are worth it and we have something to live for, they will be less committed to our defense. The thymus gland speaks to our T cells from its central command station, sending a hormone into the blood to activate them when their energy is flagging.

Since the thymus secretes its hormones under parasympathetic stimulation when you are relaxed, you can develop a meditation practice and find ways to take 20-minute relaxation breaks regularly. Bovine thymus extract and homeopathic thymuline 9CH have a modulating and strengthening effect on the gland and can be taken as directed by a naturopath or holistic doctor. Exercises that involve coordinated arm and leg movements on alternate sides strengthen the thymus — we can swing our arms as we walk and avoid carrying heavy bags on one side, and can march, swim, and do yoga.

Assisting Lymphatic Circulation

Between the breast tissue and the pectoralis major muscle that lies beneath it there is a space called the 'retro mammary space' that is extremely important, allowing for free movement of the breast over the muscle, and allowing better drainage for the breast tissue.

The skin on the surface of the breast is richly supplied with lymphatic vessels, as is the breast tissue itself. The flow of the lymph in the breast drains from superficial to deep, and toxins are carried through the breast tissue to the retro mammary space before entering the lymph tubules.

Seventy-five percent of the lymph drains to the underarm lymph nodes, while the rest drains to either the collarbone area, to below the breast, or across to the other breast. When removal of lymph nodes obstructs the flow of the lymph, we can encourage it to take an alternate route with directed massage. Lymphatic flow can also be obstructed by tight bras, poor posture, and tight neck and shoulder muscles.

Six practices that will improve lymphatic circulation are dry brush massage, contrast showers, rebounding, exercise, going braless, and breast self-massage.

Dry Brush Massage

Dry brush massage stimulates the lymphatic system to expel toxins through the skin. About one third of all body impurities are eliminated through the skin, more than one pound of waste disposal every day. If skin pores remained clogged, the body removes its waste less efficiently and the burden is increased on other detoxifying organs.

The body 'breathes' through the skin as well as the lungs, with oxygen being absorbed and carbon dioxide released through its pores. By dry brushing, blood circulation is increased to the internal organs as well as the skin, which promotes oxygenation and healing. The body's natural defenses against sickness are improved, especially when used with the hot-cold shower technique.

Dry Brush Massage Instructions

1) Buy a long handled, natural bristle brush, with a brush pad about the size of your own hand. If you can't find a natural bristle brush, you can substitute a natural plant fiber vegetable brush, a bath glove made of twisted hog's hair, or a loofah mitt.
2) Start with the soles of your feet. Brush in a circular motion as you move up your body, feet to legs, hands to arms, back to abdomen, and chest to neck. The face and inner thighs are sensitive areas and can be avoided. Brush with as much pressure as is comfortably possible until your skin feels pleasantly warm (this is usually about five to 10 minutes). The massage is best performed when you rise in the morning and before you go to bed at night.
3) You can increase the cleansing qualities of a dry brush massage if you follow it with an alternating hot-cold shower (hot for three minutes, cold for 30 seconds), repeating the hot-cold pattern three times.
4) Make sure that you wash your brush every two weeks with soap and water to remove the debris that may have moved from your skin to your brush, and then dry it in a warm place. Use a separate brush for each family member.

Contrast Showers

Alternating hot and cold showers improve blood circulation, increase cellular oxidation, enhance immunity, strengthen the nervous system, and flush cellular toxins into the blood. When we shower in hot water for less than five minutes, it has a stimulating effect on our circulation. Similarly, when we have a cold shower for less than one minute, we stimulate blood flow and metabolism. Cold applications first constrict and then later dilate blood vessels. By finishing with a short cold shower, we cause the following physiological effects: increased oxygen absorption; increased carbon dioxide excretion; increased nitrogen absorption and excretion; increased tissue tone; increased white blood cell count and thus

FACT
One of the factors that promotes tumor growth is poor microcirculation in the area where the tumor develops. Contrast showers are excellent ways to improve the microcirculation, bringing nutrients and oxygen to the cells and removing waste more efficiently.

improved immunity; increased red blood cell count; decreased blood glucose; heightened metabolism.

The supplements you take will nourish your body better if you use contrast showers. To some degree, healing is proportional to improved blood flow.

Principles of Hydrotherapy

To use the principles of hydrotherapy, stand in the shower (after dry brush massage) and shower following this sequence: 1-3 minutes hot, 30 seconds cold. Repeat 3 times. As you shower, tap the sternum with your fingertips for a minute to stimulate the thymus gland. Lovingly touch your breasts with your hands, giving them a gentle massage. Rub your whole body briskly as you shower. Always finish with cold. Rub yourself down with a towel when you finish.

Exercise
Movement of the arms, armpits, and chest assists lymphatic cleansing of the breasts. Muscular movement causes the lymphatic fluid to flow efficiently to the cleansing lymph nodes, where the white blood cells work away at keeping your body free of bacteria, viruses, toxins, and cancer cells. Exercises such as rebounding, skipping, tennis, racquetball, swimming (in non-chlorinated water), rowing, window washing, drumming, jumping jacks, wood chopping, marching, and walking while swinging your arms are extremely beneficial on a daily basis. Regular exercise enhances the metabolism of estrogen and improves blood sugar regulation.

Going Braless
Many types of bra restrict the movement of the breasts and impede lymphatic circulation. In the book *Dressed to Kill*, the authors found that women who develop breast cancer usually wear their bras more than 12 hours per day and may wear them to bed.[1] On the other hand, women who wore their bras less than 12 hours daily had a 19-fold protection from breast cancer compared with the general population of women. Red marks on the skin from a tight-fitting bra might indicate restricted lymphatic circulation.

Breast cancer incidence is much lower in cultures where women go braless.[2] Although wearing a bra probably does not cause breast cancer, it may undermine the efforts of our lymphatic system to cleanse environmental toxins and cancer cells out of the breast area. If you have large breasts and need to wear a bra, take it off when you get home and make sure it isn't too tight.

The Lymph Flush

This program came to me from a breast cancer survivor. It has been used by practitioners and cancer patients for many years to flush the lymphatic system and works well for lymphedema. The cleanse lasts for three days. Use the lymph flush when you feel sensitivity or swelling in your lymph nodes or with lymphedema

Directions: Pour the juice in a glass gallon container and fill the remainder of the container with pure water. On the first day of the flush, take 1 tbsp of epsom salts in ½ glass of water. Repeat this two more times at ½ hour intervals for a total of three repetitions. After the third glass of epsom salts and water, begin to drink the juice.

Eat no other food for the three days, excepting an orange if you are hungry. On the fourth day, begin to eat lightly — vegetable broth soups, fruit, salads. Eat normally after that.

Lymph Flush Recipe
Ingredients:
    Juice of 6 lemons,
    6 grapefruits, and
    12 oranges each day
    Pure water
    Epsom salts

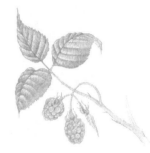

Breast Self-Massage Instructions

Breast self- massage is another way to stimulate the flow of the lymph to help remove toxins from our breasts. Two exceptional massage therapists, Pam Hammond and Sarah Cowley, provide the following guide to teaching women how to touch their breasts in a healing way. You might want to start in the shower by "washing" your breasts with your hands until you become comfortable with the idea of massaging your breasts. Also consider using the Healthy Breast Oil described later in this chapter.

1) Place your hands on either side of your neck and gently move the skin back and down towards your collarbone. Do this 15 times.
2) Place the palm of your hand under your underarm and gently pump your armpit. The movement is slightly up toward your shoulder and in towards your body. Do this 15 times.
3) With soft hands use the flat surface of three or four fingers to make small semi-circles around the outer part of your breasts working inward until you reach the areola. Do not press hard. It is very gentle work. Apply as much pressure as you would to stroke a young kitten.
4) With your hands cupped around your breast, gently pull your breast away from the chest wall and move your breasts in a circular or up and down movement. This allows breast generated lymph fluid to drain into the retro mammary space and out through the external lymph tubules in the axilla.
5) If you do find a lump, do not try to massage it away. You might irritate it. Eighty percent of all breast lumps are benign, but it is important to bring any lump to your health care professional's attention.

Rebounding Exercise Instructions

A rebounder is the equivalent of a small trampoline. Jumping on a rebounder greatly improves the circulation of lymphatic fluid within the body as muscular contractions push the fluid through the lymphatic vessels. Some of the additional benefits of rebounding include gentle massage of the liver and colon; increased oxygenation on a cellular level; improved muscle tone; improved digestion, elimination, and body detoxification; easier weight management through calorie expenditure; increased energy; improvement in cardiovascular health; stress reduction and release; and an increase in strength, stamina, balance, and agility.

Rebounding for 10 minutes has the aerobic effect equivalent to playing tennis for 40 minutes or jogging for 30 minutes. The lungs increase their efficiency and process more air, increasing the oxygen uptake of the blood. The heart muscle grows stronger and pumps more blood with each stroke, reducing the number of heartbeats necessary per minute. The aerobic effect of rebounding also increases the size and number of blood vessels in the body. There is a greater total blood volume and increased ability to bring oxygen to all body cells. Cancer cells do not thrive in a well-oxygenated environment.

Constipation is usually relieved by rebounding regularly because this exercise improves the peristaltic action of the intestines. By improving bowel movements, we can lessen our risk of breast cancer by eliminating more toxins and estrogen from the colon. If you have any weakness in your bladder you may want to wear a small menstrual pad while rebounding to catch any urine that is released while jumping. Each of the exercises below can be done anywhere from 30 seconds to 3 minutes, making your rebounding workout approximately 7 minutes to 45 minutes long. Do what you are able to depending upon your age, fitness level, and endurance. Start with a shorter time and slowly increase it. Practice once or twice daily.

1) Place an image on the wall that you face while rebounding that will act as a centering device for you. Gaze at it as you rebound. It can be a mandala, a family photograph, a symbol of something that represents all you have to live for, or a picture that symbolizes health or brings tranquility, such as a nature scene. Choose it carefully for it will help to activate your immune system as you exercise.

2) Jump straight up and down and circle the arms in a backward direction as though swimming the backstroke. Complete one backward circle of the arms for every two jumps. Then speed it up so that you complete one arm rotation per jump. Move the armpits as you jump. Then reverse the movement, rotating the arms simultaneously to the front. Imagine that you are releasing any grief, anger or unresolved emotion from the past as you move the arms backwards. Imagine that you are moving to the future that is calling you as you roll the arms forwards.

3) Jump straight up and down and alternate rotating the left arm and then the right arm to the back, as though doing the back crawl in swimming. As you do it, imagine that you are unwinding and releasing the past. Then reverse the movement, rotating the arms to the front as though doing the front crawl. Imagine that you are progressing towards your ideal future securely with each movement. You can make the journey towards your goals and ideals.

4) On the first jump clap the hands out in front of the body. On the next jump clap the hands behind the body. Continue alternating clapping in front and back. Clap for the life you have lived and the life you have yet to live.

5) Inhale as you raise the left knee up and lift the left arm above your head. Exhale on the next jump and raise your right knee up as you raise the right arm above your head. Lift the knees high. If this is too strenuous for you then include an extra jump between the raising of the knee and arm. If the breathing is difficult, coordinate the movements with a long deep breath.

6) Inhale as you raise the left knee up and the right arm high above your head. Exhale and jump with both feet on the rebounder and the arms at your sides. Then inhale as you raise the right knee up high and lift the left arm above your head. Exhale as you bring both feet down with the arms at your sides. Continue this pattern.

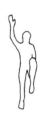

Our Lymphatic and Immune Systems

7) Jump up and down and circle the hands in front of the breasts with the palms facing forward. The left palm rotates counter-clockwise while the right palm rotates in a clockwise direction. Touch the tips of the thumbs as both hands come towards the center. As you do it imagine that you are washing any toxins or cancer cells out of your breasts and direct positive energy towards them.

8) Jump straight up and down and alternate swinging both arms in front of the body to the left. On the next jump, swing them to the right. Inhale as you swing to the left, exhale to the right. Continue one minute. Then as you swing your arms to the left twist your hips to the right so your feet land pointing to the right. On the next jump swing your arms in front of the body to the right as you twist your hips to the left and land with both feet pointing to the left. Continue alternating the twist, coordinating it with the breath.

9) Jump up and down and swing the left arm out to the left side at shoulder height as you tap the sternum firmly between the breasts with the fingertips of your right hand. On the next jump swing the right arm out to the right side at shoulder height and tap the sternum firmly between the breasts with the fingertips of your left hand. Alternate swinging one arm out to the side while the other hand taps the area of the thymus gland between the breasts. Imagine that you are programming your thymus gland for super immunity.

10) Jumping jacks. Inhale as you clap the hands above the head and spread the feet apart on the rebounder, exhale as you bring the arms down to the sides and bring the feet together. Continue this pattern. Do 26 jumping jacks or continue for 30 seconds to 3 minutes.

11) On the first jump swing the arms out to the sides at shoulder height and stretch the feet apart. On the next jump cross the arms straight out in front of the heart, pointing them in front of the body while the feet cross one in front of the other. Alternate which foot or arm is in front with each movement. Continue crisscrossing the arms and legs with each jump.

12) As you jump, inhale and throw both arms up and behind your shoulders, exhale as they come down to your sides. Then inhale as you criss-cross them in front of your chest, exhale as they swing out to the sides. Continue this pattern alternating the criss-crosses each time. Co-ordinate the movement of the arms with jumping. Breathe powerfully in and out through your nose as you jump. Imagine that you are breathing in healing energy and embracing yourself as the arms cross in front, and releasing any toxins (physical or emotional) as you throw your arms behind your shoulders.

13) Inhale the left hand forward from the shoulder and open your fingers as you stretch the arm to the front; bend your elbow and pull the arm back as you close the hand into a fist. The fist should touch the side of your chest and the elbow is bent behind you. Then exhale as you stretch the left arm forward from the shoulder, opening the fingers as though you are reaching to grab your future and your health (or whatever it is that you most want in your life); then pull the elbow back and make your hand into a fist. Continue alternating the movement of the arms with a powerful breath.

14) Jump up and down swinging the left arm to the front as the right arm swings to the back. On the next jump swing the right arm to the front as the left arm swings to the back. Coordinate the movement of the arms with the feet, bringing the right foot slightly forward as the left arm swings forward, and the left foot slightly forward as the right arm swings to the front. Find a rhythm with your breathing, either inhaling as the left arm comes to the front and exhaling as the right arm comes forward or use long deep breathing with a different pattern of jumps.

15) As you jump on the right foot, raise the left leg out to the side and lift both arms out to the sides at shoulder height. On the next jump, have your arms at your sides and jump with both feet. On the third jump, raise the right leg out to the side as you jump on the left foot while simultaneously lifting both arms out to the sides at shoulder height. On the fourth jump, have your arms by your sides as you land on both feet. Continue this four-part sequence.

Low Immunity Factors

There are many factors that negatively affect our immune status. Many of these we can change, some we cannot. Below is a list of factors that can lower immunity. Make note of the ones that apply to you and make efforts to change those that you can. These categories and examples have been derived in part from Luc De Schepper's book, *Peak Immunity*.[3]

Hereditary Factors

Immunity may be lower and thus the risk of cancer higher when there is a family history of one or more of the following diseases:

Hypothyroidism
Rheumatoid Arthritis
Scleroderma
Cancer
Manic-depression
Hashimoto's Disease
Hypoglycemia
Allergies
Diabetes mellitus
Lupus

Personality Factors

The immune system may be weaker in those with the following personality traits:

Obsessive about Exercise
Dominating
Competitive
Inability to Relax
Nervous
Insecure
Impatient
Lives in the Past
Easily Frustrated
Overly Pleasing
Easily Angered
Aggressive
Overly Analytical
Passive
Non-Assertive

Stress Factors

The following stress factors may tax the immune system:

History of Child Abuse
Divorce or Separation
Jail Term
Difficult Mortgage
Family Conflict
Unwanted Pregnancy
Marital Conflict
Change in Residence
Alcoholic Parents
Sexual Difficulties
Job Loss
Job Conflict
Death of a Loved One
Personal Injury
Empty Retirement

Nutritional Factors

These nutritional patterns result in lowered immunity:

Addiction to Sugar or Chocolate
Irregular Eating Habits
Consume Coffee regularly
Over-consumption of Bread
Eat Beef or Pork regularly
Lack of Whole Grains
Overeating White Flour Products
Consume Alcohol regularly
Consume Fried Foods
Skip Breakfast
Eat Fruit rarely
Experience Food Allergies
Eat Canned rather than
Fresh Foods
Drink Soft Drinks regularly
Drug or Tobacco Addiction

Chemical Factors

These chemical factors around your home lower immunity:

Aluminum Pots or Pans
Gas Stoves
Teflon Pots and Pans
Ammonia Cleansers
Hair Sprays
Turpentine, Paint Fumes
Fluoridated and Chlorinated Water
Kerosene
Newspaper Print
Dyes
Paint Lacquer
Nail Polish
Pesticides
Tobacco Smoke
Formaldehyde
Exposure to Insecticides
Recycled Air
Underground Parking
Ceilings containing Asbestos
Exposure to Electromagnetic
Radiation from Copy Machines
Exposure to X-rays or Computers

Health Factors

The following health factors result in lowered immunity:

History of Past Surgeries
Recurrent Infections
(more than 6 in a year)
Past Use of Chemotherapy
or Radiation
Sensitivity to Ragweed or Leaf Mold
History of Antibiotic Use
Past History of Cortisone Use
History of Birth Control Pill Use
Environmental Sensitivities

Specialized Cells of the Immune System

Complement System

The complement system is composed of proteins manufactured by the liver and spleen. These orchestrated proteins are able to destroy cancer cells, viruses, bacteria and immune complexes.

White Blood Cells

White blood cells originate in the bone marrow and are transported in the blood. About half of the white blood cells go from the bone marrow to the thymus gland, where they 'mature' and assume different functions. These are known as T-lymphocytes, and after maturity they leave the thymus, circulate in the blood, and populate the lymph nodes. The T-lymphocytes include Helper T-cells, Killer T-cells, and Suppressor T-cells, which together make up about 75% of the circulating lymphocytes. The other lymphocytes that originate in the bone marrow but do not go to the thymus become B-lymphocytes. Their primary function is to make antibodies. They also reside in the lymph nodes. Other types of white blood cells include macrophages and memory cells.

Macrophage

This cell type is able to engulf and digest debris that enters the bloodstream. When it encounters a foreign organism, it summons helper T-cells to the scene.

Helper T-Cell

This cell type identifies the foreign substance or 'enemy' and rushes to the spleen and lymph nodes where it stimulates the production of other cells to fight the infection.

Killer T-Cell

This cell type is recruited and activated by the helper T-cell and specializes in killing cells of the body that have been invaded by foreign organisms, as well as cancer cells.

B-Cell

These cells are housed in the spleen or the lymph nodes and are activated to replicate by the helper T cell. They produce potent chemical weapons called antibodies that are protein molecules. The B cell rushes to the infection site with its antibodies, neutralizing the enemy or marking it for attack by other cells or chemicals.

Suppressor T-Cell

This T cell is able to slow down or stop the activity of B cells and other T cells, playing an important role in calling off the attack once an infection has been conquered.

PREVENTION
Enhance your complement system with herbs containing inulin, which include echinacea, burdock root, and dandelion root.

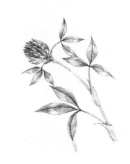

Memory Cell

This type of cell is generated during an initial infection and may circulate in the blood or lymph for years, allowing the body to respond more quickly to future infections.

Western Herbs for Improving Lymphatic and Immune Function

Western herbs have been used singly or in formulas for lymphatic circulation and cleansing — and for breast health. Ayurvedic and Chinese herbs and herbal formulas have similar applications. Calcium, iodine, and magnesium are additional minerals that help to resolve lymphatic congestion. They are found in high amounts in almonds and sea vegetables such as kelp, arame, hijiki, and dulse.

Besides the herbs described here, several others that look promising in breast cancer prevention and treatment are turmeric, myrrh, blue violet, bloodroot (Sanguinaria canadensis), mandrake, and juniper. The latter three were all found to inhibit the proliferation of both estrogen receptor positive and estrogen-receptor negative cell lines in vitro, with bloodroot having the strongest effect.[4] Follow the recommendations of a naturopathic doctor or an herbalist in using these herbs and formulas.

Phytochemicals in Herbs Active Against Breast Cancer Cells

The chart below summarizes some of the plant chemicals (phytochemicals) found in herbs that are known to inhibit breast cancer cells. See Chapter 10, 'Breast Disease Treatments,' to see how they disrupt cell division.[5]

Phytochemical	Herbs that Contain the Plant Chemical
Berberine	goldenseal, barberry, bloodroot, Coptis chinensis (Huang Lian)
Beta-sitosterol	juniper, myrrh, red clover, echinacea, turmeric, marigold
Beta carotene	goldenseal, phytolacca
Genistein	red clover, wild indigo
Lutein	European mistletoe, marigold
Quercetin	may apple (mandrake)
Curcumin	turmeric

Dosage: 25-100 drops tincture, 3 x daily. It can be used for months or even years at a time.

Contraindications: Do not use in pregnancy as it is a uterine stimulant. Begin with a low dosage otherwise, building up to a higher one if needed.

Burdock Root (Arctium lappa)

Burdock has a special affinity for the kidneys, bladder, and liver. It promotes detoxification, clears dampness, dissolves deposits and removes lymphatic congestion. It can help with breaking down benign and malignant breast tumors. Burdock clears internal heat and toxins, reducing infection, inflammation, and swelling. It is commonly used in chronic skin conditions. Burdock acts as a digestive tonic and promotes bile flow. The fresh root helps to remove heavy metals and chemicals and encourages the growth of beneficial intestinal bacteria. It is a tonic to the immune system and is found in the Essiac formula developed by Rene Caisse, as well as the Hoxsey formula. It works well in combination with red clover and dandelion.

Marigold Flower (Calendula officinalis)

Marigold is a healer for the liver, heart, uterus, skin, veins, lymphatic, system, and blood. Like burdock, it clears heat and toxins, reduces infection (bacterial, fungal, viral, and amoebic) and inflammation, relieves swelling and removes lymphatic congestion. It contains high amounts of lutein, a phytochemical that prevents breast cancer.

It has been used to reduce tumors, cysts, and cancer of the reproductive organs, breasts, and intestines. Marigold stimulates digestion and reduces liver congestion. When used before and after surgery it promotes tissue repair, decreases scarring and acts as an antiseptic to the skin.

Dosage: 50-100 drops tincture, 3 x daily. Use after breast cancer surgery for one month.
Contraindications: Do not use in pregnancy as it is a uterine stimulant.

Goldenseal Root (Hydrastis canadensis)

Goldenseal's action extends to the stomach, intestines, lung, heart, reproductive organs, bladder, kidneys, liver, and gallbladder. It clears heat, dries up excess mucous, reduces infection and inflammation, and stops discharge while soothing mucous membranes. It is used in treating cirrhosis of the liver and gallstones. Goldenseal is one of the best herbal antibiotics, being effective against a wide array of bacteria, yeast, fungi, amoeba, and parasites while seemingly sparing normal intestinal flora. Like barberry, it is a very useful herb in treating chronic candidiasis. Goldenseal helps to shrink tumors of the reproductive organs, breasts, and stomach and will assist in decreasing breast pain and swelling. It contains the anti-cancer chemical, berberine as well as beta carotene.

As a digestive tonic it stimulates hydrochloric acid production, relieving appetite loss and fatigue. As an immune tonic, goldenseal improves the ability of macrophages to engulf and digest foreign particles and bacteria. It increases the blood supply to the spleen, enhancing the function of the white blood cells in defending us against bacteria, viruses, toxins, and cancer. As it is a strong acting herb, usually only small doses are needed.

Dosage: 7-40 drops tincture, 3 x daily. In a powdered solid extract with a 10% berberine content, the dose is 250-500 mg, 3 x daily. Use it for three weeks at a time, followed by a week-long break. It has a slight cumulative toxicity. If you are using it in a formula with several other herbs, it can be taken for several months at a time.
Contraindications: Do not use in pregnancy, as it is a uterine stimulant. Do not use in persons with high blood pressure, as it will elevate it. If you experience nausea while taking goldenseal, reduce the dosage.

Echinacea Root (Echinacea augustifolia)

Echinacea has an affinity for the blood, lymph, skin, stomach, and urogenital organs. It clears heat and toxins, reduces infection, fever, and inflammation. Echinacea helps to remove lymphatic congestion and reduce tumors, and has been used in anti-cancer formulas for many generations. As an immune stimulant, it raises the white blood cell count when taken in large doses, improves macrophage activity, and increases interferon. It can be used for short periods of time to deal with acute infections, or for up to three months as a detoxifying, cancer inhibiting herb.

Dosage: 25-50 drops tincture, 3 x daily.
Contraindications: In sensitive people it can sometimes cause dizziness, nausea, throat irritation, joint pain, and canker sores.

European Mistletoe (Viscum album)

In Germany in 1995, European mistletoe was the most commonly prescribed biological medicine for cancer, used in 80% of patients.[6] European mistletoe promotes urination and detoxification, dissolves deposits, stimulates immunity, and reduces tumors (benign and malignant). It contains the phytochemical lutein as well as proteins called lectins, which are similar to anti-tumor proteins found in medicinal mushrooms.[7] Mistletoe also contains arginine, an amino acid that inhibits tumor growth and increases the activity of T-Killer cells. To be effective, mistletoe preparations should be made from the fresh green or freshly-dried plant. Mistletoe is a mild herb and can be used for years.

A fermented preparation of the European mistletoe called 'Iscador', once associated with Rudoph Steiner and the Anthroposophical movement, now is marketed by Weleda AG. It combines fermented mistletoe with homeopathic dosages of silver, copper, and mercury. When injected into rabbits, it caused an increase in natural killer cell activity, increased numbers of other white blood cells, and improved the scavenging ability of macrophages.[8] Iscador caused a 78% increase in the weight of the thymus gland in rats when they were injected with it daily for 6 days. It caused the thymus cells to be 29 times more responsive to a stimulant. In women with breast cancer, it caused a significant enhancement in the scavenger activity of white blood cells.

Iscador is generally used for 10-14 days prior to surgery to prevent metastatic spread of the cancer from the surgical procedure. Then it is used after surgery or radiation for several years to reduce the risk of recurrence. Generally, it is injected at or near the tumor site, a typical course of treatment involving 14 injections given in increasing concentration.[9] The herb can also be taken in tincture form.

Dosage: 25-75 drops tincture, 3x daily.
Contraindications: Do not use in pregnancy, as it is a uterine stimulant. In high doses it can act as a sedative or irritate the gastrointestinal tract. If this occurs, decrease the dosage. Do not use American mistletoe, which is a different plant and can be toxic.

Poke Root (Phytolacca decandra)

Poke root acts upon the digestive, lymphatic, and musculoskeletal systems. It promotes detoxification, clears dampness and heat, reduces lymphatic congestion, and can shrink tumors. Poke root can reduce liver congestion and relieve constipation. It has a particular affinity for the breasts and reduces fibrocystic breast disease and breast swelling. It is excellent in homeopathic dosage for mastitis. Poke root is also an immune stimulant and is found in the Hoxsey formula. Eclectic physicians in the 1850s included poke root routinely in formulas for breast disease.

Dosage: 1 drop of tincture daily for 6 weeks; or 3 pellets of a 6X homeopathic potency once daily for 6 weeks; or 3-25 drops on its own or in combination with other herbs for several weeks. Then break for a week. It is toxic in high doses and has a cumulative toxicity even in small doses.
Contraindications: Do not use in pregnancy as it can cause fetal abnormalities.

Red Clover (Trifolium pratense)

Red clover is a specific healer for the skin, lungs, nerves, and bladder. It promotes detoxification and urination, clears dampness, and shrinks tumors, particularly of the breasts, skin, and ovaries. It is used for chronic bladder infections and for drying up vaginal discharge. It is commonly included in formulas for clearing the skin of acne and eczema. Red clover can help us detoxify from heavy metal poisoning. Containing significant amounts of phytoestrogens, red clover is a wonderful herb to include in a breast cancer prevention

Dosage: 20-100 drops tincture, 3x daily or several cups as a tea daily. Steep flower heads for 15 minutes.
Contraindications: None.

formula. It is part of the Hoxsey formula and is included in FlorEssence, a variation of the Essiac formula made by Flora. It has a long history of use and outstanding reputation as an anti-cancer herb. Hundreds of cases of cancer remission have been documented after regular use of red clover.[9] Red clover must be taken for months to achieve its deep cleansing and tumor-reducing effects. The fresh flower tops can be added to juices or steeped to make tea.

Cleavers Herb (Galium aparine)

Cleavers has an affinity for the liver, bladder, prostate, blood, lymphatic system, and skin. It is a detoxifying herb that can relieve breast swelling, help to break down benign and malignant tumors, and remove lymphatic congestion. It also acts as a blood thinner and can dissolve clots. This blood thinning action makes it contraindicated before or after surgery, and it may increase menstrual flow. Cleavers relieves liver congestion. It is a cooling, refreshing herb and can be used to lower a fever. This is a very safe herb when indicated, and best results are gained from long term use. The herb is always used fresh and is never boiled.

Dosage: 2 tsp of juice, 3 x daily; or 40-100 drops tincture, 3 x daily.
Contraindications: Do not use while you have excessive menstrual bleeding or for three days before or after surgery.

Wild Indigo Root (Baptisia tinctoriae)

I have been preoccupied with this herb since I found out that it had a very high content of genistein, the phytoestrogen also found in soy (see phytoestrogen chart in Chapter 7, 'Eating Right for Breast Health.') It was in a related species, Baptisia australis, that this was measured, but the genistein content is likely to be similar in this North American herb. Baptisia relieves lymphatic congestion and has been used in treating lymphedema and breast infections (mastitis). It clears heat and toxins, reduces infection, fever and inflammation, and helps to stop discharge. It moves the blood in the liver, which when stagnant can lead to breast cysts. Baptisia is a digestive tonic and stimulates bile flow, helping to pull toxins from the liver. It improves constipation and elimination. Wild indigo promotes tissue repair, helping to stop decay, heal sores and ulcers, and has a history of use in malignant tumors of the breast. It is an immune tonic, increasing white blood cell count and activity.[10] In short, Baptisia seems to address all the areas necessary to prevent and treat breast cancer. It is a strongly acting herb, so only lower doses are necessary.

Dosage: 2-25 drops, 3 x daily.
Contraindications: It is toxic in high doses, so stay within the recommended amount. Discontinue if you experience vomiting, diarrhea or respiratory difficulties. Do not use if you have chronic loose stools.

Bloodroot (Sanguinaria canadensis)

Another herb which contains phytoestrogens, bloodroot has been shown to inhibit the proliferation of both estrogen receptor positive and estrogen receptor negative breast cancer cell lines in vitro as did mistletoe, mandrake, and juniper.[11] Historically, bloodroot has been used successfully in external salves to reduce and remove breast cancer tumors.[12] For more information on this technique, consult Ingrid Naiman's remarkable book, *Cancer Salves: A Botanical Approach to Treatment* or see the salve recipe in Chapter 10. Internally in small doses, bloodroot stimulates digestion and improves circulation, while in large doses it can cause nausea and vomiting and acts as a sedative. Small doses improve liver and

Dosage: 2-10 drops, 3 x daily.
Contraindications: Work with a naturopath when using this herb; avoid in pregnancy or when breast-feeding.

glandular function. Two of the active constituents in bloodroot that inhibit cancer cells are berberine (which is also contained in goldenseal) and sanguinarine. Use bloodroot cautiously. It is a potentially toxic herb and large doses can cause death.

Pau d'arco or Taheebo

Dosage: 50-100 drops tincture, 3 x daily; or 6-18 g in tea form 3 x daily.
Contraindications: None known.

The inner bark of this South American tree contains a plant chemical called lapachol, which has shown anti-cancer properties. It is active against solid tumors, leukemias, and several cancers, including breast cancer. Pau d'arco is used to treat candidiasis, a systemic fungal infection which lowers immunity, and is effective against bacterial, fungal, viral, and parasitic infections. Taheebo detoxifies the body, particularly through its action on the kidneys and bladder. It is a very useful herb for chronic bladder infections. It can also be helpful in lessening arthritic symptoms. It builds the blood and promotes tissue repair, helping to heal skin ulcers, eczema, and psoriasis. Pau d'arco is very safe, easy to make as a tea, and readily available.

Carnivora (Venus-flytrap)

Dosage: 1 capsule, 3 x daily, before meals.
Contraindications: None known.

Carnivora is an extract of the entire Venus-flytrap (Dionaea muscipula) in a highly purified form. In cancer it works to break down tumors by blocking the protein kinase enzymes in the cancer cell which are needed to make protein. Without protein, cancer cells die. Dr Helmut G. Keller of Germany discovered the plant and has been using it regularly with his patients. His product in capsule form is called 'Carnivora'.

Green Tea

Dosage: Two cups daily. If you have cancer, consider using an extract or pill form of green tea and take the equivalent of 10 cups of tea daily.
Contraindications: Do not use in pregnancy if it contains caffeine. Use infrequently if you have fibrocystic breasts unless it is decaffeinated.

Green tea contains polyphenols and epigallocatechin-3-gallate, which have been found to regulate cancer cell replication and induce programmed cell death (apoptosis). Green tea protects against all stages of cancer — initiation, promotion, and progression.[13] Part of its protection lies in its ability to suppress new blood vessel growth to tumors.[14] Green and black tea are harvested from the same plant, Camellia sinensis, but their difference lies in the processing of the leaves. Green tea does contain caffeine, although less than coffee. Because caffeine can increase fibrocystic breast disease, use decaffeinated green tea. Be sure your green tea is organic.

Western Herbal Formulas for Breast Health

The Hoxsey Formula

The Hoxsey formula was popularized by Harry Hoxsey, who operated a cancer clinic in Illinois and Texas.

Hoxsey's formula acts to assist digestion (berberis, burdock, prickly ash); detoxify the liver and kidneys (red clover, berberis, burdock); inhibit estradiol from binding to estrogen receptors on breast cells (licorice, red clover); improve elimination (cascara, berberis, buckthorn bark); act as an antiparasitic (berberis); encourage the growth of bifidobacterium in the large intestine and act as a deterrent to bacteria that may cause estrogen to be reabsorbed (burdock, berberis); cleanse the lymphatic system (burdock, red clover, poke root, stillingia); reduce tumors (burdock, red clover, poke, stillingia); normalize the thyroid (potassium iodide); and contains the two minerals that Dr Max Gerson also believed were invaluable in cancer treatment, potassium and iodide.

I have used the Hoxsey formula numerous times with women who have breast swelling, fibrocystic breast disease, lymph node swelling, and mastitis and am rarely disappointed in its effectiveness. Along with the Healthy Breast Formula, it is one of the remedies I most often prescribe for women with breast cancer.

A variation of this formula is used today at the Bio-Medical Center in Tijuana, Mexico, run by Mildred Nelson, who has been treating cancer patients there since 1963. The current formula does not contain prickly ash or buckthorn and cascara sagrada is used instead of cascara amarga.

Dosage: 25-100 drops (¼-1 tsp) tincture after meals and at bedtime, mixed with ⅓ cup water. (Be prepared for its awful taste). Take the lesser amount as prevention and the higher amount if you are recovering from breast cancer. Tinctures are always more effective than capsules or tablets. This is available in tincture form from St. Francis Herbs as Red Clover Combination and from Gaia and HerbPharm as Red Clover Supreme or Hoxsey Formula.

At the Bio-Medical Center the Hoxsey formula is administered in the following way: the diluted tonic is taken in ⅓ glass water, grape juice, milk, or herb tea, initially at 1 tsp, 4 x daily. It is taken in this way for at least 5 years and then every spring and fall after that for 3-4 months. Some people are advised to take larger amounts, depending on their condition.[15]

Contraindications: Do not take while pregnant or for long periods while breast-feeding. Do not use if you have a hyperactive thyroid or experience disturbing symptoms with use. It can be toxic in high doses, so use should be supervised by an herbalist or naturopathic doctor.[16]

Essiac

Another popular formula for preventing and treating breast cancer is a Native American tea called Essiac.

Renee Caisse was a Canadian nurse from Bracebridge, Ontario, born in 1888, who worked as head nurse at the Sisters of Providence Hospital in Haileybury, Ontario. While on duty one day, she received a recipe from an elderly patient who had been cured of breast cancer 30 years earlier by drinking a mixture of eight herbs given to her by an Ojibway medicine man. Soon afterwards Renee's aunt, Mireza Potvin, was diagnosed with stomach and liver cancer, and after exploratory surgery was told she had six months to live. Renee gave her the Ojibway formula daily, and at the end of a year she recovered fully. She lived another 21 years.

The original recipe contained eight herbs, which Renee eventu-

Original Hoxsey Formula (16 oz)
Ingredients:

150 mg	KI (potassium iodine)
20 mg	Chinese licorice
20 mg	red clover
10 mg	burdock root
20 mg	stillingia root
10 mg	berberis root (berberis vulgaris or berberis aquifolium)
5 mg	cascara amarga or cascara sagrada
5 mg	prickly ash bark
20 mg	buckthorn bark
10 mg	poke root (phytolacca)

Essiac Formula
Ingredients:

6½ cups	dry burdock root, cut
16 oz.	powdered green sheep sorrel
1 oz.	Turkish rhubarb root, powdered
4 oz.	slippery elm bark, powdered

To make a smaller amount for one individual, use:

1⅝ cups	cut burdock root
4 oz	powdered sheep sorrel herb
1 oz	powdered slippery elm inner bark
¼ oz	powdered Turkish rhubarb root

ally reduced to four. She administered these in tea form to cancer patients who came to her from all over Ontario and witnessed hundreds of remissions. Renee refused payment for her services, accepting instead donations of food, labor, hand-knit sweaters, and other voluntary contributions. She spent over 50 years selflessly tending to the sick and died at the age of 90, in 1978.

Essiac is available at most health food stores, manufactured by the Respirin Corporation or in a slightly different formula called FlorEssence by Flora. The latter formula includes red clover, which makes it an even better formula for breast cancer prevention.

Essiac Formula Instructions

If you are interested, here is the Essiac formula for making a large quantity of this herbal remedy.

Directions: Use one cup of dry herb mix to two gallons of pure spring water. This yields 13-15, 16-oz bottles. For the individual size mixture, use ½ gallon of water and ¼ cup of herb mix. All utensils, pots, etc. must be cast iron or stainless steel.

1) Bring two gallons of pure spring water to a hard boil.
2) Add one cup of herb mix, hard boil for 10 minutes, stirring very often.
3) Turn off burner and cover and then let the mix sit over night (12 hours) and stir about half way, if possible.
4) In the morning sterilize 15, 16-oz amber-colored glass bottles. The herbs are light-sensitive and should be stored in the dark. To sterilize the bottles, put ½ inch of water in each bottle and set one inch of water in a large roasting pan. Put the pan and bottles in a 300°F oven for 40-60 minutes, until very hot.
5) When bottles are close to being sterilized, turn on the burner under the herbal liquid and just barely bring to a boil.
6) Let the herbs settle to the bottom for a few minutes.
7) Now you can fill the hot sterilized glass amber bottles. As you empty the hot water out of the bottles, you then fill them with the liquid herb mixture. Tighten the lids on the bottles as you fill them so that you get a good seal. Wipe the inside of the lids with liquor (vodka) prior to bottling. Let them set until cool. Then store in a dark cool place. Refrigerate once the bottle has been opened.
8) Always keep Essiac refrigerated after opening but never in the freezer.

PREVENTION

As part of a breast cancer prevention program, consider taking either the Hoxsey formula, Essiac (or FlorEssence), or the Healthy Breast Formula for three months once or twice a year, the frequency and dosage being dependent upon your risk factors. Use one of them with short breaks every six weeks if you are recovering from breast cancer and continue for at least 5 years after your diagnosis.

Dosage: Do not eat or drink anything for at least one hour after taking Essiac. Take 1-2 oz of Essiac with an equal amount of hot water, 1-3 x daily or every second day at bedtime, on an empty stomach, two or three hours after supper. Sip it slowly over a four-minute period.

Different sources have recommended different dosages, the usual being 2 oz, 2 x daily mixed with an equal part of purified hot water, in the morning before breakfast and in the evening at least two hours after the evening meal.

For prevention, 1 oz daily or every other day may be sufficient. In late-stage cases of cancer, increase it to a total of 6 oz daily in three divided doses for at least 12 weeks before reducing it to the usual 4 oz dose.[17]

Contraindications: Do not use Essiac while pregnant or breast-feeding.

Our Lymphatic and Immune Systems

The Healthy Breast Formula

Women with a history of benign breast disease or at high risk for breast cancer may consider the following formula, which I have composed. It integrates some of the herbs in both the Hoxsey formula and Essiac, with a focus on the breasts and lymphatic system. Use organically grown herbs in tincture form to make this formula. You can order a ready-made preparation using the form at the back of the book.

Directions: To blend this formula yourself, purchase organic tinctures of the above herbs and mix them together in the ratios given. Pour into sterilized amber glass bottles and add the potassium iodide, which can usually be purchased from a pharmacy.

Dosage: 20-100 drops, 2-3 x daily, one half hour before or two hours after a meal. As prevention, take it for three months, once or twice a year. If you have breast cancer, use it continuously with week-long breaks every 4-6 weeks. It can be used in conjunction with one of the immune-activating formulas described elsewhere in this book plus goldenseal, echinacea, bloodroot and juniper for a stronger effect.

Contraindications: Do not use in pregnancy or if breast-feeding. Do not use or use cautiously with hyperthyroidism

Ayurvedic Herbs for Improving Lymphatic and Immune Function

Ayurveda is a vast system of knowledge thousands of years old that arose in India. Ayurvedic herbs are chosen for their ability to temper the five elements of ether, air, fire, water, and earth that exist not only in nature but in each individual. Disharmonies in the balance of the elements may result in disease. Here are two Ayurvedic herbs with strong immune enhancing effects.

Amla (Indian Gooseberry)

Amla is one of the richest sources of vitamin C (with 3,000 mg per fruit) and other bioflavonoids in the vegetable kingdom. It is also an excellent antioxidant, increasing Superoxide dismutase levels by 216%. (Superoxide dismutase helps to quench free radicals formed during Phase 1 liver detoxification). This herb is one of the best to help us adapt to stress, with anti-fungal, anti-viral, anti-bacterial, anti-inflammatory, anti-mutagenic, and yeast inhibiting properties. As a restorative herb, it strengthens the teeth and bones, causes the growth of nails and hair, improves eyesight, and stops the bleeding of gums. Amla protects the liver, improves appetite, and regulates blood sugar. Amla forms the basis of the Ayurvedic tonic, Chyavan Prash.

Ashwaganda

Another excellent Ayurvedic herb for helping us adapt to stress is ashwaganda, an immune enhancer which helps to shrink tumors, especially when it is injected directly into the tumor. It can kill some amoeba, bacteria, and fungi. Ashwaganda is prescribed for

Healthy Breast Formula
Ingredients:

20 parts red clover Trifolium pratense (fresh flower heads)

20 parts burdock root Arctium lappa (dried root)

20 parts European mistletoe Viscum album (twig and leaf, from the fresh green or freshly dried plant)

20 parts cleavers Galium aparine (fresh herb)

10 parts calendula Calendula officinalis (flower petals)

5 parts poke root Phytolacca decandra (fresh root)

5 parts wild indigo root Baptisia tinctoriae (root) potassium iodide (3% w/v)

Dosage: Use 1 tsp paste 3 x daily; or 5 g of powder in water 2 x daily as a tonic.
Contraindications: Do not use with acute diarrhea or dysentery.

Dosage: 250-1000 mg, 2-3 x daily or 3000 mg at night for insomnia.
Contraindications: Do not use if you are severely congested.

nervous exhaustion, debility, memory loss, muscular weakness, glandular swelling, fatigue, and insomnia. Its sedative action generates calmness and a restful sleep.

Chinese Herbs for Improving Lymphatic and Immune Function

Cancer prevention in Chinese medicine consists of effective means to treat depression, anger, anxiety, grief, or other emotional factors that interfere with the circulation of energy; avoidance of substances that increase the production of phlegm (such as unhealthy fats, wheat, dairy, and sweets); improving circulation so that stagnation will be kept to a minimum and elimination of toxins.

Chinese herbs are almost always used in formulas rather than alone. Herbs used in formulas for breast cancer prevention or treatment are divided into several categories.

Etiology of Breast Cancer in Chinese Medicine

In order to understand the use of Chinese herbs in breast cancer prevention and treatment, we must understand the etiology of breast cancer from an Oriental medical perspective. Breast cancer arises after a process caused primarily by the following:

1) First, there is stagnation of energy in the liver. One of the functions of the liver in Oriental medicine is to circulate the body's energy, or qi, freely in all directions. This energy flow can be blocked by suppressed emotions — holding on to anger, anxiety, worry, a long period of depression or frustration, or grief. These emotions will interfere with the smooth flow of energy in the liver, causing a blockage. Other variables that contribute to liver stagnation include lack of exercise, shallow breathing, and excess consumption of unhealthy fats. Qi stagnation may manifest as irregular periods, premenstrual breast swelling and pain, breast cysts, irritability, fatigue, and depression. Qi stagnation is also often linked to a deficiency of yin or blood in the liver and kidney.

2) Second, there is stagnation of blood in the liver. As the liver energy does not circulate freely, the blood that the liver holds becomes stagnant, not moving as it should. Energy moves the blood. If the energy flow is disrupted, the blood flow is impaired. There will be reduced circulation to the breast area. In medical terms, the blood coagulates more easily than it should, or has increased viscosity.

3) Another contributing factor to breast disease is the accumulation of dampness or phlegm. Phlegm arises from qi stagnation affecting the function of the spleen. The role of the spleen in Chinese medicine is to transform and transport food and to regulate the body fluids. The disturbance in the liver will affect the spleen so that it is unable to perform these tasks effectively. A build-up of fluids will occur, which over time can form a soft mass or lump.

4) Eventually, the combination of qi stagnation and phlegm accumulation may cause the mass to become firmer. The presence of an actual toxin encourages the mass to become cancerous. The toxins may be internally or externally generated. Toxins can include but are not limited to environmental chemicals, pesticide residues, encrusted fecal matter, and excess estrogen.

5) After a period of time, the stagnant qi turns into heat or 'fire' and becomes what is known as toxic heat. The toxic heat injures the blood and yin even further so that the mass hardens, leading to a cancerous tumor. A soft breast lump indicates the accumulation of phlegm, while a hard breast lump is indicative of blood stagnation or toxic heat. I find it interesting that thermography can pick up the presence of cancer from the increased heat in the area, generated by the higher vascular supply to a tumor.

Our Lymphatic and Immune Systems

Herbs for Removing Toxins

Generally these help to remove toxic heat or fire and include *Sophora flavescens*, *Oldenlandria diffusae*, *Isatis tinctoria*, *Solanum*, *Wikstroemia*, *Lonicera japonica*, *Prunella vulgaris*, *Lithospermum erythrorhizon*, *Scutellaria baicalensis*, *Viola yedonensis*, *Curcuma aromatica*, oyster shell *Concha ostreae*, dandelion *Taraxicum mongolicum*, garlic *allium sativa*, and sea weeds such as kelp *Laminaria* and *Sargassum*.

Oldenlandria is able to increase the white blood cell count and improve the ability of macrophages to engulf and destroy toxins. It acts to shrink tumors, particularly in the upper body, and improves liver function.

Herbs for Removing the Accumulation of Phlegm (Soften Lumps)

These herbs help to break down the fibrous protein that protects a tumor so that the cells of the immune system can get at it. For soft masses or lumps, the following are used: *Semen Coicis lachryma jobi*, *Bulbus Fritillariae thunbergii*, Chih-ko, *Carapax amydae sinensis*, *Conchae ostreae*, *Sargassum*, *Thallus algae*, *Laminaria*, and *Curcuma aromatica*. To break down hard, painless lumps, use: *Bombyx batryticatus*, *Pericarpum Citri reticulatae viride*, *Sparganium*, *Taraxicum mongolicum*, *Curcuma zedoaria*, *Semen Vaccariae segetalis*, and *Squama Manitis pentadactylae*.

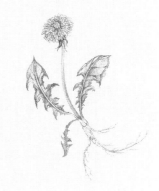

Herbs to Activate the Blood

When the blood is less 'sticky' or has a lower viscosity, circulation is improved and cancer is less likely to develop. In order for cancer cells to metastasize, they need the help of 'sticky' materials in the blood to attach to other sites. Blood-activating herbs help to prevent this from occurring. Herbs that move the blood often also help to prevent scar tissue from forming after surgery and can reduce the side-effects of chemotherapy. They dilate the capillaries, improving the microcirculation to bring nutrition to cells and remove waste. Blood-activating herbs include *Radix Salvia miltiorrhizae*, *Sparganium simplex*, Pangolin scales, Frankincense, *Flos Carthamus tinctoria*, Myrrh, *Curcuma zedoaria*, *Ligusticum wallichii*, *Paeonia rubra*, and *Semen Persica*.

Herbs that Promote the Function of the Internal Organs

Tonic herbs that promote the function of the internal organs and rebuild the body after cancer therapies include Adenophora, Astragalus, Codonopsis, Cordyceps, Coriolus, Ganoderma, Glehnia, Gynostemma, Jujube, Licorice, Ophiopoon, Royal Jelly, and Rehmannia. Together they will improve energy and stamina and tonify the immune system.[16]

Chinese Herbal Formulas for Breast Health

Chinese herbal patent medicines have been developed to perform a combination of the above functions in preventing and treating breast ailments and breast cancer. Please work with a practitioner of Traditional Chinese Medicine before using any of these formulas. Many of these formulas are available at Chinese herbal stores or from Chinese medicine practitioners. See the 'Resources Directory' at the back of this book for mail-order sources.

Formula for Liver QI Stagnation, Obstruction & Breast Distension

Formula	**Xiao Yao Wan**
Contains	Bupleurum, angelica sinensis, atractylodes, paeonia lactiflorae, poria cocos, glycyrrhizae uralensis, zinziber officianalis, herba menthae.
Action	Moves stagnant liver energy, strengthens the spleen, nourishes the blood.
Indication	For liver qi stagnation due to blood deficiency, irregular periods, breast swelling and tenderness, relaxes emotions.
Dosage	8 pills 3x daily. No contraindications.

Formulas for Breast Swelling, Inflammation, or Abscesses

Formula	**Ru He Nei Xiao Tang/Wan (Breast Kernel Inner-Dissolving Pill)**
Contains	Bupleurum, cyperi rotundi, citri reticulatae, curcuma, angelica sinensis, paeonia rubra, spica bulbus vulgaris, rhapontici seu echinops, fasciculus vascularis luffae, glycyrrhizae uralensis.
Action	Removes qi stagnation, blood stagnation and toxic heat.
Indication	For inflammatory swellings of the breasts which have become hot and painful.

Formula	**Ru Bi Xiao (Tablet for Breast Nodules)**
Contains	Laminaria, sargassum, prunella spica, moutan radicis, paeonia rubra, scrophularia, carthami tinctorii, notoginseng, taraxacum, spatholobi, cornu cervi parvum.
Action	Resolves and softens hard lumps and masses. Clears heat and promotes blood circulation.
Indication	Nodular breast masses, including gynecomastia and tuberculosis of the breast
Dosage	1.6 g 3x daily. Do not use in pregnancy.

Formula	**Gua Luo Xiao Yao San**
Contains	Trichosanthis, poriae cocos, curcuma, paeonia lactiflora, bupleurum, angelica sinensis, cyperi rotundi, glycyrrhiza uralensis, mentha haplocalycis, cornu cervi.
Action	Removes qi stagnation, dissolves lumps and opens the collateral meridians. Improves appetite and prevents weight loss.
Indication	Large, relatively soft breast lumps, phlegm accumulation in the breast collaterals.

Formula	**Chih-Ko/Curcuma Tablets (ITM Formula)**
Contains	Citri aurantii, curcuma, myrrh, fritillariae thunbergii, lonicera japonicae, ostrea concha, sargassum, sparginium stoloniferum, curcuma zedoaria, isatis, sophora.
Action	Reduces and softens masses, resolves phlegm, moves stagnant blood, removes toxins.
Indication	For abscesses and tumors.

Formula	**Gynostemma Tablets (ITM Formula)**
Contains	Citri aurantii, curcuma tuber, gynostemma, ganoderma, oldenlandria, astragalus, ostrae concha, sargassum, sparganium, curcumae zedoaria, isatis, sophora.
Action	Enhances immune function, reduces masses, improves qi, resolves phlegm, softens hardness, disperses stagnant blood, removes toxins.
Indication	Reduces swelling, bruising, abscesses and tumors.

Formula	**Blue Citrus Tablets (ITM Formula)**
Contains	Spica prunellae, radix curcuma, ostrae concha, sparganium, isatis
Action	Reduces masses, softens hardness, moves stagnant blood, removes toxins.
Indication	Reduces swelling and bruising, reduces abscesses and tumors.

Formula	**Special Cure for Hyperplasia of the Mammary Gland**
Contains	Scrophularia, scutellaria barbatae, salvia miltiorrhizae, fritillaria, radix curcuma, tinosporae, oldenlandria.
Action	Moves liver stagnation, alleviates depression, dissolves masses, improves energy and moves the blood.
Indication	Breast swelling and pain, mastitis.
Dosage	4-7 tablets 3x daily after meals with boiled water. Prolonged use may cause minor indigestion, dry mouth and dry stools.

Formula	**Xing Xiao Wan (Tumor Reversing Pill)**
Action	Dissolves lumps and masses.
Indication	Breast lumps, abscesses and tumors.

Formula	**Nei Xiao Luo Li Wan**
Action	Dissolves lumps and masses.
Indication	Fibrocystic breast disease, fibroadenomas, breast cancer.
Dosage	8 pills 3 x daily.

Formulas to Strengthen Immunity and Protect from the Side Effects of Chemotherapy

Formula	**Ji Xue Teng Jin Gao Pian (Caulis Millettia Tablets)**
Contains	Millettia reticulata benth.
Action	Increases white blood cell count, builds the blood, relaxes tendons
Indication	For the side effects of chemotherapy and lowered immunity.
Dosage	4 tablets 3 x daily. No contraindications known.

Formula	**Ling Zhi Feng Wang Jiang (Ganoderma-Royal Jelly Essence)**
Contains	Ganoderma, royal jelly, codonopsis, lycii chinensis.
Action	Tonic to strengthen energy and blood.
Indication	Helps prevent the fatigue and weight loss that occurs with cancer and chemo.
Dosage	1 10-cc vial of liquid to be taken daily in the morning. No contraindications.

Formula	**Paris-7 (ITM Formula)**
Contains	Isatis, scutellaria, oldenlandria, sophora.
Action	Removes heat and toxins and inhibits cancer.
Indication	For weakness and toxicity.

Formula	**Coriolus-3 (ITM Formula)**
Contains	Coriolus, ganoderma, cordyceps, sophora
Action	Improves immune response.
Indication	For weight loss and energy depletion.

Formula	**Astragalus/Oldenlandria Tea (ITM Formula)**
Contains	Astragalus, glycyrrhizae uralensis, oldenlandria, rehmannia glutinosa, caulis millettia, salvia miliorrhizae.
Action	Improves immune response, promotes blood circulation, improves digestion.
Indication	For exhaustion, and weakness on exertion.

Formula	**Canelim Tablets (Ping Xiao Pian)**
Contains	Radix curcumae, abrimoniae, fructus aurantii
Action	Promotes blood circulation, alleviates pain, clears toxic heat and toxins, stimulates immunity, shrinks tumors, helps prolong life. This formula is used for prevention and treatment of breast cancer. Dissolves breast masses.
Indication	Active cancer with lowered immunity.
Dosage	4-8 tablets 3x daily.

Immune Tonic Tea

Ingredients: ▶

48g astragalus (huang qi)

24g schizandra (wu wei zi)

24g white atractylodes
(bai zhu)

24g codonopsis (dang shen)

24g ganoderma
(reishi mushroom)

Dosage: 1-2 cups daily, at least one half hour before or two hours after a meal.

Dosage: 15-30 drops tincture, ▶ 3-5 x daily. Use for 6 weeks on, one week off.

Contraindications: Do not use goldenseal during pregnancy or with high blood pressure.

Dosage: 2-3 tablets, 3 x daily. ▶
Contraindications: Do not use in pregnancy.

Dosage: 2-3 tablets, 3 x daily. ▶
Contraindications: Do not use in pregnancy.

Immune Power Formula

Ingredients:

40 parts astragalus

20 parts codonopsis

10 parts ganoderma

10 parts St. John's wort ▶
flowers

5 parts pau d'arco

5 parts ligustrum

Dosage: 30 -60 drops 2-3 times daily. It may be taken long term.

Contraindications: Do not take it during chemotherapy or with medications that St. John's Wort interacts with, such as SSRI anti-depressants.

Immune Enhancing Formulas

Immune Tonic Tea Recipe

This recipe uses Chinese herbs to activate the immune system strongly. The recipe will last for approximately one week if you drink one cup daily or several days if two cups are consumed daily.

Directions: Soak the herbs in 13 cups of water for one hour. Bring to a boil, then simmer for one hour. Strain into a glass jar. Keep refrigerated. The above ingredients are enough for several days to one week of tea. Consider purchasing several bags at once from a Chinese herbal store.

Echinacea and Goldenseal Combination

A formula containing these two cancer fighting and immune stimulating herbs can be used for up to three weeks at a time to deal with an acute infection or for longer periods if dealing with cancer.

Astragalus 10+ (Seven Forests)

This formula of astragalus, eleuthero, ganoderma, ophiopogon, ligustrum, Ho Shou Wu, cistanche, atractylodes, licorice, ginseng, schizandra, and morus fruit is fabulous for nourishing the blood and activating the immune system. It can be used over a long period of time, and improves chronic fatigue and general weakness. Astragalus 10+ is available from Seven Forests Herbs and the Institute for Traditional Medicine (503-233-4907).

Ganoderma 18 (Seven Forests)

Comprised of ganoderma, astragalus, rehmannia, cistanche, peony, ligustrum, epimedium, dioscorea, Tang-Kuei, ophiopogon, atractylodes, Ho Shou Wu, lycium fruit, eucommia, ginseng, schizandra, licorice, and citrus, this formula enhances energy, nourishes the blood, and is useful for lowered immunity and general debility. Ganoderma 18 is available from Seven Forests Herbs and the Institute for Traditional Medicine (503-233-4907).

Immune Power Formula

The following formula is one that I have devised to strongly activate your immune system.

Directions: You can buy these tinctures separately and mix them together in the above ratios, or order the blend from my office using the form at the back of the book.

Herbal Oils for Breast Health

A variety of infused oils can be used to maintain healthy breasts and to alleviate breast cysts. These infused oils are made from fresh plants, except for the calendula blossoms, which are dried for two days first.

Calendula Blossom Oil

Regular use of calendula oil on the breasts will help to reduce breast cysts and prevent breast cancer. It is especially useful after breast surgery to prevent scarring, or to remove old scars and keloids.

Castor Oil

Castor oil at room temperature can be applied morning and night for several months to reduce breast cysts.

Dandelion Oil

Both the flower and the root of dandelion can be used in an oil to reduce breast cysts, clear long-held emotions, and improve liver function.

Poke Root (Phytolacca) Oil

Poke root oil will help to decrease breast swelling and breast cysts. Apply the oil to the area around a lump, cover it with a cotton flannel cloth, and place a hot water bottle on top. Keep the application on for at least an hour. Repeat twice daily until the lump has disappeared. If there is no change after three months, discontinue use.

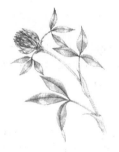

Directions for Making Herbal Oils

From Blossoms: To make an oil from blossoms (calendula, dandelion flower, red clover, St. John's wort) pick dry blossoms on a sunny day, making sure there is no moisture or dew on the flowers. Shade the blossoms from the sun after picking. Fill a dry, large-mouthed, dark glass jar almost full with blossoms. Pour extra virgin olive oil over them until all the flowers are completely covered, stirring with a stick to mix it in. Put a lid on the jar, label the lid with the date and name of the plant, and store it at room temperature. After six weeks, pour the oil through a cotton cheesecloth to remove the plant materials. Store the oil in a cool, dry place until you are ready to use it.

From Roots: To make an oil from a root (poke root, dandelion root), harvest the roots of the plant in the spring or the fall, when the leaves are not actively growing or have fallen off. Carefully dig around the roots and lift them out, shaking off as much dirt as possible. Keep the top of the plant attached. Place them overnight in a shady spot with good ventilation, brushing off more dirt the following morning. Avoid washing the roots unless they were already wet. When dry, chop the roots into small pieces and put them in a dark glass jar with a wide mouth. Cover them with extra virgin olive oil, leaving extra oil on top. Cap and label the jar and strain it after six weeks. Store in a cool dry place until ready for use.

Poke root should not be used continuously for months at a time, but can be used intermittently with other oils, such as red clover.

Red Clover Blossom Oil

Red clover blossom oil will help to remove breast lumps, discourages breast cancer, and improves lymphatic circulation. It can be used daily for breast self-massage.

St. John's Wort Oil

St. John's wort is known particularly for its ability to regenerate and repair the nerves and skin. It is useful after breast surgery (with calendula) to heal damaged tissue, relieve pain, and prevent lymphedema. It can be applied before and after radiation treatments to reduce damage to the skin and to relieve nerve and muscle pain.

Essential Oils

Several essential oils show promise in preventing or reversing breast cancer. A class of chemicals called monoterpenes is present in high amounts in palmarosa, lavender, orange, lemongrass, and geranium. There are three primary therapeutic monoterpenes — geraniol, limonene, and perillyl alcohol. Perillyl alcohol is five times stronger than limonene and is found in particularly high concentrations in palmarosa.[18,19] It is also found in peppermint, spearmint, cherries, celery seeds, and lavender.

Monoterpenes act to inhibit the formation of cholesterol; improve the liver's ability to break down carcinogens by increasing the amount of liver enzymes; stimulate programmed cell death (apoptosis) in breast cancer cells; and selectively block the division and multiplication of cancer cells. Perillyl alcohol has been found to be protective against breast, ovarian, and prostate tumors.[20,21] Other oils which have been used for breast health include Roman chamomile, marjoram, carrot, parsley seed, cypress, and clary sage.

Juniper herb has been found to prevent breast cells from replicating in a laboratory setting. It is a detoxifier for the liver and kidneys and promotes the excretion of uric acid and toxins as well as decreasing fluid retention. Rosemary is antifungal and antiparasitic and stimulates the liver's ability to manufacture the protective C-2 estrogen from estrone. It supports the nerves and is a hormone balancer. Frankincense acts as an immune stimulant, antidepressant, and activates the blood, discouraging metastases.[22]

▶ Healthy Breast Oil Formula

We can combine some of the herbal oils with essential oils to make a blend that will be healing for the breasts. Use the following oils, if available.

Directions: You can make a variation of the above mixture with whatever quality organic essential oils are available to you, or simply use 10 drops of one or more of the essential oils in one ounce (30 ml) of carrier oil. If only a small amount is necessary, use 3-5 drops of essential oil in 5 ml (1 tsp) of base oil. Extra virgin olive oil is the best choice of carrier oil for breast health. Because of its high perillyl alcohol content,

Healthy Breast Oil Formula

Ingredients:
Use 20 ml each of:
Phytolacca oil
Calendula oil
Dandelion oil
Red clover oil

Add 10 drops each of essential oils of:
Palmarosa
Lavender
Rosemary
Juniper
Frankincense
Lemon

Mix with five ounces (150 ml) of carrier oil:
Extra Virgin olive oil

palmarosa oil is your best choice of a single essential oil for protecting from breast cancer. You can also order the Healthy Breast Oil using the form at the back of the book. Women who use it, love it.

Dosage: Gently and lovingly apply the oil mixture to your breasts or body one or more times daily, and use it when you do your breast self-massage. I have the oil beside my bed and put it on just before going to sleep. If you have breast cancer, consider applying the oil several times daily to the tumor site. If using phytolacca oil, take a break from it for one week of each month.

Medicinal Mushrooms

I commonly recommend a blend of the medicinal mushrooms listed below as part of a cancer recovery program. See the 'Resources Directory' section of this book for suppliers.

Maitake (Grifola frondosa)

Maitake has been used as food in Japan for hundreds of years, in amounts up to several hundred grams daily, and is entirely safe. Compounds in Maitake mushrooms called Beta-glucans are able to shrink tumors and have a beneficial effect on the immune system by increasing macrophage activity.[23,24,25,26] The most important of these compounds is called the D-fraction constituent. In a non-randomized clinical study of advanced stage (III-IV) breast cancer patients, tumor regression or significant symptom improvements were observed in 11 out of 15 women.[27] It also inhibits the formation of metastases.[28] Maitake lessens the side effects of chemotherapy, helping to decrease nausea, keep the white blood cell count high, and reduce pain. One manufacturer is Maitake Products, Inc. (www.maitake.com), which produces a Maitake D-fraction extract in liquid form. The dosage is 1 mg per kg of body weight per day, which for a 150-lb woman is 34-68 drops daily.

Shitake (Lentinus edodes)

Shitake mushrooms have been well-studied since the 1960s and possess constituents that have anti-tumor properties and enhance immune function. They contain two compounds called lentinan and LEM which increase macrophage and natural killer cell activity as well as interferon levels. A derivative of lentinan has been used as an injectible anti-cancer drug in Asia. This mushroom also exerts anti-viral and anti-bacterial effects and reduces cholesterol. It has been used as a tonic for chronic fatigue syndrome.[29,30] Shitake mushrooms taste delicious and can be added to stir fries and soups or made into a spread for vegetables and sandwiches. They are a staple in the macrobiotic diet, which has long been used in cancer recovery. Shitake mushrooms are available in dried form in Chinese herbal stores or fresh in supermarkets.

Reishi (Ganoderma lucidum)

Also known as the 'Mushroom of Immortality', Ganoderma has been consumed for almost 2,000 years in China. Its cancer-fighting con-

FACT
Medicinal mushrooms have been traditionally used in China and Japan for their immune and energy enhancing effects. They are now more frequently used in North America during cancer treatment to offset the effects of chemotherapy and radiation.

stituents are B-Glucans, Hetero-B-Glucans, and Ling Zhi-8 Protein. These act to shrink tumors, enhance the immune system by increasing T-cell function, strengthening stamina, and reducing cholesterol, and are anti-viral.[31] This mushroom also has anti-oxidant and anti-inflammatory properties and has been used effectively for arthritis. Reishi mushrooms increase the absorption of oxygen by the lungs and have a positive benefit to patients with chronic fatigue syndrome. They have very low toxicity even at very high dosages but should not be used during surgery as their vasodilation effect can result in excess bleeding. Use cautiously in women with heavy menstruation.

Zhu ling (Polyporus umbellatus)

This mushroom contains B-Glucan, which has anti-tumor and immune-enhancing properties.[32] Zhu Ling has antibiotic, anti-inflammatory, diuretic and liver protecting action. Studies have demonstrated that it improves immune function after chemotherapy and radiation and decreases cancer recurrence.[33]

Royal Sun Agaricus (Agaricus blazei)

This mushroom has very strong anti-tumor properties and contains more B-glucans than most, if not all, other mushrooms. It is immune enhancing and has caused complete recovery in cancer infected laboratory animals.[34] It also acts as an anti-viral and reduces cholesterol levels. It is available in tincture form.

Turkey Tail (Trametes coriolus versicolor)

Compounds from this mushroom have been shown to inhibit the growth of cancer cells and to increase the immune system's number of natural killer cells, which directly target cancer cells.[35] It has been used clinically in the treatment of cervical, breast, colon, stomach and lung cancer. Breast cancer patients who were positive for the HLA B40 antigen derived the greatest benefit. Trametes is the source of the anticancer drug known as 'Krestin', which has been demonstrated to increase the disease-free survival rate of cancer patients in Asia.[36,37] Also available in tincture form.

MGN-3

Dosage: 250-750 mg daily. Contraindications: Do not use if you are allergic to mushrooms.

MGN-3 is an extract of the outer shell of rice bran combined with extracts from the following three mushrooms: Shitake, Kawaratake, and Suehirotake. It improves the ability of T-killer cells to destroy cancer cells by increasing the number of explosive granules in the T-killer cells. MGN-3 increases the body's levels of interferon and tumor necrosis factors, both of which help to destroy cancer cells. In one study involving 24 cancer patients who took the product for two months, the T-killer cells became 27 times more effective at killing cancer cells than they had been prior to treatment.[38] Used with chemotherapy, MGN-3 lessens toxic side effects of the chemo and fortifies the white blood cells.

Our Lymphatic and Immune Systems

Summary

Your lymphatic and immune systems are your body's defense system. Their fundamental role is to protect the life of the body by distinguishing 'self' from 'non-self' and recognizing what needs to be eliminated or destroyed (a cancer cell, virus, bacteria, environmental toxin, internal toxin). The stronger your immune system is, the more resistant to breast cancer you are.

1) Activate you lymphatic system with one or more of the following daily practices: dry brush massage, contrast showers, rebounding, going braless, and breast self-massage.
2) Watch your breathing throughout the day and deepen it to improve the flow of the lymph.
3) Make up a blend of herbal and essential oils for your breasts, keep it by your bed, and apply it nightly.
4) As prevention, consider using both a lymphatic formula, such as the Healthy Breast Formula or the Hoxsey Formula, as well as an immune activating formula or tea for 1-3 months per year, particularly during the winter. If you are recovering from breast cancer, use both formulas continuously with short breaks every 6 weeks.
5) Drink pau d'arco tea and decaffeinated green tea regularly, and use Chyavan Prash when you can.
6) Use the herbs burdock root, goldenseal, echinacea, astragalus, and codonopsis to nourish the spleen if you are dealing with a bacterial infection, rather than antibiotics.
7) Sugar and excessive sweets decrease immunity — limit your sweet intake to occasional use.

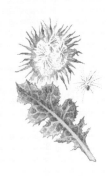

Eating Right for Breast Health

CONTENTS

EXERCISES, CHARTS, CHECKLISTS & WORKSHEETS

Each of us has a unique biochemistry, constitution, and dietary needs. In my naturopathic practice, I recognize that there is no one diet that suits all people. Some of us are fine as vegetarians; others seem to need animal protein now and then. Some individuals are reactive to carbohydrates, others to beans, tofu, or nuts and seeds. Raw food is easily digested by certain individuals but too much causes diarrhea or flatulence in others. Many of us gain weight easily and need to monitor our fat intake closely, while the lucky few may be able to feast on avocados with no weight gain. You know your body best and will be able to tell how it responds to a particular diet.

Having said that, there are foods we can eat and foods we can avoid to help prevent breast cancer. Adopt as much of these dietary recommendations as agree with you. Work with a health professional to create a dietary program tailored for you using some or all of the recommendations in this chapter. In creating guidelines for a diet that protects us from breast cancer, I have considered many healing traditions. These include the macrobiotic diet as outlined by Michio Kushi, the Hippocrates health diet promoted by Ann Wigmore, the Gerson diet, the Hallelujah diet promoted by George Malkmus, Dr Joanna Budwig's use of flaxseed oil with sulphur-containing protein, food combining, an anti-candida diet, rotation diets to improve immunity, and scientific research into the field of breast cancer. Although my recommendations are not true to any of the above traditions, they integrate some of their best principles.

Organic Food

Organic food by definition is food that has not been sprayed with chemicals and is not genetically engineered – in other words, it's just the way nature made it. Here are some of the reasons why we should eat organic food. Women farmers around Windsor, Ontario are nine times more likely to get breast cancer than women from other occupations, and women living in areas of Canada where lindane was used on canola (Marquette, Manitoba) have the highest incidence of breast cancer in the country. Pesticides (endosulfan, propazine) commonly used on our lettuce, carrots, and cucumbers promote breast cancer in animals. Israel's breast cancer rate dropped 8% after they banned the use of three pesticides – lindane, DDT and alpha-BHC. Two or three pesticides acting together on our food can have a synergistic estrogenic effect 1000 times greater than either pesticide alone, and an average Canadian peach contains 31 pesticides. If we want to keep our breasts and the breasts of our children, we need to eat organic food.

Organic food has fewer of these dangerous chemicals and is richer in cancer-fighting nutrients.[1] An Italian study done in 2002 found that vitamin C and E levels were higher in organic peaches and pears than in non-organic ones.[2] Organic crops contain significantly more vitamin C, iron, magnesium, and phosphorus than their chemically grown cousins.[3]

Transform your lawn by growing your own vegetables in a front or backyard garden. (My tiny front yard garden provides my family and the neighbors with lettuce and tomatoes all summer long.) Ask makers of your favorite brands of foods to use organically grown crops in their products. Insist on an organic section in local supermarkets. Push your city governments into establishing community gardens and investigate the principles of permaculture to transform our cities into green oases.[4]

Vegetarianism

A vegetarian diet is one that does not include meat, poultry, or fish, but may include dairy and eggs. A lacto-ovo vegetarian will include dairy products and eggs as part of their diet. A vegan is a vegetarian who avoids dairy, eggs, and all animal products.

The vitamins, minerals, fiber, and phytochemicals in vegetables and fruit offer significant protection from breast cancer, particularly when eaten raw, as enzymes and vitamins are destroyed through heating, as are the indoles in the brassica family of foods. For example, the incidence of cancers of all types is 30-40% lower in Seventh Day Adventists, who are strict vegetarians.[5,6] The present trend to early onset of puberty in young girls can be reversed when a vegetarian diet is eaten rather than the standard North American diet.[7] Eating lower on the food chain decreases the quantity of environmental chemicals that we ingest. We saw in Chapter 3 that a low fat, high fiber vegan diet was best for managing our estrogens. In Chapter 5, we found that animal protein creates strong acids that use up our alkaline mineral reserve.

FACT
A 2003 study published in the *Journal of Agriculture and Food Chemistry* showed that levels of antioxidants and other cancer-fighting compounds were over 50% higher in organically grown food than in conventionally grown food.

PREVENTION
Eat and grow organic food.

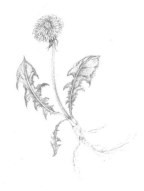

FACT
Research shows that a vegetarian diet prevents 20-50% of all cancers.

PREVENTION
Consume a primarily vegetarian diet of at least 50-80% raw vegetables and fruit. Eat 6-9 servings daily, where one serving is equal to $1/2$ cup of vegetables or one cup of salad or one large piece of fruit.

Cancer Fighting Phytochemicals

The following chart shows the 'phyto' or plant chemicals in common foods that are effective in fighting cancer.[9,10] Try to eat at least one food from each of these categories daily.

Phytochemical	Effect
Allyl sulfides	Increases liver enzymes to detoxify carcinogens.
Capsaicin	Prevents carcinogens from binding to DNA.
Carotenoids	Act as antioxidants that neutralize free radicals, enhance immunity, and high intake is associated with low cancer rates. They promote cell differentiation.
Polyphenols	Act as antioxidants; reduce damaging effects of nitrosamines. Kills human cancer cells.
Flavonoids	Prevents the attachment of cancer-causing hormones to cells by blocking receptor sites.
Curcumin	Assists the liver in detoxifying carcinogens. Arrests cancer cells.
Ellagic acid	Neutralizes carcinogens in the liver, antioxidant, inhibits cancer cell divisions.
Isoflavones (genistein and daidzen)	Bind to the estrogen receptor so that harmful estrogens can't bind; block the formation of blood vessels to tumors, inhibit enzymes that might cause cancer; inhibits activation of breast cancer genes.
Indoles	Induce protective enzymes, stimulate C2 estrogen production. Decreases the estrogen that initiates breast cancer.
Isothiocyanates	Prevents DNA damage; blocks the production of tumors induced by environmental chemicals, act as antioxidants, assist liver detoxification.
Limonoids	Induce protective enzymes in liver and intestines that fight cancer.
Linolenic Acid	Regulates production of prostaglandins in cells.
Lycopene	Protects from cell damage.
Lutein	Protects against cell damage.
Monoterpenes	Antioxidant properties, induce protective enzymes, inhibit cholesterol production in tumors, stimulate the destruction of breast cancer cells, inhibit growth of cancer cells.
Phenolic Acids	Block the effects of free radicals; inhibit the formation of nitrosamine, a carcinogen.
Plant Sterols (beta-sitosterol)	Prevent cells from becoming cancerous . and lowers fat levels in the body.
Protease Inhibitors	Block the activity of enzymes involved in the growth of tumors.
Quercetin	Slows down cell division.
Quinones	Neutralize carcinogens.
Sulforaphane	Increases the ability of the liver's detoxifying enzymes to remove carcinogens. Is an antioxidant.

Food Sources

garlic, onions, leeks

chili peppers

parsley, carrots, spinach, kale, winter squash,
apricots, cantaloupe, sweet potatoes

broccoli, carrots, green tea, cucumbers,
squash, mint, basil, citrus

most fruits and vegetables, including parsley, carrots, citrus,
broccoli, cabbage, cucumbers, squash, yams, eggplant, peppers, berries

turmeric

red raspberries, walnut skin

soybeans, tofu, miso, lentils, dried beans, split peas, garbanzo beans,
green beans, green peas, mung bean sprouts, red clover sprouts

raw cabbage, broccoli, Brussels sprouts, kale, cauliflower,
bok choy, kohlrabi, mustard, turnips

mustard, horseradish, radishes, turnips, cabbage, broccoli, cauliflower,
Brussels sprouts, kale, bok choy, watercress, garden sorrel

citrus fruit rind, essential oils of lemon, orange, celery, lemongrass

flaxseeds and flaxseed oil

tomatoes, red grapefruit, guava

spinach, kiwi, tomato, grapes

cherries, lavender, parsley, yams, carrots, broccoli, cabbage,
basil, cucumbers, peppers, squash, , eggplant, mint, tomatoes, grapefruit

berries, broccoli, grapes, citrus, parsley, peppers, soy, squash,
tomatoes, grains

broccoli, cabbage, soy, peppers, whole grains

beans and soy products

onions, apples, green cabbage

rosemary, pau d'arco tea

broccoli sprouts, broccoli, cauliflower, Brussels sprouts

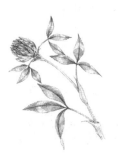

Cancer Fighting Phytochemicals

A broad class of constituents known as phytochemicals work synergistically in fruits and vegetables to prevent breast cancer. Particularly good vegetable choices are those in the brassica family, as well as onions, garlic and leeks, sprouts, and sea vegetables. These should be consumed daily. Foods high in beta carotene are protective against breast cancer. These include orange fruits and vegetables and leafy greens. Many fruits and vegetables are naturally high in anti-oxidants, which protect us from cancer.[8]

Raw Foods

Because enzymes are destroyed at temperatures higher than 129°F or 50°C, we should focus on eating foods rich in enzymes, including raw fruits and vegetables, sprouted seeds and grains. Many vitamins are also destroyed through heating, as are the indoles in the brassica family of foods. If you cannot digest raw food, cook it lightly through steaming or the use of a slow-cooker. Consider the use of supplemental plant enzymes before meals if cooked food is the mainstay.

Beneficial Brassicas

Particularly potent healing vegetables include members of the brassica family, which are cabbage, broccoli, cauliflower, Brussels sprouts, bok choy, kale, kohlrabi, turnips, rutabagas, garden sorrel, radish, watercress, and collards. We can enjoy the beneficial effects of brassicas by eating coleslaw several times a week, adding cabbage to salads, consuming raw broccoli and cauliflower with hummus or other bean dips, and adding broccoli sprouts to our main dishes and salads. We can drink fresh vegetable juices daily, including cabbage, kale, bok choy, garden sorrel, watercress, or collard juices. Kale, Brussels sprouts, and the other brassicas can be lightly steamed and served as a side dish or mixed in a tofu stir-fry. Use the brassicas with seaweeds or dulse powder whenever possible.

Animals eating diets supplemented with vegetables from the brassica family develop far fewer breast tumors than animals that do not eat these vegetables.[11] A phytochemical in these called indole-3-carbinol helps to inactivate potentially harmful estrogens and prevent breast cancer.[12] Indole-3-carbinol is present in cabbage juice as well as cabbage itself, so the simplest way to get our daily dose of 300 mg might be to juice ⅓ of a cabbage daily along with carrots and beets. To have the greatest effect, the brassicas should be eaten raw or only lightly steamed. Heavy cooking destroys indoles.

Thiols and isothiocyanates are sulfur-containing phytochemicals that help to prevent DNA damage and block the production of tumors induced by environmental chemicals. Sulforaphane is a particular isothiocyanate that increases the effectiveness of Phase 2 detoxification enzymes in the liver. It is highest in three-day-old broccoli sprouts.

For people with an underactive thyroid or goiter, caution is advised when consuming raw brassicas, although they are fine when cooked. In some people they may interfere with thyroid function. This is ameliorated in part by ingesting sea vegetables daily.[13]

Sprouts and Cereal Grasses

Sprouts and cereal grasses are powerhouses of minerals, vitamins, and enzymes. Sprouts can be grown in your kitchen or purchased at supermarkets, while cereal grasses are present in many powdered green supplements, such as Greens+, Pure Synergy, and Barley Green, to name a few. All of these help to alkalinize the body, and are especially rich in beta-carotene.

Mung bean sprouts have the highest content of the phytoestrogen coumestrol and also contain significant amounts of genistein and daidzen. They are inexpensive and versatile — we can use them in salads, stir-fries, mixed into bean and rice dishes, or juiced with vegetables. Clover sprouts contain high amounts of the phytoestrogens genistein and daidzen and are simple and inexpensive to grow at home.

Three-day-old broccoli sprouts have the highest amount of sulforaphane in broccoli's growth cycle. The amount of sulforaphane available from only 5 g of three-day-old sprouts is equal to what we would get from 150 g of adult broccoli. Sulforaphane has been found to inhibit chemically induced cancers in rats.[14,15]

Sprouts are best consumed at the beginning of the meal because their enzyme power will assist in digesting food.

FACT
Significant amounts of phytoestrogens that protect us from breast cancer are available in mung bean, red clover, soybean, yellow pea, green lentil, chick pea, fenugreek, adzuki bean, alfalfa, and fava bean sprouts.

PREVENTION
Aim to eat at least six cups of sprouts weekly. Consume 2-3 tsp twice daily of a cereal grass supplement, mixed in water or juice, such as spirulina, Greens+, Pure Synergy, or Barley Green.

Directions for Sprouting Broccoli Seeds

We can provide ourselves with a natural form of chemotherapy by ingesting a few tablespoons of broccoli sprouts daily. We can even grow them in our kitchen laboratories! Add them to soup, stir-fries, bean dishes, salads, and tofu dishes, have them on toast or use them in juices. Sprout other seeds in the same way.

1) Seeds should be untreated with pesticides and organic.
2) Place 3 tsp of seeds in a glass jar with a wide mouth. Cover the seeds with one cup of distilled or filtered water and soak for 8-12 hours.
3) Cover the mouth of the jar with a piece of cheesecloth or screen secured with a rubber band. Drain out the water and rinse the seeds again. Place the jar in a dish drainer upside down.
4) Rinse them three times daily adding 1 tsp of food grade hydrogen peroxide to the rinse water each time to prevent fungal growth, and then place the jar upside down in the drainer after each rinse. Keep them near a light source to accelerate growth and increase chlorophyll.
5) Eat after three days, or keep them refrigerated. Sulforaphane content diminishes each consecutive day after the third day of growth.
6) Prevent the growing sprouts from becoming moldy by using a wide mouth jar to increase air circulation, and by rinsing several times daily, being sure that they drain well.

Garlic, Onions, and Leeks

Garlic has been proven to inhibit the growth of both estrogen receptor positive and ER negative breast cancer cells and helps prevent the initiation, promotion, and recurrence of many forms of cancer.[16,17] Garlic is especially high in the trace minerals selenium and germanium, which reduce the risk of cancer.[18] It contains protective antioxidants, isoflavones, and allyl sulfides (see chart above). Garlic also shields us from many species of bacteria, fungi,

PREVENTION
Eat a raw onion or leek and 1-3 cloves of garlic daily or slow-cook them in soup.

parasites, and viruses especially when we consume at least 10 g or three cloves daily.[19] Garlic, onions and leeks contain sulfur bearing amino acids, which aid the liver in its detoxification pathways.

Sea Vegetables

Sea vegetables include nori, arame, hijiki, kelp, dulse, and kombu. They offer significant protection against radiation and breast cancer, are high in trace minerals, and are a very alkaline food.[20] They have long been used in Chinese medicine to dissolve tumors, particularly kelp. Animals given seaweeds as 2% of their diet were half as likely to develop chemically-induced breast cancer as animals not fed seaweeds.[21]

Sea vegetables contain substantial amounts of calcium and iron. They are also rich in iodine, an essential nutrient for the thyroid gland and one of the integral components of the Gerson therapy. Iodine is present in the cells lining the ducts and lobules of our breasts, and makes them less sensitive to stimulation from estrogen. With the farming methods used today, the soil and our foods are deficient in minerals such as iodine, zinc, and selenium.

Dandelion Root and Leaves

Dandelion root prevents and reverses breast cancer, decreases estrogen levels, promotes bile flow, and reduces lymphatic congestion.[22] In Chinese medicine, a relative of dandelion is used specifically to reduce hard breast nodules.[23] The leaves are very high in vitamin A and minerals.

Fresh Vegetable Juices

Juices supply vitamins, minerals, and phytochemicals that support good health. We need the alkaline minerals in vegetable juices to offset our body's overacidity that leads to illness. The Gerson Therapy Center regularly treats patients with advanced cancer using 13 glasses daily of various raw organic juices prepared hourly. They also serve three full vegetarian meals daily, freshly prepared from organically grown vegetables, fruits, and whole grains. Some vegetables that are particularly healthful juiced include carrot, beet, cabbage, parsley, watercress, asparagus, potato, tomato, bok choy, mustard greens, and kale.

The staple for breast cancer prevention is two parts carrot, one part beet, and one part cabbage juice. Dulse or kelp powder, ground flaxseeds, citrus peels, garlic, ginger, and sprouts (broccoli, red clover, mung bean) can be added to vegetable juice combinations for greater benefit and to decrease the glycemic load.

When you drink several glasses of vegetable juice daily, your body will quickly detoxify, and must be supported in the cleansing process with the use of liver regenerating herbs and bowel cleansers or enemas.

Lycopene Rich Tomatoes

Lycopene is a form of carotene and acts as a good antioxidant. Its structure gives a deep red color to the fruits and vegetables in which it is present, including tomatoes, watermelon, pink grapefruit, guava, and rosehip. Tomatoes are by far the highest source: approximately 85% of dietary lycopene comes from tomatoes and tomato products. Lycopene is more bio-available when tomatoes are heated and processed; there is five times more available lycopene in tomato sauces than in an equivalent amount of fresh tomatoes. Olive oil used in the cooking of tomatoes improves lycopene absorption.

In the body, lycopene is found in the liver, breasts, prostate gland, colon, and skin. It protects us from cancers of the breast, cervix, mouth, pharynx, esophagus, stomach, bladder, colon, and rectum by stalling cell division in cancer cells.[24,25,26] The benefits of lycopene can be gained by drinking about two glasses of tomato juice daily.[27]

A little caution is necessary before we consume a lot of processed tomato products. People with arthritis may find that their joints are made worse by tomatoes. My suggestion would be to include tomatoes in your diet twice weekly generally, less often if you have arthritis, are overly acidic, or have an allergy to them. Lycopene is also available in supplement form, and the recommended daily dose is 15 mg.

PREVENTION
Consume tomatoes or tomato products regularly, at least twice weekly unless contraindicated by joint pain or allergy.

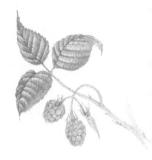

Flavonoid and Limonene Rich Citrus

Citrus juices and peel contain flavonoids and limonene, natural antioxidants that inhibit the growth and proliferation of breast cancer cells.

Limonene is an oil that assists the liver in removing carcinogens and nourishes the production of digestive enzymes. It is found in highest amounts in the peels of citrus fruit, with the juice containing lesser amounts. Limonene is also found in dill, lemon, caraway, and mint.

Animal studies have shown that limonene can prevent breast cancer caused by environmental chemicals and can shrink existing breast tumors.[28] Ninety percent of tumors became smaller and the number of new tumors was reduced by 50% when animals were fed a diet containing 10% d-limonene.[29] A phytochemical closely related to limonene is perillyl alcohol, which is over five times stronger that limonene in its action on breast tumors. It is found in high amounts in the essential oils of palmarosa, lavender and in cherries.

PREVENTION
Include fresh citrus fruits, juices, and peel in your diet regularly. Add organic citrus peel to your diet by grating a little over your salad or using the peel in your tea daily. Drink mint tea and make dill a familiar kitchen herb. Use essential oils of palmarosa, lemon, and lavender in a base of olive oil on your skin. The most effective way to use limonene and perillyl alcohol is topically through an essential oil blend. See the recipe for Healthy Breast Oil in Chapter 6, 'Activating Our Lymphatic and Immune Systems.'

Citrus Flavonoids

This chart outlines the effectiveness of citrus flavonoids in reducing breast cancer in animal studies.

Type of Citrus	Flavonoid	Effectiveness
Grapefruit	naringenin	effective
Oranges and lemons	hesperetin	more effective
Tangerines	tangeretin and nobiletin	most effective, but tangeretin interferes with Tamoxifen

---

'Good' Fats and 'Bad' Fats

Over the last decade there has been much confusion about the role of fat in breast cancer risk. It is not so much the amount of fat that is the problem, but the kinds of fats used in our diets and the ratios that exist between them. Also of importance is the way in which these fats are both processed and packaged. We still do not know all the facts about fat and breast cancer, but approximate guidelines can be made based on what we do know. [30,31,32]

'Good' Essential Fatty Acids
(alpha-linolenic acid and linoleic acid)

Our bodies cannot make the two essential fatty acids: alpha-linolenic acid, which belongs to the 'Omega 3' family; and linoleic acid, part of the 'Omega 6' family of oils. Diets that recommend no fat will make us sick, for these 'fats' are necessary for life. Together these oils promote good health. They maintain the integrity of the cell membrane, making it less vulnerable to carcinogenic substances.

Actions

Essential fatty acids are the precursors for hormones and about 50 different chemical messengers called prostaglandins. Prostaglandins are made by every one of our cells and progress down one of several pathways to either create disease or restore health. Prostaglandins regulate blood pressure and arterial function and play an important role in calcium and energy metabolism. They prevent inflammation and help to control arthritis. Certain prostaglandins inhibit cancer growth by regulating the rate of cell division and improving the function of the T-cells, the guardians of our immune systems. Others promote cancer.

Essential fatty acids are unique in that they attract oxygen, absorb sunlight, and carry a slight negative charge. Because of the negative charge, their molecules repel each other, causing them to spread out in a very thin layer over surfaces. This ability, called surface activity, allows them to carry toxic substances to the surface of the skin, intestinal tract, kidneys, or lungs where these substances can be eliminated. The negative charge allows them to bind to protein molecules.

Essential fatty acids also perform the following functions: they are able to increase the rate of metabolic reactions in the body when used in amounts higher than 15% of one's total calories, resulting in fat burn-off and weight loss; they are digested slowly and prevent hunger for as long as 5-8 hours after a meal; they help transport excess cholesterol so that it does not clog the arteries; they help to generate the electrical currents that keep the heartbeat rhythmic; they are found around the DNA where they regulate chromosome stability, preventing damage from radiation and chemical toxicity; they are required in cell membrane formation; they are essential in the health of the immune system; they are required for brain development in infants and children and a deficiency during fetal development can result in permanent learning disabilities; and they can help to buffer excess acid in the body.

FACT

Omega 3 fatty acids, found primarily in flaxseed oil, purslane, black currant seed oil, and cold water fish oils, protect us from breast cancer. Saturated fats, found in meat, butter, animal products, coconut oil, and peanut oil, increase breast cancer risk, as do hydrogenated and partially hydrogenated fats. Omega 6 oils will promote breast cancer if not balanced with at least twice as much Omega 3 oil.

FACT

Essential fatty acids help transport oxygen from the air in the lungs to each cell membrane in the body, where the oxygen acts as a barrier to viruses, bacteria, parasites, and cancer.

Omega 3 Fatty Acids

Omega 3 fatty acids play a key role in our health. Symptoms of Omega 3 fatty acid deficiency include growth retardation, poor vision, learning disabilities, tingling in the arms and legs, loss of motor coordination, defective glandular regulation, and behavioral problems. Omega 3 fatty acids are divided into four subgroups: alpha-linolenic acid (LNA), stearidonic acid (SDA), eicosapentaenoic acid (EPA), and docosahexaenoic acid (DHA). Alpha-linolenic acid is the essential fatty acid found in flaxseeds, hemp seeds, pumpkin seeds, soy beans, walnuts, purslane, and dark green leafy vegetables. Flaxseed is the finest of these, containing 57% of its oil as LNA. It also contains less than 20% Omega 6 oil as linoleic acid, the other essential fatty acid. Stearidonic acid is found in black currant seeds.

Omega 3 fatty oils possess anti-tumor qualities and are antimiotic (preventing cell division) and anti-viral.[35] Populations who consume higher amounts of Omega 3 fatty acids have lower breast cancer rates.[36,37]

Flaxseed Oil and Fish Oil

The best dietary source of alpha-linolenic acid is flaxseed oil. In his book, *Fats that Heal, Fats that Kill*, Udo Erasmus states that flaxseed oil is the only oil recommended for cancer patients.[38] In studies on rats, Lilian Thompson and her co-workers from the University of Toronto found that flaxseed oil and flaxseeds reduced the growth of established tumors in late stage cancer.[39] Other studies have verified flaxseed oil's ability to suppress tumor growth.[40] Flaxseed oil prevents cancer cells from sticking to other tissue cells, decreasing the likelihood of metastases.[41]

Flaxseed oil should never be used for cooking but can be used on food such as beans, grains, vegetables, and baked potatoes after they have been cooked. It can also be used on bread instead of butter. It should be used within six weeks of purchase and kept in the freezer (it will not freeze) or refrigerator between use. It is fine mixed with lemon as a salad dressing. If you dislike the taste of flaxseed oil, buy it in capsule form. In my family, we bring the flaxseed oil on to the table with dinner and frequently 'pass the oil, please' from one person to the next.

Another good source of Omega 3 fatty acids is fish oil. Eicosapentaenoic acid and docosahexaenoic acid are found in fish oils such as salmon, trout, white tuna, mackerel, sardines, cod liver oil, and herring oil. Because fish oils are often highly processed and can be contaminated with environmental pollutants, we should use them only if we are certain of their purity and quality. One study on mice found that even low amounts of dietary fish oil (7% of caloric intake) raised levels of Omega 3 oils in cell membranes, and after 5 weeks, fish oil supplementation was just as effective as the chemotherapy drug, Doxorubicin, in slowing tumor growth.[42]

FACT

Omega 3 fats weaken the effect of estrogen on breast cells and balance the tumor-promoting effects of Omega 6 fatty acids when used in a ratio of approximately 2:1, Omega 3:Omega 6. The most benefit of the Omega 3 essential fatty acids is obtained when their amount is greater than the Omega 6, reducing the initiation, progression, and metastasis of breast cancer.[33,34]

PREVENTION

If you are in good health, consume 1-2 tbsp of flaxseed oil daily, along with at least 2 tbsp of ground flaxseeds. Also use fish oil capsules (700 mg daily) containing EPA and DHA, but be sure they are free of contaminants. If you have a degenerative condition, like arthritis, diabetes, or cancer, take 3-5 tbsp of flaxseed oil daily with 2-4 tbsp of seeds. Individuals with cancer metastases can take 6-7 tbsp daily along with 6-7 tbsp of ground seeds daily. Only buy refrigerated flax oil and use it within 6 weeks.

FACT

Vitamin E protects from oxidative damage when consuming essential fatty acids such as flaxseed oil. Vitamin B6 is required in essential fatty acid metabolism, along with other minerals and vitamins, and should be included in your diet or supplements in the dose of 50-200 mg per day.

Consume small amounts of Omega 6 oils in the form of raw unsalted nuts and seeds (1-2 tablespoons daily). Balance this with a higher amount of flaxseed oil (Omega 3). If you have cancer, do not use these seeds — take only flaxseeds, flaxseed oil, and fish oil certified to be free of PCBs and dioxin.

FACT

In higher amounts, all Omega 6 oils promote breast cancer and its metastases when other causative factors are present, when they are used in excess without the balancing influence of Omega 3 oils, or when they are improperly processed.[44,45]

Omega 6 Fatty Acids

There are four types of Omega 6 fatty acids: linoleic acid (LA), gamma-linolenic acid (GLA), dihomogamma-linolenic acid (DGLA), and arachidonic acid (AA). Linoleic acid is found in safflower, sunflower, hemp, soybean, walnut, pumpkin, sesame, and flax. Gamma-linolenic acid is found in borage, black currant seed, and evening primrose oil. Dihomogamma-linolenic acid is found in mother's milk. Arachidonic acid is found in meats and other animal products.

We need some linoleic acid regularly, as our bodies do not make it. Adding a small amount of sunflower seeds, sesame seeds, almonds, and pumpkin seeds to our diets supplies us with this oil. However, we must be cautious not to consume too much Omega 6 fatty acids.

Evening primrose oil containing GLA is very beneficial for many ailments, including fibrocystic breast disease, menopausal symptoms, eczema, and learning disabilities.

Studies on rats suggest that GLA also inhibits breast cancer when used in amounts less than or equal to 1% of their diets (about 1/3 tsp for humans). However, in amounts higher than this, the body may convert GLA into something called DGLA, which becomes arachidonic acid with the help of an enzyme called delta 5 desaturase. This enzyme is activated by sugar in the diet and high insulin levels, which are common in breast cancer patients. Arachidonic acid promotes tumor growth. One study in mice found that 8% dietary GLA caused both an increase in lung metastases and an increase in arachidonic acid in their cell membranes.[43] Therefore I do not recommend evening primrose oil to women with a breast cancer history.

We don't know yet what the precise ratio of these oils should be to prevent or reverse breast cancer. Udo Erasmus recommends a 2:1 ratio of Omega 3 to Omega 6 essential fatty acids, present in his oil blend called 'Udo's Choice' for overall health. A ratio of 4:1 has been found to decrease mortality from heart disease by 70%; a ratio of 2.5:1 decreased growth of colorectal cancer, and a ratio greater than 2:1 was associated with decreased breast cancer risk in several studies.[46]

Omega 6 oils are commonly found in margarine, mayonnaise, and store bought salad dressings, and are added to packaged foods such as crackers. Their amounts have increased substantially in the North American diet in the last two decades, probably contributing to breast cancer incidence. One reason that Omega 6 fatty acids may be harmful in excess is that they are easily transformed into trans fatty acids through refinement and hydrogenation.

Omega 9 (Olive Oil)

The Omega 9 fatty acid (known as oleic acid) is found in olive oil. In Mediterranean countries where olive oil consumption is high, there are lower breast cancer rates than in Northern European countries.[47] Because olive oil promotes the flow of bile in the liver, and the bile carries toxins, it helps us detoxify the liver and gall-bladder more efficiently.

We can use extra virgin olive oil, purchased in a metal or opaque glass container, in moderation. It is best not to cook with olive oil, but to use it in salad dressings and on foods after they have been cooked, or on bread. One way to minimize the harm done to olive oil when it is cooked is to add 1-2 tablespoons of water to the pot before adding the oil. This will prevent the olive oil from getting too hot, as its temperature will not exceed that of the water. If the oil starts to sizzle and pop, it's too hot.

Processing of Oils

The integrity of essential fatty acids is easily destroyed by light, air, and heat, so careful processing and packaging of them are crucial. Refined vegetable oils have been distilled at 300°F, bleached at 230°F, deodorized at 450°F, and preserved with chemicals. This alters the fat molecules, creating 'trans' fatty acids that are toxic. Essential fatty acids should be packaged in opaque glass bottles where there is no exposure to light, as light speeds up the reaction of the oil to air 1000 times, resulting in rancid oil. The processing should be done in an environment with no oxygen, as the oxygen breaks down the essential fatty acids, also causing rancid oil. 'Good' oil will be pressed and packaged in the dark, with no oxygen, and stored in opaque glass containers, which exclude air and oxygen.

'Bad' Fats to Avoid

It is too simplistic to tell women to avoid all fats as a method of preventing breast cancer, for there are 'fats that heal and fats that kill', as Udo Erasmus has described in his book of the same title, but here are some basic guidelines.

Hydrogenated Fats

All oils altered by processing are toxic. Processing includes hydrogenation, deep frying, refining, deodorizing, and exposure to light, heat, or oxygen during storage.

The process of hydrogenation, used in making margarine and vegetable shortening, can shift the shape of naturally occurring cis fatty acids, which are flexible and fluid at room temperature, into their trans forms, which are more solid. Hydrogenated fats containing trans fatty acids interfere with immune function and increase breast cancer risk. Margarine contains 30-50% trans fatty acids. These are also present in potato chips, fried foods, French fries, commercial baked goods, cookies, and crackers. The more trans fatty acids that are present in the diet, the more essential fatty acids are needed to repair the cellular damage they cause.[48]

PREVENTION
Aim to make up 15-20 % of your daily caloric intake from good fats, with a higher ratio daily of Omega 3 to Omega 6 oil, and with some olive oil (from the Omega 9 family). Persons with cancer may need to take higher amounts of good quality, fresh flaxseed oil and/or pure fish oil and avoid the Omega 6 oils until the cancer retreats.

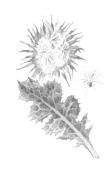

PREVENTION
Avoid all products that say 'hydrogenated' or 'partially hydrogenated' on their labels.

Fat Content of Common Foods

The amount of fat a person should consume varies with age, weight, health, gender and level of physical activity, but generally an average man (25-49 years old) needs 30 grams or less and an average woman (25-49 years old) needs 20 grams or less.

The ideal dietary fats to use, in decreasing order, are flaxseed oil, extra virgin olive oil, nuts, and seeds. Supplement with fish oil. Avoid cooked oils, fried foods, and hydrogenated or partially hydrogenated fats. Avoid or minimize saturated fat. The meat and dairy items in the chart are included for your interest only. They are not recommended.

The following chart, compiled from information available from Health Canada, the Beef Information Centre, and various restaurants, lists the fat content, in grams, for popular foods. The asterisk * indicates only trace amounts.

Type of Food	Grams of Fat	Type of Food	Grams of Fat
Fruits and Vegetables		1 cup ice cream with 10% fat	16
1 medium apple	*	1 egg, boiled	6
1 medium banana	*		
green salad	*	**Meats and Alternatives**	
4 spears of asparagus	*	*Beef:*	
1 cup of green peas	*	3 oz inside round broiled	5
1 cup of broccoli	*	3 oz sirloin steak, broiled	9
1 baked potato	*	with fat rimmed	6
1 ear of fresh corn	*	3 oz rib roast, trimmed	10
1 sweet potato	1	3 oz lean ground, broiled	13
1 slice of watermelon	3	*Chicken:*	
5 olives	3	3 oz breast, roasted	7
20 French fries, deep fried	16	with skin removed	3
1 California avocado	30	3 oz leg, skin removed	5
		breaded and fried	14
Dairy Products		*Pork:*	
1 cup of skim milk	*	3 oz tenderloin, lean, broiled	4
1% milk	3	3 oz loin, trimmed, broiled	6
2% milk	5	3 strips side bacon, fried crisp	9
homogenized milk	9	*Fish:*	
2 cups of chocolate milk shake	12	3 oz tuna, water-packed	1
½ cup of regular frozen yogurt	5	oil-packed	7
½ cup of 6% milk fat yogurt	6	3 oz haddock, baked	1
½ cup of 1.5% milk fat yogurt	2	breaded and fried	7
½ cup of vanilla ice cream	8	3 oz sockeye salmon, baked	8
premium ice cream	12	*Processed Meats:*	
1 ounce of part-skim mozzarella	5	1 oz turkey roll	2
regular mozzarella	7	regular ham	3
cheddar	10	corned beef	6
1 slice of processed cheddar	10	summer sausage	9
1 ounce of ricotta	3	1 wiener, beef or pork	11
½ cup cottage cheese, 2 % fat	2.5	chicken	7
1 tbsp. regular cream cheese	5		
1 tbsp. light cream cheese	1		

Saturated Fats

Saturated fats, found in red meat, milk, cheese, butter, vegetable shortening, palm and coconut oils, animal products and lard, are linked with a higher incidence of breast cancer. Saturated fats interfere with the way our cells utilize oxygen and prevent the transport of glucose from the bloodstream into muscle cells, which causes blood sugar levels to rise. This causes the body to make more insulin, increasing breast cancer risk.

The five-year survival rate of women with breast cancer in Tokyo, where dietary fat is reduced, is 15% greater than in Western countries.[49] When dietary fat is decreased, there is a drop in circulating levels of estradiol and estrone.[50] Women who consume large amounts of beef and pork double or triple their risk of breast cancer.[51]

DDT and other chemicals are found at low levels in fatty foods, especially dairy products.[52]

FACT

Breast cancer is more prevalent in countries with a diet high in saturated fat, such as Canada and the United States where most people derive 40% of their total calories from fat.

PREVENTION

Decrease saturated fat content to not more than 5% of your caloric intake, or less than 7-10 g daily, which is less than 2 tsp.

Type of Food	Grams of Fat	Type of Food	Grams of Fat
Beans and Tofu		**Cereals**	
1 cup cooked kidney beans	1	¾ cup of bran flakes with raisins	*
1 cup cooked lentils	1	1 Shredded Wheat biscuit	*
1 cup cooked split peas	1	½ cup instant oatmeal	3
1 cup cooked white beans	1	½ cup plain toasted wheat germ	6
1 cup cooked chick peas	4	½ cup granola, homemade	17
1 cup baked beans with pork	4		
½ cup tofu, extra firm	14	**Pasta and Rice**	
1 tofu hot dog	1.5	½ cup of long-grained cooked rice	*
		1 cup spaghetti	1
Nuts and Seeds		with ⅓ cup meat sauce	5
½ cup nuts	35	¾ cup of macaroni and cheese	13
½ cup pumpkin seeds	38		
½ cup sunflower seeds	38	**Fats**	
½ cup sesame seeds	38	1 teaspoon margarine	4
1 tbsp. nut butter	0.8	1 teaspoon butter	4
		1 teaspoon oil, all types	5
Breads and Baked Goods			
1 slice of whole wheat bread	*	**Fast Foods and Snacks**	
1 slice of white bread	*	pretzels	*
4 soda crackers	1	1 cup plain popcorn	*
1 bagel	1	10 potato chips	1
1 medium bran muffin	4	1 doughnut, glazed	16
2 small chocolate chip cookies	6	1 slice of pizza	16
1 croissant	12	1 beef burrito	19
1 piece apple pie	18	6 Chicken McNuggets	20
		poutine (20 fries with	24
		curds and sauce)	
		Big Mac	27

High Fiber

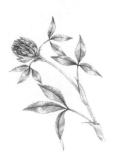

Benefits of Fiber

East Africans, who have one of the lowest rates of breast cancer in the world, consume close to 40 grams of fiber daily and eat no processed food. Their dietary staples include brown rice, potatoes, maize, and casaba.

Fiber is present in fruits and vegetables, legumes, grains, nuts, and seeds. Fiber reduces the amount of circulating estrogen in the blood and protects us in many other ways. Many plants and vegetables contain isoflavones and lignans that can be converted by bacteria in the bowel into weak estrogens that may compete with estradiol for receptor sites in breast tissue. A high fiber diet is less often associated with obesity, which tends to increase estrogen production by the body's fat cells. A high fiber diet usually has a lower content of fat and a higher content of antioxidant vitamins, which may protect against breast cancer. Diets high in fiber and complex carbohydrates stabilize blood sugar and improve insulin sensitivity, which is associated with a drop in circulating estrogen.[53] A high fiber diet modifies the composition of flora in the bowel to decrease the numbers of bacteria that can split the glucuronide conjugate, thus decreasing estrogen reabsorption.[54]

Fiber increases the feeling of fullness for a longer period, so there is less tendency to overeat. It reduces bacterial toxins and speeds up excretion of bile acids and toxins from the liver. Fiber speeds up elimination and decreases toxicity, while improving bowel disorders such as irritable bowel syndrome and colitis. Fiber stabilizes blood sugar and insulin levels by reducing the glycemic index of foods. A high fiber diet also maintains the integrity of the intestinal flora, which is necessary for the health of the immune system. Specific intestinal bacteria (Clostridia paraputreficum) are necessary to convert the phytochemicals from soy and flaxseeds into weak estrogens that protect us from breast cancer.

Soluble and Insoluble Fiber

Fiber is divided into two types — soluble and insoluble fiber. The most protection is gained when we consume equally high amounts of psyllium (soluble fiber) and wheat bran (insoluble fiber) as opposed to either one by itself.[55,56,57] Together they decrease the enzyme beta glucuronidase, which is generated by intestinal bacteria and causes reabsorption of estrogen.

Soluble fiber includes the following foods: bananas, oranges, apples, potatoes, cabbage, carrots, grapes, oatmeal, oatbran, sesame seeds, flaxseeds, psyllium seeds, and beans. Soluble fiber absorbs water and improves the motility of the bowel so that food moves more quickly through the intestinal tract. It also lowers cholesterol, triglycerides, and sugar levels in the blood.[58]

Insoluble fiber includes wheat bran, unpeeled apples and pears, tomatoes, strawberries, canned peas, raw carrots, bran cereals, whole grain breads, beets, eggplant, radishes, and potatoes.[59] Insoluble fiber also improves the transit time required to move fecal matter through the colon, decreasing the likelihood of constipation. It absorbs little water. Insoluble fiber is beneficial in that it encourages regular bowel movements. One study has shown that women with two or less bowel movements per week had 4.5 times the risk of precancerous breast changes than other women who had bowel movements more than once daily.[60]

High Fiber Diet

We can follow a high fiber diet by eating a cooked cereal for breakfast such as oatmeal, quinoa, buckwheat, amaranth, rye flakes, 7-grain or millet meal with added wheat bran (which is better tolerated than wheat), and freshly ground flaxseeds. Wheat bran rather than oatbran has been found to be more beneficial in preventing breast cancer because it is highly insoluble and helps to draw estrogen bound to the glucuronide complex out of the body, preventing its release back into the blood-stream.[61] Wheat bran significantly decreased the levels of estradiol and estrone circulating in the blood when used daily as part of the diet.[62]

Grains that can be included in lunch or dinner are brown or basmati rice, wild rice, millet, quinoa, buckwheat, barley, and kamut. Wheat (other than the bran) and corn are common food allergens, and should be used infrequently, perhaps once weekly, or not at all. Psyllium can be taken in powdered or capsule form for additional benefit and bowel cleansing. Beans are a wonderful source of fiber and can be consumed daily in soups, spreads, or with grain dishes. Fruit can be consumed by itself as an alternative to grain at breakfast, or as a snack between meals.

Beans

Beans are very high in fiber, particularly kidney beans. Dried beans, especially lentils, contain cancer-inhibiting enzymes that prevent the development and recurrence of breast cancer. Many beans contain phytoestrogens that are converted into active hormone-like compounds by bacteria in the colon. These competitively inhibit estradiol uptake by attaching to estrogen binding sites in breast tissue.[63] Diets high in soybeans, mung beans, and adzuki beans in Asian populations are associated with reduced cancer risk.[64]

Phytoestrogens

Phytoestrogens are a varied group of substances with a chemical structure similar to estrogen. So far about 15 different phytoestrogens have been discovered in human urine. The two main classes of phytoestrogens are isoflavones and lignans. Isoflavones are found in soy products, some legumes and their sprouts, and several herbs. Lignans are highest in flaxseeds, pumpkin seeds, berries, some vegetables, and grains. Coumestrol, a third class, is a less common phytoestrogen found in mung bean sprouts.

Genistein and Daidzein

Genistein and daidzen are two isoflavones, of which genistein is the stronger phytoestrogen. Isoflavones act like weak estrogens (similar

PREVENTION
Part of a breast cancer prevention program includes encouraging at least two bowel movements daily, preferably three.

PREVENTION
Eat 30 g or 1.06 oz of fiber daily, using beans, bran, ground flaxseed, raw fruits and vegetables, and whole grains to do so. Minimize flour products such as bread, baked goods, and pasta. Focus on whole grains instead. Consume wheat bran (if tolerated) and psyllium daily, approximately one tablespoon of each.

FACT
Phytoestrogens increase the production of SHBG (steroid hormone binding globulin), the transport system that carries estrogen in the blood before it attaches to a receptor. The more SHBG, the less estrogen is available — which is good for preventing breast cancer.

Evaluating the Fiber Content of Your Diet

We should aim to eat at least 30 grams or just over 1 ounce (1.06) of fiber each day to help prevent breast cancer and promote good health. This is equivalent to one serving of high fiber cereal; one cup of cooked beans; two pieces of whole grain bread; one serving of cooked whole grains such as brown rice, quinoa, or millet; and six servings of fruit or vegetables.

Using the following chart, estimate what your daily fiber intake has been each day over the last three days. My average daily fiber intake is: _____ grams or ounces. How close do you come to 30 grams or 1 ounce?

Grams / Oz Fiber	Food Item	Day 1	Day 2	Day 3
15 g / .53 oz	1 cup kidney beans			
10 g / .35 oz	½ cup wheat or oat bran 1 cup split peas 1¼ cup lentils ¾ cup navy beans ¼ cup ground flaxseed			
5 g / .18 oz	½ cup cooked dried beans, peas or lentils 1 serving of a high fiber wheat bran cereal			
2 g / .07 oz.	1 serving of a fruit or vegetable 1 serving of any whole grain food 1 cup oatmeal 1 slice of whole grain bread ½ cup whole grain pasta ½ whole grain bagel 1 slice rye crisp cracker ½ cup cooked brown rice			
1 g / .035 oz.	1 serving of refined grain 10 almonds 20 filberts			
		Total:	Total:	Total:
		3-day Average:		

to the body's estriol) and bind to breast cell receptors so that the body's strong estrogens (estradiol and estrone) are blocked from doing so.[65] They act paradoxically as anti-estrogens opposing the body's strong estrogens that might cause breast cancer, and as weak estrogens that have the ability to prevent osteoporosis. When present in the diet, isoflavones manipulate the breakdown products of estrogen, helping to increase the 'good' estrogens. Studies on premenopausal women have shown that when they consume 65 mg of isoflavones daily, they can increase the C2/C16 hydroxyestrone ratio, and decrease the urinary excretion of the C4 hydroxyestrone, meaning they are producing less of it. Both of these effects are protective and will reduce breast cancer risk.[66]

Genistein slows down or reverses the cancer process and deactivates breast cancer genes. Genistein influences enzymes that regulate cell growth and division and has antioxidant properties.[67] It inhibits platelet aggregation, which means that the blood is less 'sticky'. It lowers production of LH and FSH by the pituitary gland and decreases estrogen production by the ovaries in pre-menopausal women. Genistein reduces the bioavailability of sex hormones, so that there is less circulating estradiol and estrone. It induces differentiation in cancer cells, which means they become more clearly defined, so that they are more similar to normal cells; and inhibits protein tyrosine kinases, which are enzymes that encourage the transformation of normal cells to cancer cells and increase their ability to multiply. Protein tyrosine kinases also activate breast cancer genes.

Intestinal bacteria convert genistein and daidzen to equol, and convert the lignans, secoisolariciresinol (SECO) and matairesinol, to enterodiol and enterolactone, respectively. Equol and enterolactone bind to estrogen receptors and exhibit weak estrogenic activity while their precursors do not. Equol has a slightly higher protective effect than enterolactone as a phytoestrogen. Equol and enterolactone excretion in urine is significantly lower in women with breast cancer than in healthy women.[68] An Australian study found that women who excreted the highest amounts of equol had one quarter the breast cancer risk of women excreting the lowest levels of equol, while with enterolactone the risk reduction was one third.[69] Excretion is higher in vegetarians and highest in those who follow a macrobiotic diet. Those of us who consume a macrobiotic diet have approximately a tenfold higher excretion of dietary estrogens than those eating a typical North American diet.[70] A diet high in fat and meat significantly decreases equol production. Some people are unable to produce equol, despite soy consumption, or produce it in very low amounts.[71] This is most likely linked to the health of the intestinal flora, and an absence or deficiency in the bacteria that convert the isoflavones to equol and the lignans to enterodiol and enterolactone.

Foods and Herbs with Genistein and Daidzen

Genistein and daidzen are found in higher amounts in the sprouts and roots of legumes (particularly mung bean and red clover), being more concentrated in the root. We would do well to consume the living sprouts of these legumes on a regular basis.

Genistein is found in the following herbs in significant amounts: Indian breadroot (*Psoralea corylifolia*), wild indigo (*Baptisia australis*), red clover (*Trifolium pratense*), licorice (*Glycyrrhiza glabra*), fenugreek, and alfalfa, being particularly high in Baptisia australis. Traditionally used to decrease liver stagnation, stimulate immunity, and remove lymphatic congestion, Baptisia may become a staple ingredient in alternative breast cancer prevention and treatment. Red clover and licorice are already commonly used. Phytoestrogens are also found in decreasing amounts in mandrake (*Podophylum peltatum*), bloodroot (*Sanguinaria Canadensis*), thyme (*Thymus vulgaris*), yucca, turmeric (*Curcuma longa*), hops (*Humulus lupulus*), verbena (*Verbena hastate*), yellow dock (*Rumex crispus*), and sheep sorrel (*Rumex acetosella*).[72,73] Yellow dock and sheep sorrel are present in the Essiac formulas.

FACT
There is a lowered breast cancer risk in women who have high dietary intakes of the isoflavones genistein and daidzen. Genistein is invaluable for its ability to help prevent and reverse breast cancer.

FACT
Genistein induces apoptosis, or programmed cell death, which is a form of suicide by damaged or cancerous cells, and inhibits DNA topoisomerase II, helping to prevent cancer cells from multiplying. It also inhibits the formation of blood vessels that feed cancerous tumors (angiogenesis), helping to starve tumors.

FACT
Genistein and daidzen are found in the following foods in decreasing amounts: tofu, soy milk, miso, red clover sprouts, fava beans, Indian potato, yellow peas, pinto beans, green lentils, garbanzo beans, black turtle beans, mung beans and mung bean sprouts, adzuki beans, bush beans, navy beans, baby lima beans, black-eyed peas, and kidney beans.

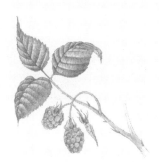

Bacteria, Antibiotics, and Phytoestrogens

We need the activity of certain intestinal bacteria to convert the isoflavones and lignans into weak estrogens. This conversion happens in the first part of the large intestine and is followed by recirculation of the weak estrogens from the large intestine to the liver. When we use antibiotics, the activity of the intestinal bacteria on the isoflavones and lignans is reduced or absent, sometimes for as long as one month after stopping antibiotic use.[74]

The higher incidence of breast cancer in North America and Northern Europe might also be linked in part to our overuse of antibiotics and the damaging effect that this has on intestinal flora. We have done to our bodies what we have done to the soil — used 'heroic' measures to conquer organisms while destroying the natural ecology that has existed in equilibrium through generations. We must replenish the balance of microorganisms in our intestines as we replenish the land upon which we grow our food.

Fabulous Five Phytoestrogens

For about $2.00 a day, you can help protect yourself from breast cancer with these phytoestrogen-rich foods.

Phytoestrogen	Suggested Amounts
Flaxseeds, freshly ground	2-4 tablespoons daily
Tofu and soy products	½ cup tofu or 1 ½ cups soy milk daily
Raw pumpkin seeds	1-2 tablespoons daily
Clover sprouts	3 or more cups weekly
Mung bean sprouts	3 or more cups weekly

Soy Products

Soy products (particularly miso) protect cells from the cancer-promoting effects of radiation and chemicals. In Asian countries where breast cancer rates are at least two thirds lower than in Canada and the United States, the average consumption of soy products is 35-60 g per day. The urinary excretion of phytoestrogens in Japanese women is 20-30 times higher than in Finnish women.[77]

Of all foods, soy also has one of the highest amounts of the amino acid cysteine, which allows more glutathione to be manufactured in the liver and body. Glutathione is the liver's great detoxifier and is an immune enhancer. Additional benefits of soy foods are its ability to lower cholesterol levels and to decrease the LDL:HDL ratio, which reduces our risk of heart disease.

We need to ensure that soy products are organic and non-genetically modified, since the common pesticides used on soy are ones that can promote breast cancer. Be sure your soy milk has no added oil or sugar. Include miso in your diet several times a week, perhaps as miso soup. You may also supplement with quality soy

Phytoestrogen Content of Various Foods

The mean (ug/100g) isoflavonoid and lignan concentrations (after removing the water content) of various foods is provided here. These amounts will vary for each sample tested depending upon environmental conditions, soil quality, attack by pathogens, and genetic makeup.

PHYTOESTROGEN	ISOFLAVONES		LIGNANS		COUMESTROL
Food Source	**Genistein**	**Daidzein**	**Seco**	**Matairesinol**	**Coumestrol**
Soybean Flour	96,900	67,400	130		
Kikoman Firm Tofu	21,300	7,600			
Nasoya Soft Tofu	18,700	7,300			
Hatcho Miso	14,500	13,700			
Soy Milk	2,100	700			
Soybean Sprouts	4,290	6,270			small amount
Soybeans	241	376			
Flaxseeds			369,900	1,087	
Clover Seeds	323	178	13	4	
Clover Sprouts	11,000	7,360			high amount
Yellow Peas	458	4			
Yellow Pea Sprouts	6,150				*
Green Lentil Sprouts	3,340	1,650			*
Pinto Beans	223	232			
Black Turtle Beans	451	4			
Small Lima Beans	401	4			
Large Lima Beans	344	3			
Red Lentils	250	52			
Adzuki Beans	212	46			
Adzuki Sprouts	1,300	910			*
Fava Beans	199	50			
Black-Eyed Peas	233	3			
Wheat Bran	7	3	110		
Rye Meal			47	65	
Rye Bran			132	167	
Sunflower Seeds	14	8	610		
Oat Bran			24	155	
Chick Peas	76	11	8		5
Chick Pea Sprouts	4,610				*
Urid Dahl Beans	60	30	240	79.4	
Mung Beans	365	10	172	0.25	2
Mung Bean Sprouts	1,902	745	468		1,032
Fenugreek Sprouts	910	2,310			
Pumpkin Seeds			21,370		
Carrots	2	2	192	3	
Garlic	2	2	379	4	
Broccoli	7	5	414	23	
Cranberry			1,510		
Alfalfa Sprouts	730	720			51
Baptisia australis	35,070	3,400			
Glycyrrhiza sp.	5,190				
Japanese Green Tea		2,460			
Converted to:	*Equol*	*Daidzein*	*Enterodiol*	*Enterolactone*	

Information on the coumestrol value of these sprouts was unavailable. This information was derived from a study by the Finnish Medical Society called 'Phyto-oestrogens and Western Disease' and from the report 'A Comparative Survey of Leguminous Plants as Sources of the Isoflavones, Genistein and Daidzen' published in the *Journal of Alternative and Complementary Medicine*.[75,76]

protein powder, mixed with fruit to make a shake. Balance the high salt content of miso with high potassium foods eaten in the same day. If you have high blood pressure or kidney disease, have miso only once or twice per week. If you have a problem with candidiasis, avoid miso and minimize tofu until you clear the excess yeast from your body. The isoflavones in miso are more easily absorbed from the small intestine than those from other tofu products and lead to a higher urinary output of equol, meaning that miso exerts more activity as a weak estrogen than other soy products. This is because genistein and daidzen exist in miso in an unconjugated form, whereas they are conjugated and less bio-available in tofu, soy milk, and soybeans.[78]

Calorie, Protein, Isoflavone, and Fat Content of Soy Foods

Food	Calories (Kcal)	Protein (grams)	Isoflavones (mg)	Fat (grams)
½ cup soybeans	149.0	14.3	70	7.7
½ cup tempeh	165.0	15.7	60	6.0
¼ cup soynuts	202.0	15.0	60	10.9
½ cup tofu	94.0	10.0	38	5.9
¼ cup soy flour	81.7	12.8	25	0.3
½ cup soymilk	79.0	6.6	10	4.6
½ cup texturized soy protein	59.0	11.0	28	0.2

FACT

Soy products contain phytoestrogens that prevent the initiation, promotion, and recurrence of breast cancer. Along with flaxseeds, they can be thought of as a natural, non-toxic Tamoxifen.

PREVENTION

Each day eat either ½ cup of firm tofu or tempeh, 1 ½ cups soy milk, ¼ cup soy nuts, or some combination of these, aiming for 35-60 g of soy protein daily and at least 65 mg of isoflavones. We should introduce our children to moderate but not extreme amounts of soy products early in life, with higher amounts before and through puberty.

Soy Consumption in Infants and Daughters before Puberty

Short-term exposure to dietary isoflavones found in soy is especially beneficial for newborns and girls who have not yet reached puberty. This early exposure may increase the proportion of differentiated breast cells and decrease risk of breast cancer caused by carcinogens later in life. The diet of Japanese and Chinese women may confer part of its protective effect early in life.[79]

There has been concern that infants exposed to a regular diet of soy milk and soy foods may be getting too much. However, one study found that although four-month-old infants were fed soy, there was an absence of equol in their urine. This means that they do not yet have the intestinal bacteria to convert genistein and daidzein to equol, so that the soy has a limited estrogenic action.[80] Pregnant women, on the other hand, would make this conversion, and pass on the phytoestrogens to the fetus. Because soy products lengthen the menstrual cycle, they decrease fertility slightly. Therefore, we should be cautious about the amount of soy we consume while pregnant or when trying to conceive.[81]

Soy's Effect on the Menstrual Cycle

Breast cancer risk is in part linked to the total estrogen exposure and the cumulative number of menstrual cycles a woman experiences in her lifetime. Because of their higher consumption of soy foods, Japanese women have an average menstrual cycle length of 32 days as opposed to 28-29 days for North American women. In Japanese women, the follicular (pre-ovulation) phase of the menstrual cycle is longer than in Western women, resulting in reduced breast-cell division over their pre-menopausal years. As the length of the menstrual cycle increases, the duration of the follicular phase (pre-ovulation) increases, while the luteal phase (post-ovulation) decreases, causing less breast cell division over the pre-menopausal years. Breast cells proliferate 2-3 times more rapidly in the luteal phase than in the follicular phase.

Soy Allergies and Thyroid Function

There are several reasons to be cautious when using soy products regularly. One of them is that soy is a relatively common food allergy. Dr Max Gerson asked his patients to avoid soy because many people had allergic reactions to it and because of its high oil content.[82] Allergic reactions to soy include fatigue, bloating, and gas. We should avoid or limit our exposure to any foods to which we are sensitive.

The second area of concern is that soy may have a negative impact on the thyroid gland. The phytoestrogens found in soy (genistein and daidzen) block an enzyme (thyroid peroxidase) that is responsible for attaching iodide ions to the amino acid tyrosine to form the thyroid hormones, T4 and T3. Instead, the iodide ions attach to either genistein or daidzen, causing a deficit of thyroid hormones.[83] When iodide is added to the diet along with soy, this effect on the thyroid is diminished substantially or eliminated.

Infants in particular, when fed soy formula without the addition of iodine or seaweeds, are more likely to develop autoimmune thyroid disease later in life.[84]

We must incorporate sea vegetables in our diets or take a kelp supplement regularly to offset the potential of soy and the raw brassicas for interfering with thyroid function. If soy formulas are given to infants, and the evidence suggests that they may protect infants from breast cancer later in life, then the formula should also contain small amounts of iodine or seaweed, such as kombu.[85]

Flaxseeds and Other High Lignan Foods

Lignans have been shown to have anti-viral, anti-bacterial, and anti-fungal properties. These properties help protect our digestive tracts from invading organisms and exert a sparing effect on our immune systems. Lignans also contain two phytoestrogens, known as secoisolariciresinol (SECO) and matairesinol. Like the isoflavones in soy, these are converted by intestinal bacteria to weak estrogens (enterodiol and enterolactone, respectively).[86] Enterodiol is converted by gut bacteria to enterolactone, which acts as the weak estrogen. Enterodiol and enterolactone stimulate

FACT
Japanese women have fewer menstrual cycles over their life span than North American women, have lower levels of estradiol overall, and are less likely to be diagnosed with breast cancer.

FACT
While soy is an extremely beneficial food in breast cancer prevention and treatment, it should be used judiciously with annual monitoring of thyroid function through blood tests and tracking body temperature.

FACT
Like soy, flaxseed influences the way we manage our estrogens, helping to decrease the amount of harmful C4 and C16 estrogens while increasing the protective C2. Flaxseed oil protects us from all cancers, particularly when tumors have already been established.

PREVENTION

Eat flaxseeds any way you can. Aim to eat 2-4 tablespoons (25-50 g) of freshly ground flaxseeds daily. If you have more than 2 tbsp. daily, use extra vitamin B6.

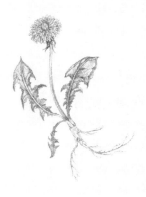

PREVENTION

Eat mung bean sprouts several times a week, aiming for 3 cups weekly.

FACT

High protein diets that encourage weight loss may promote cancer by causing excess acidity. Excess protein causes narrowing of the terminal capillaries, obstructing the transportation of oxygen, which then favors formation of cancer cell colonies.

PREVENTION

Consume approximately 30-50 grams of vegetarian protein daily.

the production of progesterone receptors, which helps to protect us from breast cancer.[87] Women with breast cancer excrete lower amounts of urinary lignans than healthy women.[88] Vegetarians excrete more lignans than non-vegetarians, and vegetarian women who do not consume dairy or eggs excrete the most.[89]

Flaxseeds contain hundreds of thousands more amounts of SECO than any other food studied so far. Ninety-five percent of the lignans are present in the fiber of the seeds, while less than 5% is present in flaxseed oil.[90] Animal studies have shown that flaxseed was able to reduce the size of breast tumors by 67% when fed to animals with breast cancer, reduced the likelihood of metastases, and was effective at preventing cancers induced by chemicals.[91] Women who used flaxseeds in their diets between the time of diagnosis and the time of surgery to remove a breast tumor were able to decrease their tumor size before the surgery.[92,93]

Flaxseed can be eaten whole or ground in a small electric coffee grinder and added to pancakes, muffins, cookies, breads, cereals, or even sprinkled in salad. Grind them daily so that the oil does not become rancid with storage. Freshly ground flaxseeds should be consumed within 15 minutes of grinding.

Lignans are found in smaller amounts in berries, fruit, legumes, pumpkin and sunflower seeds, and the outer bran of wheat, rye, and oats.

Mung Bean Sprouts and Coumestrol

Another lesser known phytoestrogen is coumestrol, which has a stronger estrogenic effect than the isoflavones and the lignans. Coumestrol is found in high amounts in mung bean sprouts, with lower amounts found in the sprouts of the following seeds: red clover, alfalfa, soybean, yellow pea, green lentil, chick pea, fenugreek, adzuki bean, and fava bean. Coumestrol is found in small amounts in the following legumes: chickpeas, urid dahl beans, and mung beans. Mung bean sprouts can be eaten on their own, added to salads, on top of bean dishes, or mixed in juices.

Protein

Protein should be sufficient but not excessive to prevent cancer in general, and needs to be combined with quality oils for optimum health. Although individual needs for protein may differ, the average adult requires approximately 30-50 g per day. More is required if you are very athletic or physically active, because exercise causes the body to use protein at a faster rate.

During the breakdown of amino acids in high protein diets by intestinal bacteria, toxins produced in the colon are linked to increased cancer risk. High protein diets also cause more calcium to be lost, promoting osteoporosis and a deficiency of alkaline minerals.

Adequate vegetarian protein would include 2-3 servings a day, where one serving equals, for example, 1 cup of cooked legumes, 1/2 cup tofu, 2 tbsp nut butter, or 3 tbsp of nuts or seeds. Protein-rich legumes include kidney beans, soybeans, chickpeas, split peas, and lentils. Soy foods are rich in protein.

Vegetarian Sources of Protein

Soy Food	Protein Content in Grams	Quantity Required
Miso	5.9	½ cup
Tofu, silken	8.1	½ cup
Tofu, firm	15.6	½ cup
Soybeans, boiled	16.6	½ cup
Soybeans, dry-roasted	39.6	½ cup
Soy milk	5.6	1 cup
Tempeh	19.0	½ cup
Soy protein powder	58.1	1 ounce
Kidney beans	15.0	1 cup, cooked
Lentils	16.0	1 cup, cooked
Split peas	17.0	1 cup, cooked
Chick peas	14.5	1 cup, cooked
Almond butter	5.0	2 tbsp.
Almonds	2.8	12
Sunflower seeds	6.5	1 oz.
Pumpkin seeds	7.0	1 oz. (142 seeds)
Sesame seed butter	2.6	1 tbsp.

Sulphur-Bearing Protein in Combination with Flaxseed Oil

Dr Joanna Budwig, who pioneered studies on fats and oils in the early 1950s, found that the combination of flaxseed oil with sulphur-containing protein prevented or helped to heal cancer. When sulphur-containing protein and Omega 3 oils are taken together, there is increased oxygen uptake in tissues.

Linoleic Acid Deficiency

Dr Budwig analyzed blood from cancer patients and found that it lacked linoleic acid, which helps to form phospholipids that maintain the integrity of cell membranes. A deficiency of linoleic acid would prevent the formation of healthy cell membranes and cause incomplete cell division. She also found that cancer patients lacked lipoproteins, which contain linoleic acid combined with sulphur-rich protein. Their blood contained a yellow-green protein instead, which disappeared when she added linoleic acid and sulphur-rich protein. The red blood pigment, hemoglobin, appeared in its place. This explains why many cancer patients are anemic and lack oxygen and energy. Linoleic acid deficiency prevents hemoglobin from being made and the blood can't carry enough oxygen.

In practice, Dr Budwig found that flaxseed oil (which contains alpha-linolenic and linoleic acid), combined with skim milk protein, helped cancer patients. Her mixture was 20 parts by weight skim milk protein, 8 parts flaxseed oil, and 5 parts milk to liquefy it.

FACT

Sulphur-bearing amino acids include cysteine and methionine. These two amino acids are very important for liver detoxification and for inactivating the toxic C4 estrogen, as well as playing a role in increasing cellular oxygen.

PREVENTION

Aim to eat 500 mg twice daily of sulphur-containing protein in combination with at least 2 tbsp of flaxseed oil daily. If you are unable to get it from food, organic whey powder, soy protein powder or the supplement N-acetyl-cysteine can be used.

Sulphur-Containing Protein (Cystine and Methionine) Rich Foods

Because many of us are allergic to dairy, we can choose alternate sources of sulphur-containing protein, and combine them in our meals with flaxseed oil in approximately a 5:2 ratio. In foods, cysteine is found in the form of cystine, which consists of two cysteine molecules joined together. To prevent breast cancer, vegetarian sources are best, which include soy nuts, pumpkin seeds, sunflower seeds, oatmeal, beans, tofu and all soy products, broccoli, kale, kelp, and spirulina.

Food	Cystine	Methionine	Total
Nuts and Seeds			
1 cup coconut milk	108	103	211
24 almonds	102	64	166
1 tbsp almond butter	43	28	71
47 pistachios (1 oz)	146	108	154
142 pumpkin seeds (1 oz)	85	156	241
½ cup dry roasted soy nuts	549	459	1008
1 oz sunflower seeds	128	140	268
Vegetables			
½ cup cooked broccoli	16	28	44
½ cup boiled Brussels sprouts	12	19	31
½ cup cabbage, shredded, raw	6	3	9
½ cup cabbage, boiled	14	8	22
½ cup chopped, boiled kale	16	12	28
Grains			
⅓ cup dry oatmeal	112	75	187
Beans			
1 cup boiled aduki beans	161	182	343
1 cup baked beans	157	218	375
1 cup black beans	165	229	394
1 cup pinto beans	152	212	364
1 cup chick peas	195	190	385
1 cup hummus	155	101	256
1 cup kidney beans	166	230	399
1 cup boiled lentils	234	152	386
1 cup boiled mung beans	125	170	295
1 cup boiled navy beans	173	238	411
Soy			
1 cup boiled soybeans	461	385	846
½ cup miso	131	206	337
½ cup tempeh	265	220	485
½ cup raw, firm tofu	275	255	530
1 cup defatted soy flour	757	634	1391

1 cup full fat soy flour	473	396	869
Dairy			
1 cup 1% fat cottage cheese	259	843	1102
8 oz 2% fat milk	75	204	279
1 large poached egg	144	195	339
1 duck egg	199	403	602
8 oz breast milk	48	48	96
Fish			
3 oz Atlantic cod	162	448	610
3 oz haddock	221	610	831
3 oz halibut	243	672	915
3 oz herring	210	580	790
3 oz lobster	196	490	686
3 oz mackerel	218	600	818
3 oz sockeye salmon	249	687	963
3 oz sardines	53	181	234
3 oz cooked shrimp	199	501	700
3 oz tuna (water packed)	269	745	1014
Meat			
99 g beef	167	441	608
99 g chicken	191	390	581
99 g lamb	207	471	678
99 g turkey	185	472	657
Other			
3.5 oz kelp	98	25	123
1 tsp barley, rye, or wheat grass	8	15	23
3.5 oz Spirulina	662	1149	1811

Low Sodium/High Potassium Foods

Sodium and potassium exist in a 'teetottering' balance in our bodies: sodium is present in the extracellular fluid, while potassium is found inside each of our cells. When one is low, the other will be high. If sodium levels are high, the body's cells swell and trap toxins. Dr Max Gerson counseled his patients to restrict salt so that there would be less fluid retention and fewer toxins in the body generally. He believed that it was important to eliminate salt if one wanted to detoxify fully. One of the ways he encouraged elimination of sodium was through supplementation with potassium.[94] Potassium preserves alkalinity of the body fluids and encourages the kidneys to eliminate poisonous waste products.

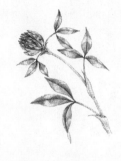

PREVENTION
Eat 3000-6000 mg of high potassium fruits and vegetables daily to help with cellular detoxification.

Potassium Content of Common Foods

Food	Quantity	Potassium Content in mg	Food	Quantity	Potassium Content in mg
Juices			Sweet potato	1	397
Prune juice	8 oz	706	Carrot	1 medium	233
Carrot juice	6 oz	538	*Beans*		
Orange juice	8 oz	436	Adzuki beans	1 cup	1224
Tomato juice	6 oz	400	White beans	1 cup	1003
Grapefruit juice	8 oz	400	Lima beans	1 cup	955
Grape juice	8 oz	334	Tofu, raw, firm	½ cup	298
Pineapple juice	8 oz	334	Soybeans	1 cup	886
Apple juice	8 oz	296	Soymilk	1 cup	338
Apricot juice	8 oz	286	Soy meal, defatted	1 cup	3038
Fruit			Black turtle beans	1 cup	801
Dried figs	10	1332	Pinto beans	1 cup	800
Papaya	1	780	Lentils	1 cup	731
Raisins	⅔ cup	746	Kidney beans	1 cup	714
Dried prunes	10	626	Great northern beans	1 cup	692
Canteloupe	1 cup pieces	494	Navy beans	1 cup	669
Banana	1	451	Black beans	1 cup	611
Mango	1	322	Mung beans	1 cup	536
Apricot	3	313	Chick peas	1 cup	477
Kiwi	1	252	*Grains*		
Orange	1	250	Dark rye flower	1 cup	1101
Pear	1	208	Carob powder	1 cup	852
Apple	1	159	Pearl barley	1 cup	320
Vegetables					
Avocado	1	1097			
Potato	1	844			
Squash	½ cup	445			

These values are taken from Jean Pennington's *Food Values of Portions Commonly Used.*

Shitake and Maitake Mushrooms

PREVENTION

Eat shitake mushrooms daily (or at least twice weekly) for a month, followed by a 7-day break.

Shitake mushrooms have traditionally been used to treat cancer, rheumatoid arthritis, poor circulation, parasites, lack of stamina, and cerebral hemorrhage. Michio Kushi recommends shitake mushrooms as a regular part of a macrobiotic diet, and undoubtedly they account for part of the success that some macrobiotic practitioners have had in reversing cancer

An experimental medicine called Lentinan has been made from shitake mushrooms and used in treating advanced cancer patients. It increases numbers of macrophages, T-killer cells and T-helper cells, and prolongs the lives of some cancer patients.[95] It improves the helper-suppressor ratio and significantly lowers the level of T-suppressor cells when used for four weeks duration. This effect is lost by eight weeks, implying that we should use shitake mushrooms for one month and then take a break before continuing their use. An extract of shitake has demonstrated ability to inhibit breast cancer in women.[96] When mice with breast cancer were given shitake extracts that composed 20% of their feed, there was a 78.6 tumor inhibition rate.[97] Other health benefits derived from intake of extracts of shitake include lowered cholesterol levels, improved liver function in patients with hepatitis B, and improvement of candidiasis symptoms in AIDS patients.[98]

Our Kitchen Pharmacies

Many herbs and spices found in our kitchens help to prevent cancer, including turmeric, rosemary, sage, thyme, and ginger.

Turmeric

Turmeric powder has been traditionally used as a spice in East Indian cookery, and as a medicinal in Traditional Chinese Medicine as well as Ayurvedic medicine. It has antioxidant, anti-tumor, and anti-inflammatory activity.[99] It stimulates bile production in the liver, improves the ability of liver enzymes to detoxify, relieves intestinal gas, is cleansing to the blood and skin, and may be helpful in treating epilepsy and arthritis. It has a cooling effect and breaks up stagnation in the liver.[100]

Curcumin, the main active ingredient in turmeric, helps to prevent the formation of a blood supply to cancerous tumors so that they aren't able to grow.[101,102] It reduces the growth of both hormone-dependent and hormone-independent breast cancer cells, as well as cells that were resistant to chemotherapy.[103]

Both curcumin and genistein (derived from soy) have been shown to reduce the proliferation of breast cancer cells caused by estrogenic pesticides or estradiol. When used together, curcumin and genistein were able to completely inhibit cell growth caused by the mixture of pesticides or estradiol. They demonstrated a synergistic action together greater than the sum of their actions individually.[106] One of the reasons for this is because they disrupt the cell cycle in different phases of cell division.

Rosemary and Sage

Rosemary and sage contain the essential oil eucalyptol, which helps to kill Candida albicans, bacteria, and worms. Rosemary contains a phytochemical called a quinone that acts to neutralize carcinogens. It blocks the initiation of cancer, interfering with the transformation of normal cells to cancer cells. It is more effective if taken with oil. Add rosemary to your salad dressing. Sage is a glandular balancer and immune tonic. When you heat these two herbs at 200°F for longer than 20 minutes, their potency is lost. Add them to your foods after they are cooked, just before eating.[107] Avoid sage while pregnant.

An extract of rosemary leaves increased the 2-hydroxylation of estradiol and estrone by 150% in mice to form more of the 'good' C-2 estrogen and decreased the formation of C-16 estrogen by 50%. It also increased the linking of estradiol and estrone to form the glu-

FACT
Curcumin has been shown to cause apoptosis (self-destruction) in breast cancer cells in a laboratory setting.[104] During radiation treatments, curcumin strongly protects the skin from burns and inflammation. Curcumin also protects breast cells from the effects of cancer-inducing pesticides.[105]

PREVENTION
Ingest 1-2 teaspoons of turmeric powder daily, or supplement with curcumin. Add it to stir-fries, soups, and bean dishes, or boil it with basmati rice. Make a paste by simmering 1 part turmeric with 5 parts water until it thickens to the consistency of toothpaste. Keep this mixture in a glass jar in the fridge and stir 1 tsp in a warm glass of soy milk before bed to get your turmeric/soy fix. Do not use turmeric or curcumin during chemotherapy treatments.

PREVENTION
To improve digestion, maintain the health of the intestines and protect from parasites, use rosemary, sage, thyme, and ginger regularly to season your foods.

curonide complex in the liver during Phase 2 detoxification, allowing estrogen to be eliminated more effectively.[108]

Do not use rosemary during chemotherapy treatments – it may reduce its effectivness.

Ginger

Ginger is a digestive tonic, anti-inflammatory, immune stimulant, tonic to the nervous system and aids detoxification of toxins in the liver. It should not be used in early pregnancy, during labor, or in someone with excessive internal heat.

Low Glycemic Index Foods

When we eat carbohydrates, they are broken down into glucose, a form of sugar that provides energy to our cells. Certain carbohydrates dramatically raise blood sugar levels after we eat them, which in turn elevates insulin levels. The degree to which a carbohydrate raises blood sugar two to three hours after eating is called its glycemic index and has been measured for different foods.

The pancreas secretes insulin into the blood in response to elevated blood glucose levels. Insulin's job is to move into the cell and facilitate the transport of glucose from the blood into the cell for energy production. The trace mineral chromium enhances insulin's ability to enter the cell. Insulin also helps to move other nutrients, such as vitamins, minerals, and amino acids, into the cell. A diet high in carbohydrates with a high glycemic index will cause consistently high blood levels of insulin (and IGF-1), which leads to increased fat deposition. Increased fat storage means increased estrogen, since fat cells help to make a particular form of estrogen. Together, the combination of estrogen and IGF-1 strongly promotes breast cancer.

If we consistently eat foods that trigger hypersecretion of insulin we may develop what is known as 'insulin resistance', whereby insulin does not enter the cell. This causes the pancreas to produce higher amounts of insulin, and insulin, glucose, vitamins, minerals, and amino acids will remain outside of our cells, rather than nourishing them. Eventually this can lead to diabetes. Weight loss, regular exercise, chromium, alpha lipoic acid, and flaxseed oil help to improve insulin resistance.

However, some carbohydrates do not elevate blood sugar levels. Generally, we should eat carbohydrates with a low glycemic index and avoid or minimize those with a high glycemic index. Foods high in fat or protein don't cause elevations in blood sugar, and fiber slows down the rise in blood sugar levels. Fiber, quality oils, and protein also contribute to a feeling of satiety after eating, and decrease cravings and the tendency to overeat.

Foods to Avoid

In addition to the fats we should avoid in our diet, there are other food groups that should be consumed in small amounts, if at all.

FACT

When we have higher amounts of insulin and IGF-1 in our blood, we are three to seven times more prone to breast cancer.

PREVENTION

Let most of your diet consist of foods with a low glycemic index. If you do consume foods from the high category, combine them with fiber, healthy oils, such as flaxseed and olive oil, or protein.

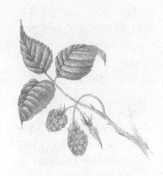

Meat

Due to its high saturated fat content, presence of pesticides, organochlorines, antibiotics, hormones, and slow transit time, which allows for more fermentation and putrefaction in the digestive tract, red meat should be avoided. Meat is difficult to digest and decreases the utilization of plant estrogens that might protect us from breast cancer. A high meat diet promotes the growth of a specific intestinal bacteria that causes more reabsorption of estrogen through the intestinal wall. Avoid beef, pork, ham, bacon, liver, and processed meats.

A breast cancer prevention diet is a meatless diet. If you must eat meat, choose organic or wild meat and balance this with a higher intake of vegetables, alkaline minerals, fiber and flaxseed oil or fish oil.

Fish

Although fish oils protect us from breast cancer, fish act as reservoirs of toxic environmental chemicals that circulate on global air currents and fall into our rivers and oceans as rain. Organochlorines such as PCBs, lindane, DDT, and dioxins accumulate in the oil of fish from polluted ocean waters.

If we won't drink the water they swim in, why would we eat the fish? Although fish have often been recommended as part of a breast cancer prevention diet due to their Omega-3 oils, I cannot include them here. Michio Kushi also advises avoidance of fish as part of a breast cancer prevention plan, unless there is a strong craving for them. Then he suggests a small amount of white-meat fish, no more than once weekly.[114]

Dairy

Although dairy products are high in calcium, they are reservoirs of environmental toxins, are difficult to digest, and many people's immune systems are stressed by them. Cows are treated with hormones and antibiotics and are fed grains that may have been sprayed with pesticides. These accumulate in the fat of the cow over its life span and are discharged into its milk. We ingest these when we consume dairy products and accumulate them in our tissues over our life spans, passing them on to our children in utero and when we breast-feed. The natural and unnatural hormones in the dairy products, and the pesticides, PCBs and dioxins, can't help but have a stimulating effect on the growth of the fetus, and we know that fetuses with a faster growth rate in utero have a three-fold increased risk of breast cancer later in life.

Cow's milk contains roughly four times as much calcium, three times as much protein, two thirds as much carbohydrate, and much more fat than human milk. These nutrients are important in these ratios for the development of a calf, but not for a human infant. Goat milk is closer to human milk in its composition. Cholesterol and fatty acids from dairy products build up in our organs and tissues, adding to heart disease, cancer, and other degenerative conditions.

Processing of milk products involves pasteurization, homogenization, and sterilization that devitalize dairy products further, rob

PREVENTION
Unless you know it is not contaminated with chemicals, avoid fish, and then eat it seldom. If you have breast cancer, do not eat fish.

FACT
Dioxins, which are extremely carcinogenic, have been found in the bodies of fish at concentrations 159,000 times higher than the water they swim in.[110,111,112] Similarly, a 10,000 times greater concentration of PCBs is found in fish tissues than in their surrounding waters.[113]

FACT
A 1979 study found that dairy products as a class increased the risk of breast cancer. A large case-control study in France in 1986 found that women who ate cheese regularly had 50% more risk than women who didn't eat cheese and those who drank milk regularly had 80% higher risk.

Glycemic Index of Various Foods

This chart demonstrates the glycemic index of various foods. The numbers refer to how fast the carbohydrate of a particular food is converted to glucose and enters the bloodstream, and are compared to the action of glucose itself. On the scale, glucose equals 100, so anything above 100 raises blood sugar faster than glucose, and any food below 100 does it that much slower.

Low Glycemic Index 7-45		Medium Glycemic Index 46-60		High Glycemic Index 61-115	
Grains & Pasta					
Burgen Soy Lin Bread	19	Macaroni	46	Rye Bread	64
Pearl Barley	25	Linguini	46	Semolina Bread	64
Rice Bran	27	Bulgur	47	Couscous	65
Chick Pea Flour Chapati	27	Red River Cereal	49	Rolled Barley	66
Fettucine	32	Pumpernickel Bread	50	Crackers	67
Vermicelli	35	Cracked Barley	50	Gnocchi	67
Spaghetti	6	Special K	54	Taco Shells	68
Whole Rye	37	Corn	55	Cornmeal	69
Barley Kernel Bread	39	Brown Rice	55	Melba Toast	70
Wheat Bran	42	Oatbran	55	Cream of Wheat	70
Barley Chapati	43	Buckwheat	55	Shredded Wheat	70
		Linseed Rye Bread	55	White Flour Products	71
		Popcorn	55	English Muffins	71
		Muesli	56	Millet	71
		Wild Rice	57	White Bagels	72
		Pita Bread, White	57	Puffed Wheat	74
		White Rice	58	Cheerios	74
		Rice Vermicelli	58	Puffed Cereals	74
		Oatmeal	60	Rice Cakes	77
		Rice Krispies	82	Corn Chips/Cornflakes	83
				Brown Rice Pasta	92
				French Baguette	95
Beans					
Chana Daal	8	Romano Beans	46	Broad Beans (fava)	79
Soybeans	17	Baked beans	48		
Red Lentils	25				
Kidney Beans	29				
Green Lentils	29				
Butter Beans	30				
Black Beans	31				
Chick Peas	33				
Navy Beans	38				
Mung Beans	38				
Pinto Beans	38				
Black-eyed Beans	41				

Low Glycemic Index 7-45		Medium Glycemic Index 46-60		High Glycemic Index 61-115	
Protein					
Plain Yogurt	14			Ice Cream	61
Nuts	15				
Skim Milk	32				
Fruit					
Cherries	22	Canned Peaches	47	Raisins	64
Grapefruit	25	Orange Juice	52	Pineapple	66
Dried Apricot	31	Kiwi	53	Dried Fruit	70
Pear	37	Banana	54	Watermelon	72
Plum	38	Mango	56		
Apple	38	Blueberry	57		
Peach	42				
Orange	44				
Vegetables					
Peas	<15	Raw carrots	49	Beets	64
Green Beans	<15	Yams	51	Mashed Potatoes	70
Tomato	<15	Sweet Potatoes	54	Rutabaga	72
Brassica Family	<15	White Potatoes, Boiled	56	French Fries	75
Sea vegetables	<15			Pumpkin	75
Herbs	<15			Cooked Carrots	85
Powdered Greens	<15			Parsnips	98
Green Vegetables	<15				
Other					
Fructose	22	Lactose	46	Sucrose	65
Stevia	N/A	Chocolate	49	Soft Drinks	68
Licorice Root	N/A	Honey	58	Glucose	100
				Maltose	105
				Alcohol	>100

(Most of these values are extrapolated from the book *The G.I. Factor: The Glycaemic Index Solution*, by Dr Jennie Brand Miller, Kaye Foster-Powell and Dr Stephen Colagiuri.)[109]

them of enzymes, and make them even more difficult to digest. Many of us are deficient in lactase, the enzyme that digests lactose, or milk sugar. Our bodies can react to dairy products by producing excess mucus. Mucus tends to accumulate in particular areas and be linked to certain conditions: in the eustachian tubes it leads to chronic ear infections; in the sinuses, sinusitis; in the lungs it can result in asthma; and in the breasts, uterus or ovaries, it may cause tumor formation.

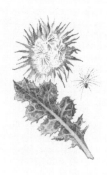

Cancer Risk

Several studies have shown a link between dairy consumption and cancer risk, including two Harvard University studies of milk from hormone treated cows published in 1998.[115,116] The Physicians' Health Study and the Nurses' Health Study found that insulin-like growth factor 1 (IGF-1), a protein that is elevated in the milk of cows treated with bovine growth hormone, increases risk of both breast cancer and prostate cancer. We all have IGF-1 circulating naturally in our bodies but its levels are increased slightly by consuming hormone treated milk and carbohydrates with a high glycemic index. The Nurses' Health Study reported that pre-menopausal women with high levels of IGF-1 in their blood were seven times more likely to get breast cancer than women with low levels. The Physicians' Health Study found that men with the highest levels of IGF-1 in their blood were four times as likely to develop prostate cancer as men with the lowest levels. A 1995 study on rats published in the *Journal of Endocrinology* found that casein, a protein found in milk, slows down the breakdown of IGF-1, allowing it to circulate in blood at higher levels for longer periods of time.[117] It makes sense, then, to avoid hormone treated milk and products containing casein so that our levels of IGF-1 might be lower.

Alternative Sources of Calcium

Women in their menopausal years are often given estrogen replacement therapy and told to drink milk to replenish their calcium levels depleted by this therapy. Calcium supplements should contain calcium, magnesium, vitamin D3, boron, molybdenum, vanadium, manganese, copper, zinc and vitamin K — some of the brands that have most of these include Bone-Up, Osteoprime and OSX by Genestra. Walk an hour a day. If you do have osteoporosis or metastatic cancer to the bone, use the supplement Ipriflavone, at 200 mg 3 times daily to help with either of these conditions. By eating right, exercising, and supplementing you can maintain your bone mass without endangering your breasts.

Sweets

When we consume sweets, a type of white blood cell called the phagocyte decreases its numbers within 30 minutes, and this decline lasts for over five hours, with a 50% reduction in phagocytes approximately two hours after ingestion. This leads to a poorly functioning immune system. This effect occurs after glucose, fructose, sucrose, honey, and orange juice.[118] Sweets will also promote an overgrowth of unwanted organisms in the intestinal tract, such as yeast and parasites. Included in the category of restricted sweets are soft drinks, juice-flavored drinks, powdered instant drinks, canned juices, candy, chocolate bars, granola bars, chocolate, donuts, and cookies.

Breast cancer susceptibility is increased if soft drinks are consumed on a regular basis. After drinking soft drinks, there is a fast and dramatic increase in both glucose and insulin levels within the first hour. This response is more pronounced when body mass is lower, in children, for example. Therefore, children who consume soft drinks regularly increase their breast cancer risk later in life.[119]

Calcium Content of Various Foods

Type of Food	Calcium Content
Fish	
Sardines + bones	325 mg/ 3 oz
Pink salmon + bones	179 mg/ 3 oz
Chum, Coho salmon + bones	300 mg/ 4H oz
Sockeye salmon + bones	300 mg/ 3H oz
Chinook salmon + bones	300 mg/ 7 oz
Beans	
Kidney beans, boiled	50 mg/ 1 cup
Broad beans, boiled	62 mg/ 1 cup
Mung beans, boiled	55 mg/ 1 cup
Lentils, boiled	37 mg/ 1 cup
Black turtle beans, boiled	103 mg/ 1 cup
Black-eyed peas, boiled	130 mg/ 1 cup
Soybeans, boiled	175 mg/ 1 cup
Tofu, raw, firm	258 mg/ $\frac{1}{2}$ cup
Soybeans, boiled	175 mg/ 1 cup
Miso	92 mg/ $\frac{1}{2}$ cup
Adzuki beans, boiled	63 mg/ 1 cup
Great northern beans, boiled	121 mg/ 1 cup
White beans, boiled	161 mg/ 1 cup
Pinto beans, boiled	82 mg/ 1 cup
Navy beans, boiled	128 mg/ 1 cup
Chick peas, boiled	80 mg/ 1 cup
Hummus	124 mg/ 1 cup
Vegetables	
Broccoli, steamed	89 mg/ $\frac{1}{2}$ cup
Turnip greens, chopped, raw	53 mg/ $\frac{1}{2}$ cup
Turnip greens, chopped, boiled	99 mg/ $\frac{1}{2}$ cup
Bok choy, raw, shredded	37 mg/ $\frac{1}{2}$ cup
Bok choy, steamed	79 mg/ $\frac{1}{2}$ cup
Rutabagas	100 mg/ 1 cup
Lambsquarters, steamed	232 mg/ $\frac{1}{2}$ cup
Dandelion greens	150 mg/ 1 cup
Collards, boiled, chopped	148 mg/ 1 cup
Rhubarb	266 mg/ 1 cup
Radish, long greens	60 mg/ $\frac{1}{2}$ cup
Radish root, dried	400 mg/ 100 g
Mustard greens, steamed	52 mg/ $\frac{1}{2}$ cup
Parsley, chopped	39 mg/ $\frac{1}{2}$ cup
Beet greens, steamed	82 mg/ $\frac{1}{2}$ cup
Spinach, chopped, raw	28 mg/ $\frac{1}{2}$ cup
Spinach, steamed	122 mg/ $\frac{1}{2}$ cup
Watercress, chopped	20 mg/ $\frac{1}{2}$ cup
Shepherd's purse	300 mg/ 100 g

Type of Food	Calcium Content
Collard greens	220 mg/ 1 cup
Kale leaves	210 mg/ 1 cup
Broccoli	150 mg/ 1 cup
Seaweeds	
Hijiki	300 mg/ 1 cup
Wakame	300 mg/ 1 cup
Kombu	800 mg/ 100 g
Arame	1170 mg/ 100 g
Agar-agar, dried	625 mg/ 3.5 oz
Irish moss, raw	100 mg/ 3.5 oz
Nori, raw	70 mg/ 3.5 oz
Kelp or kombu, raw	150 mg/ 1 tbsp
Seeds and Nuts	
Brazil nuts	169 mg/ 100 g
Sesame seeds	630 mg/ 100 g
Sunflower seeds	140 mg/ 100 g
Sweet almonds	282 mg/ 100 g
Almond butter	43 mg/ 1 tbsp.
Hazel nuts	186 mg/ 100 g
Carbohydrates	
Millet	20 mg/ 3.5 oz
Cornmeal, enriched	140 mg/ 1 cup
Carob flour	359 mg/ 1 cup
Soybean flour, defatted	241 mg/ 1 cup
Amaranth, boiled	138 mg/ $\frac{1}{2}$ cup
Dark rye flour	69 mg/ 1 cup
Fruits	
Papaya, raw, medium sized	72 mg
Figs, dried	269 mg/ 10 figs
Dairy Products	
Milk, 2%	297 mg/ 1 cup
Evaporated skim milk	344 mg/ $\frac{1}{2}$ cup
Plain yogurt (2-4%)	396 mg/ 1 cup
Swiss cheese	272 mg/ 1 oz
Cheddar cheese	150 mg/ 1 oz
Blue cheese	300 mg/ 3 $\frac{1}{2}$ oz
Cottage cheese	300 mg/ 1$\frac{1}{3}$ cups
Miscellaneous	
Blackstrap molasses	150 mg/ 1 tbsp
Soy milk (not Ca fortified)	50 mg/ 1 cup

Most of these values are extrapolated from Jean A.T. Pennington's *Food Values of Portions Commonly Used.*

PREVENTION

Avoid white flour products. Use instead whole grains and a limited amount of whole grain baked goods.

PREVENTION

Avoid processed food and food packaged in plastic.

PREVENTION

Drink less than two to three alcoholic beverages weekly, preferably drink none.

PREVENTION

Avoid or minimize salt.

PREVENTION

Avoid coffee.

White Flour Products

White flour robs the body of B vitamins and minerals, which are essential for healing. Refined flour is quickly converted into sugar in the blood, which raises insulin levels. Chronic high levels of insulin increase breast cancer risk and cause weight gain. A diet high in refined flour products can disturb the balance of bacteria within the large intestine that normally exerts an immune-enhancing and protective function.

Processed Food

Processed food is devoid of enzymes, vitamins and minerals, lacking in fiber, and often contains colorings and preservatives that are harmful to us. Plastic containers and cans in which processed food is packaged can also be hazardous to our health. Avoid processed food as much as possible. Buy simple ingredients and make your food from scratch.

Alcohol

Alcohol use causes a woman to be more susceptible to breast cancer. A weekly intake of four to seven drinks or more will increase risk. In one study, the risk increase was 250% for women who drank two or more drinks daily. Women who have even one drink a day have an 11% higher risk of breast cancer. Alcohol may interfere with the liver's ability to detoxify both chemicals and excess estrogen in the body.[120] Moderate consumption of alcohol increases the production of insulin-like growth factors by the liver, which promote the development and/or growth of breast cancer.[121]

Salt

Dr Max Gerson believed that salt and excess sodium in general were a major cause of cancer. He theorized that chronic disease begins with a loss of potassium from cells followed by a flow of sodium and water into the cell. This causes a loss of electrical potential, poor enzyme formation, and decreased cellular oxidation. A low-salt diet withdraws water from the cells, whereas a high potassium diet is beneficial. Potassium is a highly alkaline mineral that reduces acidity in the body.

Coffee

Coffee is an adrenal stimulant that causes a short-lived output of adrenal hormones followed by a depletion in them, creating the desire for another coffee. It is high in chemicals that have been used both in the growing and the processing of it. These burden the liver so that it is less able to detoxify both internally generated and external toxins. If you are a coffee drinker, you will need more alkaline minerals to compensate for the overacid state that coffee causes. Use Greens + to help kick the coffee addiction.

Recommended Healthy Breast Daily Diet

If you were to succeed in adopting all of the breast-friendly recommendations outlined in this chapter, here is what your daily diet might look like. I have you eating every 2 hours to normalize the adrenal glands and thyroid, to keep blood sugar levels stable, and to decrease cravings.

On Rising	Green drink — either 1-3 tsp Greens +, Pure Synergy, Barley Green, spirulina or other green powder in water (or 1-3 oz of wheatgrass juice) — followed by two glasses filtered or spring water, with a little lemon or lime juice added plus a pinch of cayenne pepper.
Breakfast	1 cup whole grain cereal (use barley, oatmeal, buckwheat, quinoa, millet meal, amaranth, brown rice) with 2-3 tbsp freshly ground flaxseeds, 1 tbsp wheat bran (if tolerated), small amount of stevia if desired, plus ½ -1 cup soy milk or fruit by itself.
Snack	2 cups fresh vegetable juice, especially carrot, beet, and cabbage, with 1 tsp dulse or kelp powder or 1-2 pieces fruit, especially, cherries, apple, pear, banana, orange, grapefruit, tangerine, or berries. 2 glasses filtered or spring water or herbal tea (green tea, licorice, immune tonic tea, red clover, fenugreek, pau d'arco, mint, dandelion, rosehip).
Lunch	1-2 cups salad with cabbage (eaten at the beginning of the meal so their enzymes will aid digestion). ¾ cup vegetables (at least 50% raw, including ½ cup brassicas). ½ cup mung bean, red clover, sunflower or broccoli sprouts (in salad or in bean and rice dish). 1-2 tbsp. flaxseed oil, as salad dressing, and over beans and grain. ½ -1 cup beans, with onion and garlic (hummus, bean dips, bean soup, or bean and grain dish). ½ -1 cup grain, preferably whole grain rather than flour products (rice, millet, barley, quinoa, buckwheat). 3-4 shitake mushrooms.
Snack	1-2 tbsp raw almonds, pumpkin seeds, soy nuts and/or sunflower seeds. 2 cups vegetable juice (especially carrot, beet, cabbage, dulse powder with added watercress, parsley, kale, mustard greens, garlic, ginger, sprouts, dandelion greens, or apple). 2 glasses filtered or spring water or herbal tea, as above.
Dinner	Green drink (as before breakfast, taken ½ hour before dinner). 1 cup salad with fresh sprouts, onions and garlic, raw sunflower or pumpkin seeds, and grated citrus peel. ½ cup firm organic tofu or tempeh. ½ -1 cup whole grains (wild rice, quinoa, millet, rice, barley, and buckwheat — omit this if you are food combining or wanting to lose weight). ¾ cup vegetables, raw or lightly steamed. ½ cup red clover, sunflower, mung bean or broccoli sprouts. 2 tbsp sea vegetables (hiziki, arame, wakame, nori, dulse, kelp). 1-2 tbsp flaxseed oil and 1 tablespoon olive oil as part of salad dressing or over grain or vegetables.
Snack	2 glasses filtered or spring water or decaffeinated green tea. 1 cup Healthy Breast Drink (1 cup soy milk, 1 tsp. turmeric paste, optional banana, blended or warmed).
Notes:	One serving of fruits or vegetables is, for example: 1 cup of raw leafy vegetables ½ cup of other vegetables or fruit (cooked or raw) or I cup vegetable or fruit juice 1 medium apple, banana, or orange ½ cup fruit or 2 tbsp dried fruit Six servings in a day might include two pieces of fruit, one cup of salad, and one and a half cups of steamed or raw vegetables.

Weekly Diet Diary

Record your weekly intake of food to determine the approximate number of servings of fruits and vegetables, fiber, soy products, calories from fat, etc. you are consuming.

	Monday	Tuesday	Wednesday	Thursday	Friday	Saturday	Sunday
Breakfast							
Snack							
Lunch							
Snack							
Dinner							
Snack							

14-Day Dietary Routine Worksheet

Over a two-week period, assess how well you are maintaining a breast health/cancer prevention diet. Aim for an increased number of check marks over time. Be patient. Change takes time. Some of us may be able to make a diet transition in a few weeks; others of us will do a little more each year. Respect your pace while making your best effort. If you are in a group, share your successes, difficulties and recipes with other women. Repeat this assessment every three months or more to help you stay on track.

From (date)_____ to _____

Daily Food (Check Daily)	1	2	3	4	5	6	7	8	9	10	11	12	13	14
Vegetarian Diet														
Organic Food: fill in what %														
Raw Food : 50% or more														
Broccoli Sprouts (3 x weekly)														
Mung Bean Sprouts (3 x weekly)														
Red Clover Sprouts (3 x weekly)														
Dandelion in season (3 x weekly)														
Vegetable Juice: 2 or more														
Cabbage: $\frac{1}{3}$, juiced or raw														
Tomato Products (2 x weekly)														
Fruits: 2 or more														
Citrus Juice: organic (3 x weekly)														
Vegetables: 4 or more servings														
Brassica Family: 1 cup														
Onion: 1														
Garlic: 2 cloves, raw is better														
Sea Vegetables: $\frac{1}{3}$ cup														
Shitaki Mushrooms (2 x weekly)														
Low Salt/High Potassium														
< 15 % saturated fat/ total calories														
Flaxseed Oil: 2 or more tbsp														
Olive Oil for cooking, low heat														
Fiber: 30 g														
Whole Grains: 1 cup														
Beans: 1-2 cups daily														
Flaxseeds: 2-4 tbsp, ground														
Pumpkin Seeds: 2 tbsp, raw														
Wheat Bran: 1 tbsp														
Protein: 30-50 g daily														
Tofu: $\frac{1}{2}$ cup														
Soy Milk: 1 cup														
Miso: 1 tbsp (3 x weekly)														
Citrus Peel: 1 tsp organic grated														
Turmeric: 1-2 tsp powder														
Rosemary, Sage, Thyme, Ginger														
Water: 8 glasses filtered														
Alcoholic Drinks: < 2 /week														
Coffee: none														
Sugar: none														
Canned or Processed Food: none														
Dairy: none														

Food Rotation

When we eat the same foods day after day we can develop sensitivities to them that may result in weakened immunity. Food sensitivities can manifest as headaches, chronic ear, eye, or throat infections, fatigue, digestive upsets, arthritis, allergies, asthma, persistent cough, chronic congestion, nausea, abdominal cramps, irritability, hyperactivity, insomnia, palpitations, eczema, itching skin, joint pain, edema, frequent urination, depression, and learning disabilities. The most common food sensitivities are to dairy, wheat, brewer's and baker's yeast, eggs, sugar, peanuts, citrus, corn, and tomatoes. Many people react to foods that are healthy but which they have overused.

An accurate test for food sensitivities is the ELISA blood test, which measures immunoglobulin response to specific foods and can be ordered through your naturopathic or medical doctor. Generally, a period of avoidance of three to six months for the foods you are sensitive to plus a 5-day rotation diet help to restore digestive and immune health.

Summary

Using food as medicine and being conscious of the effects of food on our bodies and minds are integral steps in preventing or recovering from breast cancer. However, you may feel overwhelmed at such a drastic diet shift, and at a loss as to how to use some of these foods. There are many resources available. Look for a vegetarian cooking class in your neighborhood, or get together with some friends and experiment with new dishes. Go to the library or look on the internet for recipes – you will find a ton of them. This diet change will take time, and you may need some coaching, so find a healthcare professional or vegetarian friend to help you get started. The main thing is to start now, and make a little progress each month. To begin the process, try these basic dietary changes:

1) Use 2 tbsp ground flaxseeds with your breakfast.
2) Have soy milk with turmeric paste most evenings.
3) Eat at least 3 fruits, 2 cups of salad, and 1 cup of steamed vegetables daily.
4) Reduce your intake of sweets and desserts by 50%.
5) Reduce your consumption of animal protein by 50%.
6) Reduce your coffee intake by 50%.

Because we are inundated with environmental contaminants, and because the soil has been depleted and food does not contain as many minerals and phytonutrients as it used to, we need to add nutritional supplements to our breast cancer protection program. These supplements are discussed in the next chapter.

CHAPTER EIGHT

Nutritional Supplements for Breast Health

CONTENTS

EXERCISES, CHARTS, CHECKLISTS & WORKSHEETS

There are some healthcare practitioners who believe that we should get all our nutrients from food sources, while others believe that supplements are necessary for health preservation and for healing illness. My belief is that most of us suffer from at least some nutritional deficiencies due to depletion of nutrients from the soil and thus from our food. The mineral content of our foods is much less than it was 100 years ago. Our bodies need more nutrients to detoxify the pollutants in our air, water, and food; and our diets are often deficient in vital nutrients. The stress of living at this time, with its fast pace, uses up nutrient reserves; most of us don't absorb the nutrients we do take in because we are always on the go, interfering with the digestive process that needs us to relax for it to work properly. Supplementation of at least some nutrients is beneficial.

The following information is meant as a guide but not a prescription for some of the many supplements available to assist in the prevention and treatment of breast cancer. Get as many of them as you can through diet and find quality supplements from natural sources for the others. Work with a naturopath, nutritionist, or other professional in determining how to best use this information and what dosages to take.

Vitamins

All vitamins are naturally present in our food. Our bodies are unable to make most vitamins, so we must get them from what we eat or ingest. Vitamins assist enzymes in their tasks; without vitamins enzymes don't work. Enzymes are proteins that act as catalysts for almost every biochemical reaction in the body — they govern growth, metabolism, cellular reproduction, digestion, hormone production, liver detoxification and many other functions. Without enzymes, biochemical reactions would occur too slowly to support life. And without vitamins, enzymes are sluggish and inefficient. We need replacement vitamins every day for optimal vitality, either from our food or a supplement.

Vitamin A

Vitamin A, also known as retinol, is an important nutrient for maintaining the integrity of the body's skin — the outer skin as well as the mucous lining in the digestive and intestinal tract — which promotes improved intestinal health, digestion and immunity. When this layer is healthy, it is less vulnerable to chemical carcinogens and parasitic or yeast infections. Vitamin A prevents cancer from occurring on the inner lining of the stomach, lungs, skin, and in the epithelial lining of the ducts and lobules of the breast. It helps cells repair themselves when they have been exposed to cancer-causing substances. It improves our body's ability to destroy tumors and increases the number of white blood cells. It causes phagocytes, a particular kind of white blood cell, to be more efficient at digesting toxins and potential carcinogens.

Vitamin A also prevents and reverses the effects of stress on the thymus gland by promoting its growth and reducing its shrinkage, which commonly occurs when we are stressed for long periods of time. The thymus coordinates the activity of our white blood cells, the warriors of our immune system.

Vitamin A is more effective when taken with zinc and adequate vitamin E. Sufficient vitamin A has a sparing effect on vitamin C. Pre-formed vitamin A (animal derived) is fat soluble; it is stored in the liver and can be toxic when the liver's capacity to store it has been exceeded.

Contraindications: Chronic ingestion of over 100,000 IU of vitamin A daily in a susceptible person may result in toxicity. Only low doses should be used during pregnancy.

Beta-carotene, Other Carotenes, and Carotenoids

A recent Australian study of 153 newly diagnosed breast cancer cases and 151 controls found that women with the highest beta carotene levels in their blood were 47% less likely to be diagnosed with breast cancer than women with the lowest levels.[1,2]

Derived from vegetables, beta-carotene is converted to vitamin A in the body. It is only one member of a large group of over 600 different carotenes, many of which are therapeutic. Each carotenoid has a slightly different effect, and may have a preferred site of action in our bodies. Some of the other carotenes are alpha-carotene,

FACT
Vitamin A will help to improve the tissue tolerance for women undergoing chemotherapy or radiation so there is less damage to healthy cells, particularly those lining the inside of the mouth and intestines, which have a fast turnover time and are affected most by chemotherapy.

◀ **Food Sources:** butter, cream, egg yolks, fish liver oil from cod, halibut, salmon, shark. **Dosage:** 5,000-35,000 IU daily.

FACT
Beta-carotene, which is more effective than vitamin A in breast cancer prevention and a better antioxidant, has been shown to reduce the risk of pre-menopausal breast cancer by up to 90%.

gamma-carotene, lycopene, cryptoxanthin, zeaxanthin and lutein. Instead of just supplementing our diets with beta-carotene, we can consume a diet rich in vegetables which will contain other carotenes that collectively block the initiation and promotion of cancer by binding free radicals; increase the level of cytokines (interferon, interleukin, tumor necrosis factor) in the body, which help fight cancer; protect DNA from chemicals and radiation; help to produce anti-cancer enzymes in the digestive tract; increase the ratio of helper to suppressor T-cells, which improves the ability of the immune system to attack cancer cells; and increase the size, weight, and function of the thymus gland.

Beta carotene in produce is destroyed when exposed to light, oxygen, storage, and processing. Fresh and locally grown is best. Surprisingly, when foods high in carotenoids are cooked, they are up to five times more active in inhibiting cancer than when they are raw.[3]

Contraindications: Do not use during chemotherapy with 5-fluorouracil or methotrexate. It may decrease their effectiveness.[4]

Vitamin B Complex

The B complex vitamins include B1 (thiamine), B2 (riboflavin), B3 (niacin), B5 (pantothenic acid), B6 (pyridoxine), B12 (cyanocobalamin), B15 (pangamic acid), biotin, choline, folic acid, inositol, and PABA.

The B complex vitamins are needed to convert carbohydrate into glucose, giving us energy. The B complex also helps strengthen cell membranes so they are less vulnerable to stress and is needed for the health of our nerves. Irritability, impatience, depression, and many psychological disorders can often be helped with the B complex. A deficiency in the B complex will depress immunity and cause shrinkage of lymphatic tissue. An excess of estrogen, such as when women take the birth control pill, can deplete some of the B vitamins. Many of the B vitamins are needed in liver detoxification and the breakdown of estrogen into its harmless forms. If any single B vitamin is taken, the B complex should be taken along with it to prevent a deficiency of some of the other B vitamins.

Contraindications: Any excess is excreted and not stored. Be cautious of using a high potency B complex during chemotherapy, as B1 and B3 may speed up Phase 1 detoxification, breaking down drugs more quickly. Amounts present in a multivitamin are probably safe.

Vitamin B3 (Niacin)

Niacin, niacinamide, and inositol hexaniacinate are all forms of vitamin B3 that are useful in the prevention and treatment of breast cancer. Niacin assists enzymes in the breakdown and use of proteins, fats, and carbohydrates. It is also utilized in blood sugar regulation and for detoxification in the liver. It improves circulation, delivering more nutrients to the cells and removing waste more efficiently. It reduces cholesterol levels in the blood and is necessary for the synthesis of adrenal and sex hormones.

As niacin helps to break down estrogen, a deficiency will lead to an excess of estrogen and an increased breast cancer risk.[5] Some studies indicate that niacin is a common deficiency among cancer patients.[6] Niacin is required to make the enzyme ADP ribose polymerase, used in DNA replication and repair.[7] ADP ribose polymerase is made from the cell's NAD, which contains nicotinamide, a form of niacin. When animals were fed a diet low in niacin, they showed a deficiency of both NAD and ADP ribose polymerase.[8] In humans, a deficiency of niacin can lead to 70% less NAD in the cell, which would mean that cells would be 70% less capable of fixing damaged DNA.[9]

Niacin plays a role in the activation of the p53 tumor suppressor gene, which acts as a kind of gatekeeper to prevent damaged cells from dividing and replicating themselves.[10] Niacin is required to make the important breast nutrient, coenzyme Q10, from the amino acid, tyrosine. In one study, two groups of human cells were treated with carcinogens. The group given adequate niacin developed tumors at only one tenth of the rate as the group deficient in niacin.[11,12]

Dr Max Gerson used niacin as an important part of his therapy with cancer patients. He used 50 mg six times daily with his patients for four to six months. To prevent the niacin 'flush', he advised dissolving the tablet on the tongue after a meal or glass of juice.[13] The niacin flush causes the capillaries to dilate, producing a short-lived red flushing and tingling of the body similar to a sunburn. It can be very alarming for some people, but is harmless.

Niacin is also an important nutrient in sauna detoxification programs and is used in increasing amounts up to 4000 mg daily for approximately 20 days, with medical supervision. See Chapter 5, 'Detoxifying Our Bodies,' for more information on sauna detoxification and niacin supplements.

Contraindications: It can cause liver damage at dosages higher than 2000 mg daily, so anything above this should be monitored with liver function tests. It is contraindicated in persons with gout, liver disease, peptic ulcers, and possibly diabetes. If the dose is too high, nausea will be experienced, sometimes followed by vomiting. Do not use doses above 50 mg daily during chemotherapy as it may speed up Phase 1 detoxification in the liver.

Vitamin B6 (Pyridoxine)

Vitamin B6 is important for fat and protein metabolism and overall immune function. It is needed in the metabolism of essential fatty acids and in the breakdown of estrogen. Laboratory studies have demonstrated that B6 inhibits the growth of both estrogen receptor positive and ER negative breast cancer.[14] A deficiency of B6, common in cancer patients, causes lowered immunity, with shrinkage of lymphatic tissue, and a decrease in numbers of white blood cells and activity of the thymus gland.[15] B6 helps keep the balance of sodium and potassium, which regulates body fluids. It allows linoleic acid to function better in our bodies and is needed for the production of hydrochloric acid so that we digest our food better, with better absorption of protein and minerals. Alcohol, excess protein, and the use of the birth control pill can all trigger a deficiency of B6.

Contraindications: Use with caution if you have stomach ulcers. Do not exceed 200 mg daily.

FACT

Vitamin B3 (niacin) is crucial in preventing the initiation of the cancer process — and in reversing it. When niacin is administered before radiation treatments, it increases its effectiveness. Niacin suppresses tumor growth.

◀ **Food Sources:** lean meats, poultry, fish, eggs, peanuts, sunflower and sesame seeds, pine nuts, brown rice, brewer's yeast, wheat germ and bran, liver.
Dosage: 25-2000 mg daily. Higher dose to be used with supervision.

FACT

Supplementation with vitamin B6 results in the production of more protective estrogens (C2) and fewer harmful estrogens (C4, C16), as well as higher levels of progesterone — which all decrease breast cancer risk.

◀ **Food Sources:** brewer's yeast, sunflower seeds, wheat germ, tuna, beans, salmon, trout, brown rice, bananas, walnuts, hazelnuts, avocados, egg yolks, kale, bee pollen, liver, whole grain cereals.
Dosage: 50-200 mg daily.

Food Sources: green, leafy ▶
vegetables, liver, brewer's
yeast, black-eyed peas,
wheat germ and bran, beans,
soy, lentils, asparagus,
broccoli, Brussels sprouts,
whole wheat, oatmeal,
barley, almonds, split peas,
and walnuts.
Dosage: 400 mcg daily in
adults, 800 mcg during
pregnancy and breast-feeding.

FACT

Vitamin B12 has a particular
role to fill in alleviating some
of the side effects of
chemotherapy.

Food Sources: liver, kidney, ▶
meat, fish, egg yolks, poultry,
yogurt, milk.
Dosage: 50 mcg daily.

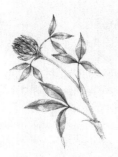

Folic Acid

Deficiency of folic acid can trigger megaloblastic anemia and degeneration of the intestinal lining, leading to poor nutrient absorption. Folic acid helps block the division of rapidly dividing cells, such as occurs in cancer formation, and is specifically used to prevent cervical dysplasia. When folic acid is deficient, there will be shrinkage of lymphatic tissue and depressed immunity. A deficiency of folic acid exists in women with breast cancer who consume alcohol.[16] Folic acid is needed for the production of DNA and for mental and emotional health. It stimulates hydrochloric acid production in the stomach, which helps to prevent intestinal parasites and assists liver function. It is destroyed by high temperatures, exposure to light, and when foods are left out at room temperature for long periods, as in salad bars.

Contraindications: None known.

Vitamin B12

Vitamin B12 is important in protein, carbohydrate, and fat metabolism. It helps the conversion of beta-carotene to vitamin A and assists in the production of DNA and RNA, the genetic material in each cell. It assists the action of vitamin C and is essential for longevity. Vegetarians are sometimes deficient in B12, as it is uncommon in vegetarian diets, and they should take a B complex that includes B12 regularly. The absorption of B12 decreases with age and the use of laxatives will deplete B12 reserves. A recent study found that if postmenopausal women had serum B12 levels below a certain threshold level, their breast cancer risk was increased.[17]

Women receiving the chemotherapy drugs Taxol, Taxotere, or Vincristine may develop peripheral neuropathy, with symptoms of numbness and tingling in their arms and legs. Weekly intramuscular injections of 1000 mcg of B12 along with a fish oil supplement may reduce these symptoms.[18] Another common side effect of chemotherapy is a drop in the white blood cell count, which must be maintained at a level of 2000 (with the normal range being 4000-10,000), for chemotherapy to continue. Weekly injections of 1000 mcg B12 can raise white blood cell counts, as B12 stimulates the bone marrow to make new ones.[19]

Contraindications: None.

Inositol and Inositol Hexaphosphate (IP6)

Inositol is part of the B complex found naturally occurring in high fiber foods, such as wheat bran, rice bran, and legumes. When bound to hexaphosphate, it forms IP6 or phytic acid. When properly combined with inositol, inositol hexaphosphate or IP6 forms two molecules of IP3 in the body. IP3 acts to prevent cancer by regulating cell division. When IP3 levels are low, cancer cells replicate out of control, whereas when there are high amounts of IP3 available, they cease to divide. In addition, IP6 promotes cell differentiation, a process whereby cancer cells become more normal. IP6 is located within all cell membranes, which allows it to receive and direct biochemical messages to regulate cell division.

Animal studies have shown that the effects of IP6 occur within 24 hours of administration and persist for several days after a single dose.[20] Rats given 0.4% IP6 in drinking water, equivalent to a diet containing 20% bran, showed a 33.5% reduction in tumor incidence and 48.8% fewer tumors.[21] Evidence suggests that IP6 has a positive effect on tumor suppressor genes such as p53, which encourages genetically damaged cells to self-destruct.[22] The combination of inositol and IP6 enhances the ability of natural killer cells to target cancer cells and acts as an antioxidant. Studies have shown this combination to be effective against breast, prostate, lung, liver, skin and brain cancers, as well as leukemia and lymphomas.

The maximum benefit is obtained from products that contain four parts IP6 to one part inositol. Zinc, iron, and calcium will be poorly absorbed if ingested with IP6, so take these supplements at a different time of day.

Contraindications: None. Take it 2 hours away from other minerals.

Vitamin C

This vitamin acts as an antioxidant to prevent cellular and DNA damage from free radicals. Some studies concluded that the greater the amount of vitamin C that a woman routinely ingested from foods, the greater the reduction of breast cancer risk.[23] Vitamin C helps to prevent tumor growth and the formation of metastases by building dense connective tissue and assists the activity of white blood cells, improving immunity. It is important in the production of interferon.

Intravenous vitamin C therapy is a common alternative therapy for many cancers. If the plasma concentrations of vitamin C are high enough, free radicals in cancer cells are converted to hydrogen peroxide, which kills them. Depending on the type of cancer, 5-40 mg/dl is required to kill 100% of cancer cells within 3 days.[24] The highest concentration we can achieve with oral supplementation is 4.5 mg/dl. Practitioners have been able to reverse cancer some of the time with sustained intravenous therapy using doses from 50 to 100 grams at least twice weekly, given intravenously over several hours. Oral vitamin C and alpha lipoic acid can be used between i.v. treatments to keep plasma vitamin C levels elevated. This must be maintained for a minimum of 2 weeks to achieve its effect.[25]

More recent studies suggest that vitamin C treatment for breast cancer can be augmented with simultaneous use of vitamin K3.[26] Vitamin C and vitamin K3 administered in a ratio of 100:1 produced selective cancer cell death with cell membrane injury, a splitting apart of DNA, and loss of cell cytoplasm in studies on mice. When used in conjunction with chemotherapy in mice, they increased life span, improved the effectiveness of the chemo, and caused no toxicity.[27] Although both vitamin C and vitamin K3 show anti-tumor activity, high doses are required for each. When combined in the C:K3 ratio of 100:1 in a laboratory setting on human prostate cells, concentrations of the vitamins needed to kill cancer cells decreased ten to sixtyfold.[28] These two vitamins have also proven to be effective against breast cancer cell lines in the laboratory, and

◀ **Food Sources:** whole grains, bran and beans.
Dosage: 800-1200 mg IP6 and 200-300 mg inositol as prevention; 4,800-7,200 mg IP6 and 1,200-1,800 mg inositol for individuals with cancer. It should be taken on an empty stomach.

FACT
According to the lowest estimates, vitamin C can reduce the risk of breast cancer by 5-10% in menopausal and post-menopausal women. Higher estimates suggest that risk can be reduced for menopausal women by 16% and for post-menopausal women by 37%.

◀ **Food Sources:** citrus, strawberries, melon, tomatoes, green leafy vegetables, papaya, mangoes, cantaloupe, broccoli, potatoes, cabbage, green and red peppers, rose hips, and the Ayurvedic herb, amla.
Dosage: 2,000-10,000 mg daily in frequent small doses, preferably with food.

although still in the experimental stage, they seem to be a promising non-toxic combination for breast cancer in women.[29]

Contraindications: Diarrhea may result at levels of 10,000 mg daily. Always increase or decrease vitamin C incrementally. Do not use for 5 days before surgery, as it can cause increased bleeding during surgery.

Bioflavonoids (Vitamin P)

Food Sources: citrus, berries, yams, soy, dark, leafy greens, milk thistle, broccoli, cabbage, squash, carrots, amla, onions, apples.
Dosage: 100 mg of bioflavonoids for every 500 mg of vitamin C; purchase vitamin C with bioflavonoids.

Bioflavonoids assist the body in using vitamin C to stimulate detoxification of chemicals, toxins, and drugs in the liver. These are a very large group of over 4,000 antioxidants which prevent cancer-promoting substances from attaching themselves to cells and inhibit cancer cell growth and metastasis. They form the pigment in plants, as do the carotenes, concentrating in the peel, skin, or outer layer of the plant. They are also present in tea and wine. Bioflavonoids include catechin, quercetin, rutin, and silymarin. They help to remove toxic copper from the body and prevent vitamin C from being destroyed. A standard Western diet contains a daily dose of 500-1000 mg of bioflavonoids, while a vegetarian diet contains 5,000 mg, which protects us from cancer and inflammation. We need certain intestinal bacteria to activate bioflavonoids.

Quercetin, one of the bioflavonoids, shows particular promise in breast cancer treatment. It inhibits the expression of mutant P53 genes, and slows down the division of cancer cells. Quercetin, like Tamoxifen and the phytoestrogens, can bind to estrogen receptors to inhibit the growth of breast cancer cells. When used during radiation treatments it lessened damage to the skin. It does affect Phase 1 and Phase 2 liver detoxification, so is best used cautiously during chemotherapy, unless we know how it interacts with specific medications. A standard dose is 500 mg 3x daily.30

Contraindications: Do not use during chemotherapy, as they can interfere with Phase 1 and Phase 2 liver detoxification and alter drug concentrations.

Bioflavonoids and Cancer

This chart summarizes some of the important bioflavonoids and their effects in preventing breast cancer.

Bioflavonoid	What It Does	Found In
Quercetin	Toxic to breast cancer cells, indirectly improves immunity.	ginger, echinacea, pau d'arco, St. John's wort, onions, apples
Rutin	Toxic to cancer cells, strengthens capillaries.	buckwheat
Silymarin	Improves liver's ability to detoxify, increases glutathione.	milk thistle
Aglycone, Kaempferol, Myricetin	Cancer fighting ability.	green and black tea
Pycnogenol	Powerful antioxidant and cell protector, strengthens capillaries.	pine bark, grape seed

Vitamin D

Vitamin D is found mainly among dairy products such as milk and cheese. However, because these foods have been linked with increased breast cancer risk, we should consume them infrequently. The easiest way to obtain vitamin D is by spending a little time in the sun. Studies show that the closer to the equator a population is, the less risk they have for breast cancer.[31] Sunshine causes the body to make its own vitamin D, which is then synthesized by the liver to become active vitamin D. The more receptors we have in our breasts for vitamin D, the greater the effect it has on tumor prevention as well as tumor treatment (vitamin D has been shown to reduce the size of malignant tumors in women with high amounts of vitamin D receptors).[32] To prevent skin cancer, we should be cautious about too much direct exposure to sunlight. Fifteen minutes towards the end of the day is probably sufficient.

Vitamin D is also a hormone that regulates the mineral balance of calcium and phosphorus. It stimulates their absorption from the intestine, works with parathyroid hormone to draw calcium out of bone tissue, and stimulates the reabsorption of calcium from the kidneys. Adequate vitamin D is crucial during and after menopause when the decline in estrogen and progesterone can lead to bone loss and osteoporosis.

Contraindications: Overdoses of vitamin D are extremely toxic, resulting in deafness and blindness.

Food Sources: dairy products, fortified soymilk, fish oils.
Dosage: For someone who avoids the sun and dairy products, 800 IU of vitamin D daily is appropriate, while 400 IU would be adequate for those living in cloudy environments.

Vitamin E

Vitamin E refers to a group of eight fat-soluble compounds composed of four tocopherols (alpha, beta, delta, gamma) and four tocotrienols. It is stored in liver, muscle, and fat tissue. As an antioxidant, it works along with vitamin C to protect from cellular damage due to toxins, radiation, and aging. It protects the other fat-soluble vitamins and oils from oxidation. We need extra vitamin E when we consume higher amounts of unsaturated oils, such as flaxseed oil.

Working together with selenium, vitamin E improves immune function, protecting the thymus gland and T-lymphocytes. Vitamin E in the form of tocotrienols derived from palm oil inhibits both estrogen-positive and estrogen-negative breast cancer cells and is more effective than the alpha-tocopherol form of vitamin E.[34] When we use a vitamin E supplement for breast cancer prevention, we should purchase one that includes tocotrienols and mixed tocopherols.

Contraindications: It should not be taken with iron, but separated from it by 8 or more hours. (Iron can increase the growth of tumors and should be avoided unless you are anemic.) It may raise blood pressure in someone who has not used it; therefore, start at a low dosage and monitor blood pressure in anyone with hypertension. Use with caution in patients with chronic rheumatic heart disease. Do not take for several days before surgery, as it can thin the blood and cause increased bleeding. Do use after surgery for wound healing.

FACT
Vitamin E as alpha-tocopherol has been shown to decrease risk of breast cancer in pre-menopausal women with a family history of the disease.[33]

Food Sources: cold-pressed vegetable oils, fresh wheat germ, raw seeds and nuts, egg yolk.
Dosage: 400-800 IU daily.

Vitamin K

Vitamin K has demonstrated effectiveness in attacking the energy packets (ATP) of cancer cells. It is usually manufactured in the intestines in the presence of healthy bacteria, yet another reason for avoiding antibiotics and supplementing regularly with acidophilus and bifidus. A synthetic form of vitamin K, vitamin K3, was developed to treat people who were incapable of producing their own vitamin K. This form of the vitamin reduces the risk of breast cancer more than the original form.[35] Vitamin K acts as a clotting agent, and is necessary to make blood clotting factors in the liver. When it was used with the anticoagulant warfarin, its effectiveness in breast cancer treatment increased. Vitamin K and warfarin can be used in combination with conventional breast cancer drugs to reduce their toxic effect. This combination greatly increased life expectancy of cancer patients. An alternative to warfarin may be to use fish oil supplements along with digestive enzymes containing high amounts of protease and bromelain to offset vitamin K3's clotting effect.

Combined with vitamin C in a 100:1 ratio, vitamin K3 has been shown to be effective in killing breast cancer cells.[36]

Contraindications: Excessive amounts of synthetic vitamin K may build up in the blood and cause toxic reactions. Use under supervision.

Minerals

Minerals are essential for overall health and well-being, forming the skeleton and teeth, present in our muscles, blood, nerve cells, and in all of our body fluids. Like vitamins, they act as catalysts for many biological reactions and are necessary components of enzymes. Our mineral balance determines how substances flow in and out of our cells and sets the pH of various fluids and tissues, upon which biochemical reactions depend. The health of our glands is related to mineral concentrations of zinc, selenium, iodine, boron, magnesium, and others. Calcium, chlorine, phosphorus, potassium, magnesium, sodium and sulfur are known as the 'macrominerals' because they are present in relatively high amounts, while other 'trace minerals' are present in only minute amounts.

Calcium

Animal studies have shown that a low intake of calcium and vitamin D combined with a high fat diet can cause an increase in tumors of the breast from 37-75%, or approximately double. The tumors in the low calcium group also tended to be larger than those in animals fed a high fat diet with sufficient calcium.[37] Girls with low calcium levels during puberty may be at more risk for breast cancer later in life.[38]

A reasonable but difficult to achieve dietary level is 800-1500 mg daily depending upon age, pregnancy or lactation and sex, while the therapeutic dose range is between 1000-2000 mg. The majority of a calcium supplement is best taken at night because more calcium is lost at night and foods may interfere with absorption. However, if an individual has deficient stomach acid, it will not be absorbed on its own and would be better taken with a meal.

Calcium should be taken with magnesium (in a 2:1 ratio) and vitamin D for proper absorption. Other minerals that enhance its absorption and utilization are boron and silica. High protein and high phosphorus intake (meats, soft drinks) promote calcium loss. Cereal grains and fiber high in phytates decrease calcium absorption. Salt, sugar, and caffeine cause calcium loss.

Chelated minerals (aspartates, picolinates, amino acid chelates) are more bio-available than metallic minerals such as gluconates, lactates, sulphates, carbonates, and oxides. Hydrochloric acid production can be stimulated with bitter herbs such as wormwood, gentian, goldenseal, and pippali. Lemon and/or apple cider vinegar taken before a meal also may boost hydrochloric acid production.

Contraindications: Although calcium acts to protect against breast cancer, there are divided opinions regarding taking high amounts if you have cancer. Dr Max Gerson found that calcium caused tumors to grow but was unclear why this would be so. The only minerals he advised taking if one had cancer were potassium and iodine.[39]

Magnesium

Magnesium reduced the incidence of malignant breast tumors by 50% in studies on rats. When used with vitamin C, selenium, and vitamin A, the number of tumors declined even further. Magnesium is a common nutritional deficiency.[40] It is needed in the metabolism of glutathione, an important amino acid complex used by the liver and white blood cells.

Magnesium is responsible for chlorophyll's green color, so any green vegetable or seed will have some magnesium.

Contraindications: High amounts of magnesium can cause diarrhea in some individuals. If this happens to you, cut your dosage down and then gradually increase it to tolerance levels, or use magnesium glycinate.

Potassium

Potassium is found in the body's intracellular fluid; only a small amount occurs in the extracellular fluid. Sodium and potassium help regulate water balance in the body, maintaining the fluids on either side of the cell wall. It is necessary for normal growth, muscle contractions, and stimulates the kidneys to eliminate waste products. It is one of the body's detoxifiers. As part of a cancer prevention program, we want to keep a low sodium and high potassium balance to prevent the accumulation of toxins in the cells.

Alcohol, coffee and excess sugar cause potassium to be lost through the kidneys, so these should be avoided. Long periods of stress can result in potassium deficiency. Signs of potassium deficiency include insomnia, slow, irregular heartbeat, poor reflexes, dry skin and muscle weakness.

Contraindications: Do not take high amounts of potassium if there is kidney damage. Kidney failure will cause potassium levels to build and become too high.

Food Sources: seaweeds, sesame seeds, almonds, sunflower seeds, dairy, soy products, parsley, kale, broccoli, beet greens, shepherd's purse, kidney beans, lentils, nettle, horsetail, sage, barley, millet, quinoa, figs, and molasses. For the calcium content of other foods, see Chapter 7, 'Eating Right for Breast Health.'
Dosage: 800-2000 mg daily.

Food Sources: pumpkin seeds, nuts, brewer's yeast, soy, dried apricots, collards, seafood, whole grains, dark green vegetables, molasses.
Dosage: 300-800 mg daily.

FACT
Potassium keeps the body fluids more alkaline, which is important because cancer prefers an acid environment.

Food Sources: navy beans, caraway seeds, dark cherries, dried apricots, lentils, walnuts, oranges, almonds, apple, avocado, peaches, banana, grapefruit, pineapple, potatoes, soybeans, squash, tomatoes, sage, and mint. For the potassium content of other foods, see Chapter 7, 'Eating Right for Breast Health.'
Dosage: 3000-6000 mg daily from foods.

Food Sources: sea salt, sea ▶ vegetables, fish, asparagus, garlic, lima beans, mushrooms, sesame seeds, soybeans, spinach, summer squash, and turnip greens.

Dosage: A reasonable dietary level is 150 mcg of iodine, while the therapeutic dose range is 100-1000 mcg daily. Start with a small dose of kelp and increase gradually. A 575 mg capsule of Norwegian kelp contains 359 mcg of iodine. Do not exceed 3 tablets daily. Increase dosage only if you are exposed to radiation.

Food Sources: None known. ▶
Dosage: 1000 mg taken 3x daily at the end of each meal, along with at least 1000 mg vitamin C. Selenium, zinc and extra potassium should be taken daily along with it.

Food Sources: legumes, ▶ whole grain cereals, kidney, liver, milk, and dark green vegetables.
Dosage: 100-500 mcg daily.

Iodine

Iodine is naturally present in the epithelial cells that line the ducts and lobules of the breast and makes them less sensitive to the stimulating effect of estrogen. Iodine is needed as a raw material to synthesize thyroid hormones and there is a link between an unbalanced thyroid and breast cancer risk. Iodine is commonly deficient in our diets because it is deficient in the soil that is inland from the sea. Japanese women traditionally use kelp in their cooking, and it may be one of the nutrients (along with soy, fish oil and no dairy) that gives them roughly one quarter of the breast cancer rates present among women in the United States. In animal studies, kelp has been shown to prevent breast tumors.[41]

Dr Max Gerson used a form of iodine called Lugol's solution, half strength in a dosage of three drops, six times daily, as well as dessicated thyroid, in treating his cancer patients, believing that it restored the electrical potential of the cell and enhanced cellular activity.

Contraindications: Side effects of too much iodine are weight loss, insomnia, anxiety, heart palpitations, acne, headaches, water retention, metallic taste in the mouth and skin sensitivities. Do not use iodine if you have a hyperactive thyroid or sensitivity to it. Dosages need to be monitored by someone experienced with thyroid disorders. Kelp is safer to use.

Cesium Chloride

Cesium is an alkaline mineral found in trace amounts throughout the earth's crust. Unlike radioactive cesium released from nuclear radiation, cesium chloride is non-radioactive and may protect an individual exposed to radioactive cesium. It has a high pH level and can change the acidic pH of the cancer cell to being alkaline. At a pH of 8 or so, cancer cells are non-viable. Cesium limits the cellular uptake of glucose in the cancer cell, helping to starve it. The high pH of cesium neutralizes the weak lactic acid that cancer cells produce and helps to decrease the pain commonly associated with malignancy. Mice fed cesium and rubidium showed a decrease in tumor sizes within two weeks.[42]

Contraindications: Should be supervised by a health care practitioner experienced in using cesium. Side effects may include tingling around the lips, nausea and vomiting, circulatory disturbances, flu-like symptoms.

Molybdenum

This trace mineral is a free radical scavenger and provides protection against chemical carcinogens. When molybdenum and vitamin C were added to the food supply in the Taihang Mountain range in northern China, the once prevalent esophageal cancer decreased its occurrence in that area. It also exerts a protective effect against stomach cancer. Molybdenum is needed in Phase 1 and 2 liver detoxification of estrogen. Animal studies have shown it to inhibit breast cancer.[43]

Contraindications: Toxicity can result in diarrhea, anemia, copper deficiency and low growth rate.

Nutritional Supplements

Chromium

Chromium is a common deficiency in North America because the soil does not contain an adequate supply and therefore neither does our food. A diet high in sweets and refined foods, North American staples, causes chromium to be used up quickly. Chromium deficiency will cause sweet cravings to increase, creating a vicious cycle of binging with further depletion of the mineral. The blood level of the insulin related hormone, insulin-like growth factor-1, is also probably decreased by chromium, although I have not found this theory tested in any studies. The Harvard Nurses' Study found that when the levels of insulin-like growth factor-1 were higher in a woman's blood, her risk for breast cancer increased sevenfold. Therefore, if chromium can help keep the levels of insulin and insulin-like growth factors low, it may help to prevent breast cancer.

Chromium is an ingredient (along with niacin and amino acids) in a substance that the body makes called glucose tolerance factor, or GTF. It increases the sensitivity of cells throughout the body to insulin. Without chromium, insulin's activity at a cellular level is blocked, causing its levels to rise in the blood, and blood sugar levels to go up. It is a critical nutrient used in treating both hypoglycemia and diabetes.

One of the strategies involved in facilitating weight loss is to increase the sensitivity of cells to insulin, since high insulin levels in the blood lead to fat deposition and weight gain. Chromium supplementation has been found to increase lean body mass and decrease weight, and to lower cholesterol and triglyceride levels. Weight loss in itself will decrease breast cancer risk as there is less estrogen available when there is a decrease in body fat.

Several forms of chromium can be found on the market, including chromium polynicotinate, chromium enriched yeast, and chromium picolinate, which is the most effective.[44]

Contraindications: Do not exceed 600 mcg daily. Very high doses can cause kidney damage.

Selenium

Selenium is toxic at high doses but deficiencies are linked to a higher cancer incidence. Many geographic areas have soil deficient in this trace mineral. Its anti-cancer effects include the inhibition of the action of chemical substances, minerals, and viruses that cause cancer by repairing DNA damage; protection against UV light; reduction in tumor volume; and stimulation of the activity of natural killer cells to directly annihilate cancer cells. It also protects the thymus gland from free radical damage. Selenium is essential for the conversion of the thyroid hormone T4 to the more active hormone, T3. Selenium improves the synthesis and activity of glutathione, along with magnesium and zinc.

Selenium can be accurately measured through hair analysis. Selenium is more effective when there are high amounts of vitamin E in the blood and works with it to protect cell membranes.[47]

Contraindications: Symptoms of selenium toxicity include hair, tooth and nail loss and dermatitis.

FACT
Chromium is essential for the maintenance of proper blood sugar levels and for keeping blood levels of insulin low. When insulin levels are increased, the risk of breast cancer is increased threefold.

Food Sources: brewer's yeast, liver, beef, whole wheat bread, beets, mushrooms.
Dosage: 200-600 mcg daily.

FACT
The higher the selenium present in a person's tissues, the lower the breast cancer incidence, providing a toxic level has not been reached.[45] One study revealed that breast cancer patients had serum selenium levels of 41-51 ug/L, while healthy subjects had levels of between 73-89 ug/L.[46]

Food Sources: Brazil nuts, sunflower seeds, barley, brown rice, red Swiss chard, tuna, swordfish, lobster, oysters, herring, brewer's yeast, wheat germ and bran, whole grains, and sesame seeds.
Dosage: 100-300 mcg daily.

Food Sources: pumpkin seeds, sunflower seeds, almonds, walnuts, garlic, turnips, split peas, potatoes, lima beans, seafood, organ meats, mushrooms, brewer's yeast, soybeans, oysters, herring, eggs, and wheat germ.
Dosage: 20-100 mg daily.

Food Sources: whole grain cereals, egg yolks, nuts, seeds, green vegetables, pineapple.
Dosage: 5 mg daily.

Zinc

Zinc is a common deficiency in our diets today because the soil has become deficient. Zinc is necessary for numerous enzyme systems in the body, including the detoxifying systems of the liver. It is essential for the metabolism of vitamin A, stabilizes cell membranes so they are less vulnerable to damage, and is needed for growth and repair. The pineal, pituitary, and thymus glands need sufficient zinc for proper function. Zinc increases thymus hormones and decreases shrinkage of the thymus due to stress or free radical damage. It increases the number of T-cells and improves phagocytosis, or the ability of certain white blood cells to digest toxins. It inhibits the growth of viruses. Zinc is important in the utilization of insulin, the hormone that regulates blood sugar. A zinc deficiency can manifest as an inability to taste with a subsequent loss of appetite. Zinc competes with copper for absorption in the small intestine, so if too much zinc is given, there will be a copper deficiency, and vice versa. Copper toxicity results in zinc deficiency.

One study found that zinc levels were decreased in women with breast cancer.[48] Another study found that women with breast cancer have higher serum copper and lower zinc levels that healthy controls.[49]

Zinc levels can be monitored yearly through an oral zinc test or hair analysis. Supplementation of zinc should generally be taken away from meals, as eggs, milk, and cereal will decrease its bioavailability.

Contraindications: Excessive zinc may result in a copper deficiency, so if you don't have cancer, consider supplementing a small amount of copper if zinc is used long term.

Manganese

As a trace mineral, manganese activates numerous enzymes, including those necessary for utilization of vitamin C. It nourishes the nerves and brain and is essential in the formation of thyroid hormone. The largest amounts of manganese are found in the pituitary gland, kidney, bones, liver, and pancreas. Manganese has been found to increase the activity of natural killer cells in mice through increased interferon production.

Contraindications: Toxicity results in weakness, irritability, psychological and motor disturbances, and impotence.

Other Nutrients

There are many other nutritional supplements that help to prevent breast cancer or assist in recovery. Some of the most important ones are described below.

Coenzyme Q10

Coenzyme Q10 is a naturally occurring molecule similar to vitamin K and is necessary for the health of all human tissues and organs. Highest concentrations of it are found in the organs that need the most energy, such as the heart, liver, muscles, and cells of the immune system.[50] Its synthesis requires the presence of the amino acid, tyrosine, vitamins B2, B3, B5, B6, B12, folic acid, and vitamin C. Deficiencies of these nutrients (particularly B6) will lead to a deficit of coenzyme Q10.

CoQ10 maintains the effectiveness of vitamin E and helps to prevent the breakdown of cell membranes. It works synergistically with the amino acid carnitine.[51] It is a component of the cellular respiration cycle from which metabolic energy is derived. It is used therapeutically in gum disease, cardiovascular disease, diabetes, and immune disorders. It activates immune responsiveness and functions as an antioxidant. With aging, the body loses its ability to make CoQ10 from foods. In animals, it was able to prevent shrinking of the thymus gland and extended lifespan.[52] People with heart disease and cancer have a very low supply of CoQ10 in their tissues. CoQ10 is helpful in preventing damage to the heart caused by chemotherapy drugs such as adriamycin.[53] As a supplement it strengthens the heart, normalizes blood pressure, improves energy and extends life

In one study, 32 node-positive breast cancer patients were treated with conventional allopathic therapy as well as antioxidants (beta carotene, vitamin C, vitamin E, and selenium), essential fatty acids, and 90 mg of CoQ10 for 18 months. None of them died or showed evidence of metastases. Six showed partial tumor regression.[54] In one patient, the dosage of CoQ10 was increased to 390 mg; in one month, the tumor was no longer palpable, and in another month, mammography confirmed that it was gone. Another patient who had non-radical surgery with a proven residual tumor in the tumor bed was also treated with 300 mg of CoQ10. After three months, there was no residual tumor tissue. One patient experienced disappearance of multiple liver metastases after 11 months on the therapy.[55] CoQ10 is a promising therapy in breast cancer prevention and treatment.[56]

A study of 200 women with breast tumors (80 malignant and 120 benign) found that CoQ10 concentrations in plasma were reduced both in patients with cancer and in women with benign lesions, compared to the control population of women with normal breast tissue. There was lower CoQ10 when the tumor volume was large, when the tumor grade suggested a bad prognosis, and when there were no hormone receptors in the breast tissue.[57]

Contraindications: None, other than the high cost for high dosages.

N-acetyl cysteine (NAC)

Cysteine is a sulfur-containing amino acid that helps our bodies make toxic chemicals and carcinogens harmless, as we learned in Chapter 5, 'Detoxifying Our Bodies.' A thiol compound on the cysteine molecule helps to prevent the oxidation of sensitive tissues, which protects us from aging and cancer. In the liver, cysteine helps the small protein called glutathione detoxify carcinogens and chemicals, including some of the organochlorines. In the rest of the body it acts as a free radical scavenger. Cysteine works synergistically with vitamin C and is an essential element in many parts of the immune system.

N-acetyl cysteine is a modified form of cysteine that is converted back into cysteine in the body. It helps clear the cells of toxins,

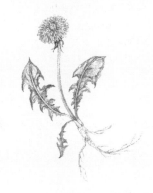

Food Sources: soy products, whey powder, black beans, adzuki beans, chick peas, lentils, split peas, dried spirulina, nori, kelp, beef, avocados, almonds, sunflower seeds, butternuts, cottage cheese, fish, eggs, organic yogurt, wheat germ, oat flakes.
Dosage: 500 mg, 1-2 times daily.

Food Sources: None. The body synthesizes it from three amino acids. Soy or pumpkin seeds are helpful.
Dosage: For prevention, 75-300 mg. With breast cancer, 1,600-2,000 mg daily, or use NAC to make it.

FACT
Alpha lipoic acid reduces the cancer-stimulating effect that environmental toxins have on breast cells and inhibits the ability of cancer cells to become invasive or to metastasize.

Food Sources: red meat, liver, yeast, potatoes, leafy vegetables. For more foods with the sulphur-bearing amino acids, cysteine and methionine see Chapter 7, 'Eating Right for Breast Health.'
Dosage: 50-100 mg daily for prevention; 300-600 mg daily with breast cancer.

increases glutathione production and reduces the toxicity of chemicals. Glutathione is necessary for melatonin to work effectively. It is safe in doses of up to 3-4 g daily, even in pregnancy, but has a nauseating taste and smell.

Contraindications: Dosages higher than 7 g daily can be toxic. Do not use with the chemotherapy drugs doxorubicin (adriamycin), or epirubicin, as it may make them less effective.[59]

Reduced Glutathione

Glutathione is made up of only three amino acids — cysteine, glutamic acid, and glycine. Glutathione is a powerful antioxidant and detoxifier, and the amount of cysteine present determines how much glutathione will be produced.

Glutathione has five main functions in the body. Briefly, it protects the body against natural and man-made oxidants, which destroy cell membranes; helps the liver to detoxify poisonous chemicals and metals such as lead, cadmium, arsenic and mercury; is necessary for immune function, increasing the numbers and efficiency of various white blood cells; protects the integrity of the red blood cells; and acts as a brain neurotransmitter. The liver manufactures glutathione whenever extra cysteine is available.

Magnesium and zinc deficiencies reduce glutathione levels. Selenium, milk thistle and alpha lipoic acid enhance glutathione synthesis and activity. Glutathione itself is poorly absorbed but 'reduced glutathione' can be used as a supplement instead.

Contraindications: Do not use during chemotherapy with doxorubicin (adriamycin), as it may decrease its effectiveness.[60]

Alpha Lipoic Acid

The amino acids cysteine and methionine help to synthesize alpha lipoic acid from linoleic acid. Alpha lipoic acid is produced in high amounts by the liver and in lower amounts by every cell. It has the extraordinary ability to prevent damage to the cell at the genetic level.[61] It decreases our susceptibility to the damaging effects of ionizing radiation.[62] It is an excellent free radical scavenger and antioxidant, and enhances immune function by increasing the number of helper T-cells. Alpha lipoic acid increases the effectiveness and lifespan of other antioxidants, including vitamins C and E, quercetin, and coenzyme Q10.[63,64] It promotes the production of glutathione, a powerful antioxidant, immune stimulant, and detoxifier. It decreases the toxic side effects of chemotherapy and regenerates the liver.

Alpha lipoic acid is one of the few substances that can chelate, or bind to, toxic metals such as lead, aluminum, mercury, copper, cadmium, and arsenic, and help to remove them from our bodies. This nutrient works synergistically with selenium, so we must ensure adequate amounts of selenium for optimal output.[65,66,67]

By consuming foods high in the sulphur-bearing amino acids along with flaxseed oil, we maximize the amount of alpha lipoic acid that our bodies produce and protect ourselves from breast cancer.

Contraindications: None; it is very safe with no adverse reactions reported.

Ellagic Acid

Ellagic acid, found primarily in red raspberries, offers powerful protection against cancer. Like curcumin, it inhibits Phase 1 and activates Phase 2 detoxification in the liver.[68] It is an antioxidant that prevents the binding of carcinogens to DNA and clears damaging free radicals. It causes apoptosis, or cell death in breast cancer cells and stimulates the immune system to destroy cancer cells.[69,70,71,72]

Contraindications: Do not use during chemotherapy.

Food Sources: in decreasing order, Meeker red raspberries, other red raspberries, strawberries, walnut skins, pecans, cranberries.
Dosage: 40 mg ellagic acid daily, or 2 (1000 mg) capsules daily of Meeker red raspberry seed extract.

Bromelain

Bromelain is an extract from pineapple that contains enzymes which digest protein. These enzymes reduce inflammation, decrease fibrin in the blood, lower plasma viscosity and help to prevent metastases. It inhibits growth and invasiveness of tumor cells and improves the activity of particular white blood cells called monocytes against cancer cells.[73]

Contraindications: Do not use with pharmaceutical blood thinners without medical supervision.

Food Sources: pineapple.
Dosage: 600 mg or more per day, taken between meals.

Beta-sitosterol

Beta sitosterol is found in seeds, seaweeds, fruits and vegetables. It modulates the immune system and can increase T cells 9 fold. When mice were fed beta-sitosterol as 2% of their diet over 8 weeks, breast cancer tumor size was 33% smaller and there were 20% fewer metastases to the lymph nodes and lungs in the beta-sitosterol group than in a control group.[74]

Contraindications: It may reduce insulin requirements if you are diabetic.

Food Sources: caraway and cumin seeds, seaweeds, soy, kiwi, most fruits and vegetables.
Dosage: 600 mg daily, taken with water or fruit juice, 45 minutes before or 2 hours after eating.

Proanthocyanins and Anthocyanins (Grape Seed Extract)

Grape seed extract contains high amounts of bioflavonoids, including what are known as proanthocyanins and anthocyanins. These act as potent free radical scavengers, apparently 50 times more effective than vitamin E and 20 times stronger than vitamin C in neutralizing free radicals. They help to slow down the rate of DNA mutation when cells are exposed to carcinogens. Grape seed extract helps prevent free radical damage to polyunsaturated oils, such as flaxseed oil. It maintains the integrity of the arterial walls and circulation, improves eyesight, and helps to restore the elasticity of the body's connective tissues.

Contraindications: None known.

Food Sources: None.
Dosage: 60-300 mg daily.

Indole-3-carbinol and DIM

Indole-3-carbinol is one of the protective ingredients in raw cabbage and the other brassicas that helps to break down estrogen in the liver and promote the formation of the 'good' C2 hydroxyestrone. Once in our bodies, indole-3-carbinol is broken down into several metabolites, the most important one being diidolylmethane, or DIM. I-3-C and DIM can bind to estrogen receptors, displacing the body's estrogens.

Food Sources: brassica family, raw — cabbage, Brussell's sprouts, broccoli, cauliflower, kale, etc.
Dosage: 150-400 mg daily of either I-3-C or DIM.

FACT

Lower levels of GL have been associated with a high risk for cancer. Calcium-D-glucarate is available in supplement form, and when converted into GL, it releases slowly into the bloodstream.

Food Sources: oranges (highest), apples, grapefruit, broccoli, Brussels sprouts, potatoes and mung beans.
Dosage: 1500-2000 mg daily.

Chemically-induced breast cancers have been inhibited by both I-3-C and DIM in animal studies, with I-3-C being slightly more effective. Indole-3-carbinol has a threefold greater stimulation of the liver's Phase 1 cytochrome P450 system than DIM, as demonstrated in one animal study. While this will speed up detoxification of environmental chemicals, if the Phase 2 system isn't able to keep up, it could potentially expose an individual to the dangerous intermediate epoxides for a longer period. Therefore, caution should be exercised in using I-3-C after known toxin exposure. In these cases, DIM may be a better choice. If curcumin were used concurrently with I-3-C, the Phase 2 enzymes would be encouraged to keep up to Phase 1, and this may be a wise practice.

When used with Tamoxifen, I-3-C was found to inhibit the growth of estrogen-receptor positive breast cancer cells in a separate yet cooperative way. I-3-C also causes apoptosis in estrogen receptor negative breast cancer cells, while Tamoxifen does not.[75] Therefore, I-3-C is a safe complement to Tamoxifen, and can be used along with it.

Contraindications: Do not take either of them while pregnant or during chemotherapy. Use curcumin or ellagic acid with I-3-C to speed up Phase 2 detoxification, and take other antioxidants.

Calcium-D-Glucarate

Glucuronidation is a Phase 2 liver detoxification process whereby toxins, carcinogens, and tumor promoters are attached to a water-soluble compound (called glucuronic acid) which can be carried out of the body through bile or urine. The glucuronidation process detoxifies aromatic and heterocyclic amines, polycyclic aromatic hydrocarbons, nitrosamines, steroid hormones (estrogens) and fungal toxins. The enzyme beta glucuronidase, produced by certain intestinal bacteria, reverses glucuronidation by breaking apart the joined compound of a toxin from glucuronic acid. It releases carcinogens, toxins and harmful estrogens back into circulation. Beta glucuronidase has been found to be elevated in cancer patients.

D-glucar-1,4 lactone (GL) is the active substance necessary for glucuronidation, which inhibits beta glucuronidase activity. It is found in oranges, apples, grapefruit, broccoli, Brussels sprouts, potatoes, and mung beans. In animal studies calcium-D-glucarate has been shown to inhibit beta glucuronidase activity in the blood, liver, colon, lungs and flora of the small intestines by 70%.[76,77] As far as I know, there are no completed studies on the effectiveness of calcium-D-glucarate in humans. For the time being, it may be best to get GL from oranges and apples.

Contraindications: None known.

Modified Citrus Pectin

Modified citrus pectin is a special form of pectin that has been shortened through a laboratory process so that it can be absorbed through the intestinal wall. Otherwise, citrus pectin, obtained from the peel and pulp of citrus fruits, acts as a soluble fiber that is not broken down or absorbed.

Research has shown that certain cancer cell types have specific carbohydrate-binding protein molecules on their cell surfaces called galectins. The more advanced the cancer, the more galectins are produced. Higher galectin levels allow greater adhesion of cancer cells to each other so that they form colonies and facilitate the binding of cancer cells to distant sites, promoting metastases. Modified citrus pectin works by blocking the galectins on the surface of cancer cells so that they cannot adhere to other cells.

Modified citrus pectin has an affinity for various cancer cell types, including breast, prostate, larynx, and melanoma. It is able to bind to cholesterol in the bloodstream, helping to prevent arteriosclerosis, and attaches to heavy metals, facilitating their excretion from the body.[78]

Contraindications: Well tolerated and safe, although there may be mild gastrointestinal complaints.

Melatonin

Melatonin is one of the body's first lines of defense in response to malignant breast cell growth. Increased melatonin keeps abnormal breast cancer cells under control, while a deficiency of melatonin allows breast tumors to form. Melatonin has been shown to prevent chemically caused breast tumors in studies on rats. It inhibits the replication of breast cancer cells in the laboratory by regulating cell division and multiplication.[79] It's as though it flips a breaker switch to turn off estradiol's activity on the breast cell and may lower estrogen levels.[80]

Some scientists believe that melatonin competes with estrogen for the estrogen receptor sites, thus negating estrogen's activity. Women with late stage breast cancer achieved partial remission lasting an average of eight months when they were given high doses of melatonin in the evening (20 mg per day). Melatonin has been found to be highly effective at inhibiting estrogen-sensitive breast cancer cells but only minimally effective in inhibiting cancer cells that were not estrogen-sensitive. Melatonin increases the effectiveness of tamoxifen when used along with it and improves patient response to chemotherapy. Melatonin has an added benefit of decreasing anxiety.[81]

If melatonin is prescribed, all doses should be taken at bedtime, since morning administration has been found to stimulate cancer growth in animal studies, while evening dosing inhibits cancer.[83,83] It is illegal for over-the-counter sale in Canada, but is available at health food stores in the United States.

Contraindications: Always take it before bed. Otherwise, appears to be very safe.

Supplement Packaging (Gelatin Capsules)

PREVENTION

Contact the suppliers of your supplement capsules and request veggie caps. Try to find products that do not rely on gelatin capsules.

At the second World Conference on Breast Cancer, held in Ottawa in July 1999, Dr Samuel Epstein made women aware of the fact that gelatin capsules may contain estradiol. Normally cows are given estradiol to increase growth and milk production. It is administered through an implant positioned under the skin of their ears, where absorption is low. When cows are slaughtered, their ears are cut off and sold to rendering plants for the manufacturing of glycerol and gelatin. Gelatin is commonly used to make capsules for supplements.

When to Take Supplements Guidelines

The following guidelines are designed to take some of the confusion out of when the best times are to take your supplements.

Supplement	Directions
Vitamins	Generally vitamins are taken with meals, with the exception of vitamin C, which can be taken in divided doses throughout the day between or with meals.
Minerals	Minerals are usually taken with meals, with the exception of zinc, which is better taken between meals, and calcium, which can be taken with a meal or before bed, providing you have enough hydrochloric acid to absorb it on an empty stomach. Calcium and other minerals should not be taken with a high fiber meal. Iron and vitamin E should be taken eight hours apart.
Amino Acids	As protein molecules, amino acids are best taken with meals. These include NAC and reduced glutathione.
Herbs	Herbal formulas are best absorbed on an empty stomach, either $\frac{1}{2}$ hour before or 2 hours after a meal. If herbs are used to improve digestion, they are taken 15-30 minutes before a meal.
Enzymes	If enzymes are used to digest food, they are taken immediately before or during your meal. If they are being used to control inflammation or digest toxins in the blood, they are taken between meals.
Probiotics (acidophilus and bifidus)	Depending on the type and the manufacturer, these can be taken either before or between meals.
Homeopathic Remedies	These are taken on an empty stomach, away from other supplements so that strong tastes or smells do not interfere with their subtle action, usually $\frac{1}{2}$ hour or more before or after a meal.

Daily Therapeutic Amounts of Vitamins and Minerals

Review the nutrients and guidelines below with your health care provider and fill in the column with any supplements that are recommended for you, their dosages, and product name, if known. Use food sources if you are limited financially or if you have an aversion to taking pills. You will find combinations of these in many products, making a supplement schedule simpler. Each of us can, with the help of a health professional, design a program that suits our lifestyle and is tailored to our particular needs.

Nutrient	Dosage Range	Your Personal Dosage
Vitamin A	5,000-35,000 IU	
Beta-carotene or mixed carotenoids	10,000-100,000 IU	
Vitamin B complex	50-100 mg	
Vitamin B3 (Niacin)	25-2000 mg (with medical supervision)	
Vitamin B6	50 mg-200 mg	
Folic acid	400-800 mcg	
Vitamin B12	50 mcg	
Inositol	200-1800 mg	
IP6	800-7,000 mg	
Vitamin C	2,000-12,000 mg	
Bioflavonoids	100 mg per 500 mg of vitamin C	
Vitamin D	0-800 IU	
Vitamin E	400-800 IU	
Calcium	800-2,000 mg (less if cancer is present)	
Magnesium	300-800 mg	
Potassium	food sources, 3000-6000 mg	
Iodine or Kelp	100-1000 mcg	
Molybdenum	100-500 mcg	
Chromium	200-600 mcg	
Selenium	100-300 mcg	
Zinc	20-100 mg	
Manganese	5 mg	
Green tea extract	10 cup equivalent	
Coenzyme Q10	60-400 mg	
Alpha Lipoic Acid	50-600 mg	
Grape Seed Extract	60-300 mg.	
Beta-Sitosterol	300-600 mg	
Modified Citrus Pectin	10-15 g	
Melatonin	3-50 mg	
NAC	500-1,000 mg	
Reduced glutathione	75-2,000 mg	
Digestive and proteolytic enzymes	1-5 capsules before &/or between meals	
Bromelain	600 mg	
Thymus extract	100-800 mg	
Flaxseed Oil	2-8 tbsps	
Probiotic + FOS	2 capsules	
"Clean" Fish Oil	700-3000 mg	
Psyllium Seed Powder	1 tsp-1 tbsp	
Chrysin (if ER positive)	1500-2000 mg	
Indole-3-carbinol or DIM	300 mg	
Curcumin	1500-3000 mg	
Ellagic acid	40 mg	
Quercetin	1500 mg	
Maitake D-fraction	1 mg per kg of body weight per day,	
Carnivora	1 capsule 3x daily before meals	
MGN-3	250-750 mg daily	

Nutritional Strategies for Breast Health Guidelines

This chart presents a grouping of most of the supplements mentioned in this book, plus a few more, according to their nutritional strategy in the prevention or management of breast cancer. Ideally, at some point in your healing process you want to address each strategy with one or more nutrients. Work with a healthcare professional to determine the timing and staging of these strategies.

Discourage Free Radical Damage and the Development of Cancer with Antioxidants

vitamin C, vitamin E, vitamin A and beta carotene, Coenzyme Q10, NAC, reduced glutathione, grape seed extract, ellagic acid, alpha lipoic acid, melatonin, zinc, selenium, IP6, green tea

Strengthen Cell Membranes so they are Less Vulnerable to Carcinogens

vitamin B complex, coenzyme Q10, vitamin E, flaxseed oil, pure fish oils, evening primrose oil (small amount), beta carotene, zinc

Help the Liver Convert Harmful Estrogens to Safe Estrogens and Detoxify Carcinogens

vitamin B6, B3, B complex, vitamin A, C and E, bioflavonoids, selenium, magnesium, zinc, copper, SAM, molybdenum, NAC or reduced glutathione, goat whey, brassicas, DIM (preferred) or indole-3-carbinol, MSM, calcium-D-glucarate, probiotics, alpha lipoic acid, amla, rosemary, curcumin, green tea, quercetin, ellagic acid, garlic, milk thistle, dandelion, schizandra, bupleurum, globe artichoke, chelidonium

Inhibit the Aromatase Enzyme to Block the Formation of Estrogen

chrysin (from passionflower), ground flaxseed, genistein (soy), zinc, natural progesterone

Keep the Body Alkaline

potassium, magnesium, calcium, coral calcium, sodium bicarbonate, cesium chloride, Alkali, Sanuvis, alkaline powder combinations, Basen pulver

Regulate Insulin and Blood Sugar

chromium, B3 (niacin), zinc, alpha lipoic acid, flaxseed oil, pure fish oil

Increase Tissue Oxygenation

coenzyme Q10, ozone therapy, microhydrin, deep breathing, Mucokehl (Sanum), flaxseed oil with cysteine

Decrease Blood Viscosity, Keep Blood Moving, Improve the Microcirculation

(this is especially important if you are using Tamoxifen)
fish oil, flaxseed oil, vitamin E, proteolytic enzymes, bromelain, curcumin, soy, vitamin C, Niacin (B3), Mucokehl (Sanum), Chinese herbs to move the blood — Salvia miltiorrhizae, Sparganium simplex, Pangolin scales, Frankincense, Flos Carthamus tinctoria, Myrrh, Curcuma zedoaria, Ligusticum wallichii, Paeonia rubra, Semen persica, Salvia Shou Wu (Seven Forests), Myrrh tablets (Seven Forests) — daily exercise

Normalize Fungal Stages in the Blood (Naessens, Enderlein)

Mucokehl, Nigersan, Alkali, Sanuvis and other Sanum Remedies, 714X

Help to Prevent Metastases

modified citrus pectin, indole-3-carbinol, curcumin, European mistletoe, proteolytic enzymes, bromelain, melatonin, vitamin C, bioflavonoids (catechin, quercetin, rutin), alpha lipoic acid, flaxseed oil, pure fish oils, Maitake-D-fraction, green tea, beta-sitosterol

Help to Repair the DNA

vitamin B3 (niacin), B12, vitamin A, PolyMVA

Encourage Apoptosis
(self-destruction of cancer cells)
IP6 and inositol in a 4:1 ratio, green tea, soy, melatonin (works best with ER+ breast cancer), i.v. vitamin C with vitamin K3 in a 100:1 ratio, quercetin, selenium, garlic, curcumin, beta carotene, ellagic acid, indole-3-carbinol, perillyl alcohol (in essential oil of palmarosa, lavender), limonene (in essential oil of lemon, celery, orange, lemon grass)

Block the Division of Rapidly Dividing Cells
folic acid, melatonin, IP6, soy, curcumin

Promote Cell Differentiation
(normalization of cancer cells)
IP6, soy, melatonin, PolyMVA

Break Down the
Hard Protein Coat Around a Tumor
high protease digestive enzymes (Wobenzyme, M7), bromelain, kelp, Chinese herbs – Laminaria, Bombyx batryticatus, Pericarpum citri reticulatae viride, Sparganium, Taraxicum mongolicum, Curcuma zedoaria, Ru Bi Xiao, Blue Citrus Tablets (Seven Forests), Chih-ko and Curcuma (Seven Forests)

Increase Immune Strength
vitamin A, C, E, B complex, B6, folic acid, beta carotene, zinc, selenium, magnesium, manganese, alpha lipoic acid, coenzyme Q10, NAC, reduced glutathione, thymus extract, IP6, melatonin, medicinal mushrooms (maitake, shitake, reishi (Ganoderma), polyporus umbellatus, Agaricus blazei, Trametes coriolus versicolor, MGN3, Maitake-D-fraction, RM10 (Garden of Life)), astragalus, schizandra, echinacea, goldenseal, European mistletoe, Iscador, pau d'arco (taheebo), thymic protein A, 714X, beta-sitosterol

Specific Action Against Breast Cancer Cells
juniper, bloodroot, goldenseal, barberry, Coptis chinensis, lycopene, garlic, green tea, EPA fish oil, podophyllum and mandrake (both toxic), soy, garlic, DHA, lycopene, red clover, myrrh, dandelion, artemesinin (from Artemesia annua – Allergy Research Group), turmeric, quercetin, ellagic acid, beta-sitosterol, Carnivora, essential oils with limonene and perillyl alcohol in palmarosa, lavender, lemon, orange, celery, medicinal mushrooms — maitake, shitake, reishi (Ganoderma), polyporus umbellatus, Agaricus blazei, Trametes coriolus versicolor

Block Angiogenesis
soy, turmeric, green tea polyphenols, C-Statin (Convulvulus arvensis), quercetin, high zinc to decrease copper

Remove Toxic Metals
high vitamin C, vitamin E, zinc, selenium, alpha lipoic acid, cilantro, reduced glutathione, NAC, Greens Plus, chelation therapy, modified citrus pectin, spirulina, kelp, psyllium and bentonite, red clover, burdock

Detoxify Bowel
formula containing psyllium seed powder, oat bran, rice bran, bentonite, guar gum, citrus and apple pectin, marshmallow root, plus ground flaxseeds, probiotic formula, perhaps coffee enemas

Remove Unwanted Guests
(yeast and parasites)
wormwood, black walnut, cloves, male fern, goldenseal, grapefruit seed extract, oil of oregano, garlic, Artemesinin

Help to Drain the Liver, Kidneys, Lymph
Liver: milk thistle, dandelion, chelidonium, schizandra, bupleurum, globe artichoke, curcumin, black radish, berberis vulgaris, choline, inositol, Unda 243, Unda 1, Unda 13, Chelidonium Plex (Unda), Rosemarinus, Juniperus, coffee enemas, castor oil packs

Kidneys: Unda 13, Unda 2, Unda 7, Juniperus, dandelion, horsetail, uva ursi, parsley

Lymph: Healthy Breast Formula (Healthy Breast Products), Flor-Essence, Hoxsey Formula, Essiac, Unda 21, Unda 48, Lymphdiaral (Pascoe), Lymphomyosot (Heel), Red Clover Supreme (Gaia), Cleavers Combo (St. Francis Herbs)
Phonix detox kit (C-23, C-26, C-3, C-22), Heel detox kit

Daily Supplement Schedule Worksheet

Fill in the times of day, amount of each supplement you need, and what it is doing for you. Tape this worksheet to your cupboard or refrigerator door until it becomes routine. Take a break every now and then from supplement taking when it feels like too much. Listen to your body's needs.

Time of Day	Supplement	Amount	Effect
On Arising			
Before Breakfast			
With Breakfast			
Between Meals			
Before Lunch			
With Lunch			
Between Meals			
Before Dinner			
With Dinner			
Before Bed			

Nutritional Supplements

Summary

Although foods supply many of the nutrients we need to prevent or recover from cancer, supplements can provide much additional benefit. But it is not possible or affordable for most people to use all of these supplements. Begin with a core group of supplements and then look at the rest with a health professional to decide which other ones you may want to add. Here's a list of supplements I recommend:

1) Multivitamin (with 400 mg of vitamin E, 50 mg of zinc and 200 mcg selenium).
2) Green Powder (rich in beta carotene and iodine, such as spirulina, or Greens +, or Pure Synergy).
3) Vitamin C (4000 mg or more).
4) Calcium-Magnesium.
5) CoQ10 (water soluble).
6) Curcumin.
7) Quercetin.
8) DIM (Diidolylmethane).
9) Alpha Lipoic Acid.
10) Ellagic Acid.
11) Flax Oil and Clean Fish Oil.
12) High Protease Enzymes, which include Bromelain, (taken between meals).
13) Niacin.
14) Probiotics.
15) Medicinal Mushroom Combination.
16) Green Tea (extract).
17) Herbal Formulas (taken regularly for the liver, lymph, and immune system).

Our supplements will work better for us if we are mindful as we take them. Think of them as healers. We can potentiate their action with prayer and mental imagery. Consider following this sequence as you take your supplements. Thank the organisms or elements that have become your supplement. Invoke a silent prayer or mantra that the supplement will add to your health and well-being. Take a minute to formulate one that you can use over and over again — for example, 'May I use the wellness you bring me to good end.' Envision the cells of your body accepting what you put into it and using it for your maximum benefit. Picture and feel the nutrients going to the parts of the body that need them or being directed by your body's innate intelligence to its target cells. Though not easily quantifiable, the power of visualization and imagery in activating our immune system and assisting in healing is considerable, as we shall see in the next chapter.

CHAPTER NINE

Psychological and Spiritual Means of Preventing Breast Cancer

CONTENTS

EXERCISES, CHARTS, CHECK LISTS & WORKSHEETS

Most illness, including breast cancer, has an emotional as well as a physical cause. Tumors of all types may arise after a sudden shock, loss, or conflict. Women more prone to cancer of any kind are sometimes those who put the needs of others first and are perceived as 'good, kind, and nice'. They are often unable to express their anger or other negative emotions. As part of the healing journey, women can be encouraged to resolve old conflicts, identify their own needs, believe that they deserve to have those needs met, and identify and express anger constructively. We need outlets to express negative emotions (art therapy, physical activity) and exercises to improve self-esteem. We need to focus on resolving conflict, developing assertiveness, transforming limiting beliefs, understanding communication styles, and releasing anger, as well as using imagery and visualization. There is a link between the level of stress in our lives and cancer. If we are not coping well with stress, then relaxation techniques, meditation, yoga or tai chi, time management training, and other coping techniques will help us. Our well-being is dependent upon our ability to heal ourselves psychologically as well as physically.

Nor should we separate our physical health from our spiritual health. Some of the spiritual links to breast cancer include the loss of a loved one, feelings of hopelessness and despair, an inability to be true to one's own nature, a life full of fear of what others may think, and loss of faith in God or the spiritual dimension. When a woman feels an underlying hopelessness and despair much of the time, this is filtered through the hypothalamus to affect the immune system and causes her to be more susceptible to cancer. The hopelessness may arise from perceiving that she is in an unhappy situation with no way out. Counseling is important to allow her to see positive choices available, and to encourage movement towards one of those choices. Often we need to release guilt as we establish a new direction for ourselves. We need to honor our own desires, intuition and direction. We can drop the mental script of what we 'should' be doing, and instead, carve a niche in life that reflects our unique identity. Otherwise the killing of the spirit can contribute to cancer development as the life force is suppressed.

Use your life force to recreate yourself.

Developing a Healthy Self-Image

Our beliefs define our lives. We see through the lens of our belief systems, and we attract conditions, situations, or people to our lives that fulfill our beliefs about ourselves and about life. These beliefs may be conscious or unconscious. We need to stop and ask ourselves what we really do believe about who we are and why we are alive, and then decide if these are healthy beliefs or not. If they are not, then it's time to change them. After first identifying our limiting beliefs we can begin the process of shifting towards establishing life-affirming beliefs for ourselves.

Becoming Assertive

Often difficulties with our self-image stem from mistaken beliefs about ourselves that devalue us in our own minds. We have learned these beliefs earlier in our lives, often from our parents, or have modeled our behavior on others with similar mistaken beliefs about themselves. We become passive or submissive, putting the needs of others before our own, believing that what we want does not count. When we pass up opportunities for being assertive, we are often left with feelings of anger, resentment, defeat, or depression. Our needs are not being met, our feelings are not voiced. The accumulated frustration interferes with our physical well-being, causing a depletion in energy.

When we are assertive, we feel empowered, have improved self-esteem, and more energy is freed up for living fully in the present. We aren't as likely to store our negative emotions in the tissues of the body.

Communication Styles

In learning to become assertive we can first identify the communication styles we use with one another.

Passive

A person is acting passively when she lets others take control of her actions or thoughts. She will not stand up for herself; she will do what she's told. She disregards what she really feels and believes and may be so cut off from her herself that she doesn't really know what she feels. The body can become a container for these repressed feelings and manifest them in physical symptoms. An underlying belief is that she does not deserve to have her needs met. She sees herself as being less important, less talented, than her family and friends. She often has an irrational fear of negative consequences that may happen if she expresses her needs honestly, and feels paralyzed.

Because the passive person does not put herself first, she falls short of accomplishing or experiencing all that she can in her life. She may defer to a partner or her children, look to their successes for validation, and never really seek out avenues of fulfillment for herself. She may never discover who she really can be.

FACT
The advantage of being passive is that this person rarely experiences direct rejection. The disadvantage is that she is taken advantage of, and may store a backlog of resentment and anger, much of it unconscious.

Exploring Your Beliefs Exercise

Read through the list of 'limiting' beliefs on the left column of this chart and see how many of them apply to you. Read out loud the parallel healthy belief and pause to notice how each statement makes you feel. If you are in a group, pick a partner. Have one person read the limiting belief and comment to their partner on whether it is an accurate statement for them. Ask the partner to then read the healthy belief back to the first person using the word 'you' instead of 'I' and allow time for the first person to take in its effect.

Circle the healthy beliefs that have the most impact for you. Write these phrases on small recipe cards and keep them in the bathroom or another spot you visit frequently. Each day, repeat one or two of the healthy beliefs out loud as you look at yourself in the mirror. Continue to do this for 40 days or so. Notice how your responses change to people and events as your beliefs change. After 40 days move on to a different affirmation.

Limiting Beliefs	Healthy Beliefs
1. I should always try to be logical and consistent. Once I choose a direction, I should keep to it.	I am free to change my mind and decide on a different course of action.
2. I feel ashamed when I make a mistake. I should know the right answer in every situation.	It is okay for me to make a mistake. I don't have to be perfect. I can learn from my mistakes.
3. If someone gives me advice, I should follow it or take it seriously. They are most often right.	I can take advice and filter it through my mind, heart, and intuition before deciding to act on it. I trust myself.
4. I should respect other people's opinions, especially if they are in a position of authority. I should keep my differences of opinion to myself.	I have a right to express my opinion. My opinion matters.
5. I am being selfish if I put my needs before the needs of others, such as family members.	I have a right to put my own needs before the needs of others sometimes. I deserve to enjoy myself and experience fulfillment in my life today.
6. When I do something wonderful, I should not tell anyone. People would think that I am boasting and would dislike me. I feel embarrassed when someone compliments me.	I deserve to be recognized for what I do well. I appreciate well-earned compliments.
7. I should be flexible and adjust to other people's agendas, even when it is inconvenient for me.	I acknowledge my own desires and agenda before I adjust to those of another.
8. I always try to stay on people's good side. I don't want to make anyone angry.	I communicate my feelings honestly to people and am not responsible for their anger.
9. When someone else thinks that my feelings or responses are unreasonable, then I must be wrong.	I have a right to all my feelings and responses and I accept them as being valid for me.
10. I should keep my problems to myself. No one really wants to hear them or be there for me.	There are individuals who care about me and are willing to help me sort out difficulties.
11. When things are going poorly for me I shouldn't try to change them. It could be worse.	I deserve the best possible life for myself and can change my circumstances for the better.
12. If people ask me to do something for them, I respond to them right away. I often agree to something without thinking it through.	I can take whatever time I need before I fully commit to a favor or task. I can say no.
13. If I am anti-social people will think that I don't like them. I am obliged to participate in social events even when I would rather be alone or doing something else.	I choose the social activities that appeal to me. I also choose to be alone at times to nurture myself.

Limiting Beliefs	Healthy Beliefs
14. I should always have a good reason for the way I feel and what I do.	It is all right for me not to know why I feel a certain way.
15. When someone is in trouble, I should help her.	I am not responsible for another person's problem or way of reacting. When I help, it is because I consciously choose to do so.
16. I should never interrupt people when they are speaking. If I ask questions, I appear stupid.	I have a right to interrupt in order to clarify a point or gather more information.
17. I should be sensitive to the needs and wishes of others, even if they are unable to express what they want.	I react to what is communicated to me directly.
18. I should always try to accommodate others. If I don't, they will dislike me and may not be there for me when I need them.	I have a right to say 'no' without feeling guilty.

Letting Go Exercise

Letting go is part of living and dying. When you let go of the old, you create space for the new. When you release the past, you rewrite the future. Letting go frees up time and space so that you can dwell more fully in the present. You may need to let go of a past relationship and the expectations you had for it, or of your old identity and the restrictions and responsibilities you placed upon yourself. You may have to let go of an addiction that keeps you blunted emotionally — to work, television, overeating, alcohol, sugar, smoking, or drugs. It may be your time to let go of your 'busy-ness' to create time to feel joy in being. You may feel compelled to simplify your life, to let go of your compulsion to fill your emptiness with material things.

Think about what life is asking you to let go of right now or what you could release to invite in new energy. Make a list below. Include past relationships, outdated ideas of who you are, material possessions, social obligations, emotions of anger, guilt, or grief, addictions, and any emotional baggage you carry around with you. If you are in a group, share three of the things you want to let go of with the other women.

Limiting beliefs to let go:	**Guilt to let go:**
Relationships to let go or transform:	**Social obligations to let go:**
Possessions to let go:	**Expectations to let go:**
Addictions to release:	**Old emotions to let go:**
What else to let go?	

Aggressive

Some examples of aggressive behavior are bullying, being pushy, fighting, threatening, blaming, and stepping on people without considering their feelings. The aggressive person believes that she has to be forceful to get what she wants. She has not experienced that her needs can be met through simply asking for what she wants or through dialog and compromise.

Assertive

A person who behaves assertively will stand up for herself, will not let others take advantage of her, and will express her feelings honestly. At the same time, she is considerate of others' feelings, and can acknowledge those feelings while holding her ground. Most of us are able to act assertively in some situations but not in others. We may be assertive with our children but not with our partners or employers. We may be able to express ourselves honestly with a few friends but not with our parents or siblings.

Before you can achieve assertive behavior, you must realize that your own life matters. Your needs, wants, goals, talents, and pleasures are important; you deserve to have them met. We can only be assertive when we value our own spiritual, physical, emotional, and mental well-being. We matter.

The Healing Effects of Being Assertive

Remember that our bodies and particularly our immune systems respond to what we believe about ourselves and what we present to the world. Breast cancer and most illness bring us the opportunity to adopt a new persona that is different from the one we had when we became sick. We can change our negative beliefs about ourselves with repetition of positive beliefs, practice of healthy behavioral scripts, validation, and encouragement.

Purging Anger

Another emotional influence on our physical well-being is suppressed anger. When we do not express our anger, we store it in our bodies where it can affect a particular area or cause muscle tension. This can have a paralyzing effect on us physically and emotionally, causing fatigue, lack of zest, flatness to our outward expression, and a thwarting of our impulses and intuition. We become stuck.

When we are holding in anger, we adopt a variety of tactics that express it indirectly. These include avoidance; that is, we may avoid the person we are angry at or avoid the topic that triggers our anger. We may compensate for the underlying anger by appearing sweet and/or smiling. We may become passive-aggressive, acting out our anger unconsciously by undermining another person through our actions (for example, being chronically late for engagements). We may talk about surface things (weather, work, someone else) rather than the issue that is consuming or preoccupying us. This reinforces our emotional barriers and prevents intimacy and

12 Steps for Purging Anger

The following 12 steps may assist you in transforming your feelings of anger.

1) Accept that anger is a valid emotion. It is okay to feel angry.

2) Acknowledge that you feel angry. Identify the part of the body that is holding the anger.

3) Identify whom you are angry with and/or what you are angry about.

4) Ask yourself if the anger is justified or if it has been magnified by a previous situation not fully dealt with. Are you projecting your mother, father, or sibling onto the person you feel anger towards? Own it.

5) Identify what lies beneath the anger. Usually there is an unmet need or a feeling of being hurt.

6) Explore the unmet needs or feelings of being hurt within yourself first, and then with the other person. If possible, communicate your feelings by saying, 'When you did such and such, I felt such and such.' Communicate it without blame. Communicate your unmet need specifically; for example, 'I need you to put down your newspaper and really listen to me when I speak to you.' If you are unable to do this directly, then write a letter, choosing to mail it or not, or use a chair exercise and speak to the person as though they were sitting in the chair. Honor your unmet need and create a plan to meet it as soon as possible.

7) Check in again with the body part that was holding the anger. Ask it if it needs anything more from you. Consciously relax the area.

8) Discharge the anger physically. Use aerobic exercise, rebounding, running, swimming, martial arts, kundalini yoga, rowing, dragon-boat racing, drumming — anything to release the build up of muscle tension. Do this on a regular basis — two to three times weekly.

9) Channel any residual anger creatively. Do a drawing, painting, or sculpture that utilizes the energy of the anger and helps externalize it rather than turn it inward.

10) Channel anger into a worthy cause or project. Help fight some of the injustices in the world and join forces with others who are helping to create global change for the better.

11) Recognize that by holding on to the anger you are hurting yourself. Choose to let go of it.

12) Give the outcome to the divine forces of the universe. Use prayer and meditation to help you access the state of forgiveness. Forgive the other person and pray for their well-being.

relationships of depth. When we have a backlog of anger, it finds its own way to be released, either through generalized irritability or unwarranted explosiveness. We may even become self-destructive, developing addictions, destructive behavior patterns, and perhaps suicidal tendencies.

It is not for us to judge another's actions. You can only do what is right and necessary for you to maintain your own truth and then leave the outcome to God or the universal energy field. You hurt yourself by holding on to the anger. Compose a letter of forgiveness and send thoughts of well being (as much as you are able to at this time) to the person you have the most anger towards. Create a space in you for this forgiveness to grow in time.

PREVENTION

Develop ways for transforming a potentially destructive emotion into something with healing power. Give the anger away. Recognize that the universe is a better container for injustices and negativity than your body. Practice letting it go, knowing that the law of cause and effect gives back to you what you put out and will do the same to others.

Communication Style Worksheet

Review the questionnaire below, and after reading these examples of different communication styles, record your answers.

Passive

Identify situations in which you act passively or identify people with whom you are passive. For example, Sandra was at the hairdresser's and had brought in a photograph to the hair stylist of just how she wanted her hair cut. She was excited about the 'new look' and hoped it would create a more positive self-image for her. As the hairdresser began to cut her hair, he talked to her about the kind of cut that was 'in' and how it would suit her facial shape. He began cutting more of her hair than she had intended and soon had styled it to the cut he deemed appropriate for her. She was unable to speak throughout, but could only smile sweetly as she fumed inside. When finished, he raved about the cut to the other staff and clients in the salon as she sat miserably in her chair. She thanked him, paid the cashier, and burst into tears when she got to her car.

Aggressive

Identify situations in which you act aggressively, or people with whom you are aggressive. For example, Sheila works long hours at work to support her family. Her husband is an artist who earns less than she does. Although self-employed as a massage therapist, she does not schedule enough breaks for herself and consequently feels burnt out at the end of her week. When her four children awaken on Saturday morning, she is irritable, bothered by their noise, and frequently yells to break up their bickering. This causes further tension in the air, more tears, and intensifies the 'acting out' of her children.

Assertive

Identify situations in which you act assertively, or people with whom you are assertive. For example, Janet's older sister often came to visit in the evening several times a week around dinner-time. Janet was studying for a law degree, and though she enjoyed her sister's company, she needed time for her studies. She thought about the situation and then spoke to her sister. "I enjoy you coming over to be with us but my priority for the next two months is studying for my exams. Could you limit your visits to Wednesday evenings for now? That way I can plan to be with you and won't feel stressed about squandering my study time. We'll have a more enjoyable time together.' Her sister responded positively, respected Janet's boundary concerning time, and Janet was able to do well on her exams.

Passive

Situations when I acted passively:
1)
2)
3)
4)
5)
Who are the people with whom I act passively (husband/partner, employer, children, sibling, particular friends, salespersons, etc.):
1)
2)
3)

What are the feelings in me during and after these interactions?

How would I like this to change?

Aggressive

Situations when I acted aggressively:
1)
2)
3)
4)
5)
Who are the people with whom I act aggressively?
1)
2)
3)
What are the feelings in me during and after these interactions?

How would I like this to change?

Assertive

Situations when I acted assertively:
1)
2)
3)
4)
5)
People with whom I act assertively:
1)
2)
3)
What are the feelings in me during and after these interactions?

How would I like this to change?

Assertive Behavior Worksheet

Certain guidelines will help to ensure that your assertive style works for you. Follow the steps below as you respond to a situation assertively. Start with something small and easy. It takes practice — you may feel uncomfortable at first, but keep trying. The more you do it, the easier it gets. Eventually, it will be natural for you to act assertively.

1. Examine and affirm your rights in each particular situation. Look at what you want out of it, what your needs are, and pay attention to your feelings. Release feelings of blame, the desire to hurt, and self-pity. Define your goal and keep it in mind as you negotiate for change. As you practice 'trying on' assertive behavior, write these things down for yourself before communicating to the other party so that you are clear and validate yourself.

    Situation #1:
    My rights:
    What I want out of it:
    My needs are:
    My feelings around this are:
    Situation #2:
    My rights:
    What I want out of it:
    My needs are:
    My feelings around this are:
    Situation #3:
    My rights:
    What I want out of it:
    My needs are:
    My feelings around this are:

2. Arrange a time and place to discuss your concerns with the person involved that is convenient for both of you.

    Situation #1:
    Possible time and place:
    Situation #2:
    Possible time and place:
    Situation #3:
    Possible time and place:

3. Be specific as you define the problem. State matter-of-factly how you see the situation and share your opinion and beliefs in a calm and rational way. For example, you might say, 'We have spent the last three weekends staying at home; it's time we did something adventurous together.'

    Situation #1:
    Define the problem specifically:
    Situation #2:
    Define the problem specifically:
    Situation #3:
    Define the problem specifically:

4. Describe your feelings around the situation so that the other person has a better understanding of you and what the situation means to you. When communicating your feelings, own them by saying, 'I feel _____ when_____.' Do not blame the other person as you express your feelings, but instead let them know how their actions affect you. Refer to a specific action as you express your feelings rather than generalizing. For example, you could say, 'When you arrive home late without calling, I feel discounted and unappreciated.' Do not place labels on the other person such as 'inconsiderate' or 'passive-aggressive' but stick to the specific situation and the feelings it caused in you.

Situation #1: _____

I feel: _____

When: _____

Situation #2: _____

I feel: _____

When: _____

Situation #3: _____

I feel: _____

When: _____

5. Express your wishes in a simple statement while being firm and specific. Clearly state your needs and what you want from the situation. For example, 'I would really like the two of us to spend time alone together this evening.' Communicate your thoughts about a particular situation in a factual, non-blaming way, using 'I statements'.

Situation #1: _____

Simple statement expressing your request: _____

Situation #2: _____

Simple statement expressing your request: _____

Situation #3: _____

Simple statement expressing your request: _____

6. Reinforce the other person so that they will be more inclined to give you what you want. Tell them what the return will be for both of you. Describe the positive consequences of what will happen if your request is granted. For example, 'If you put your pajamas on when I ask you to, then we will have time for a bedtime story.' If these positive outcomes are not motivating for the other person or don't work, then describe negative consequences for failure to cooperate. For example, 'If you do not put your pajamas on when I ask you to, then you'll have to go to bed without a story. I need time to myself tonight.' Be sure that the negative consequence is something you can and will follow through with. You will lose your own and the other person's respect if you do not keep to your word. Think about the negative consequence before you say it and don't threaten the other person.

Situation #1: _____

Positive reinforcement: _____

Negative consequences: _____

Situation #2: _____

Positive reinforcement: _____

Negative consequences: _____

Situation #3: _____

Positive reinforcement: _____

Negative consequences: _____

Resolving Conflict

Dr R.G. Hamer has developed a novel theory of the causes of cancer, proposing that every cancer begins with a severe, acute conflict that occurs as a shock to the individual and registers an effect in the psyche, in the brain, and in a target tissue or organ. The conflict is followed by nervous system stress that may manifest as cold hands and feet, loss of appetite, weight loss, sleeplessness and anxiety, or a dwelling upon the conflict. Dr Hamer feels that the type of cancer is determined by the characteristics of the initial traumatic occurrence, which registers in a particular part of the brain and in a specific location in the body.

Dr Hamer studied thousands of brain CT scans of cancer patients and was able to observe concentric rings around a target area of the brain that he called an HH (HAMERsche HERD). From the brain location of the HH, a trained physician can accurately predict where in the body the cancer has occurred and what type of conflict preceded it. Dr Hamer has found this to be true for over 15,000 documented cases.

A woman's emotional reaction and thought processes at the time of the conflict determine which body part is affected. When the conflict is resolved, healing begins. The physical stress symptoms abate, the brain repairs itself, and the cancer growth stops.[1]

Mind-Body Connections

Mind-body health is dependent upon our ability to acknowledge and express our feelings. Emotional links to illness are often buried in the unconscious. Techniques to access these feelings are helpful as part of the healing process.

Any means by which we can recover buried emotions through touch, images, and words will be helpful in releasing symptoms from the body. These avenues include drawing, dream-work, dialoging with the ailing part, and bodywork. If we use these techniques regularly and actively listen to our emotions, we may avoid psychosomatic illness.

Imagery and Visualization

Increasingly we are discovering the subtle and powerful linkages of mind and body through imagery. Jeanne Achterberg, author of *Imagery and Healing*, believes that the image can alter cellular mechanisms and the intelligence of the cell. Image can shift the cellular machinery so that it performs unnatural functions. What we imagine in our minds has a direct correlation to how our body responds to life.

Achterberg has found that imagery is able to deeply affect the individual in the following ways. There is an unplanned, non-deliberate body-mind shift due to an event or to external environmental sensory stimulation; for example, the biggest effect on infertility is for a woman to call a fertility clinic to make an appointment, for women often become pregnant just knowing that they may receive help. On the other hand, walking into a typical doctor's office causes most people's white blood cell count to go down and blood pressure to go up.

Imagery can positively affect the mind-body if a woman adopts a new identity. She takes on a new persona, changes her previous life-script, and recreates herself as the character in the play. She 'imagines' and embodies this new identity with the inner commitment to helping herself. This is a deliberate effort of moving the mind-body in a healing way. She becomes a different person from whom she was when she became sick. The global shift or new persona pervades much of her life and can last for a long time (until there's another shift).

For example, the cancer patient who shifts from being a 'pleaser' or 'victim' and initiates life changes to do what she's always

Visualization Exercise

Jeanne Achterberg developed a drawing exercise to assess an individual's likely prognosis with an illness. Using 14 specific parameters, she was able to predict over 90% of the time who would die and who would go into remission from cancer.

This is what she did. First, she ensured that the patient was in a comfortable position, preferably lying down. The patient listened to tape-recorded relaxation instructions and was given a brief education regarding the disease process, how treatment might be helping the patient, and how the immune system works. The listener was advised to imagine these three factors in action.

It was the listener's choice to imagine her cancer cells or white blood cells any way she chose: 'Describe how your cancer cells look in your mind's eye.' 'How do you imagine your white blood cells fight disease?' 'How is your treatment working in your body?'

The patient was then asked to draw a picture of the body, the immune system, the cancerous process, and the treatment.

The interview protocol plus the drawings were scored according to the following 14 parameters:

1) vividness of cancer cell
2) activity of cancer cell
3) strength of cancer cell
4) vividness of white blood cells
5) activity of white blood cells
6) relative comparison of size of cancer and white blood cells
7) relative comparison of number of cancer and white blood cells
8) strength of white blood cells
9) vividness of medical treatment
10) effectiveness of medical treatment
11) choice of symbolism
12) integration of whole imagery process
13) regularity with which they imagined a positive outcome
14) ventured clinical opinion on the prognosis

These parameters were scored on a '1' to '5' scale (from negative to positive). Total scores were found to predict with 100% certainty who would have died or shown evidence of significant deterioration during the two-month period and, with 93% certainty, who would be in remission.

All too often medical professionals create doubt in a patient's mind about her self-healing capacity by placing all hope in surgery, chemotherapy, or radiation. We must reclaim our innate capacity to heal, and no matter what our choice of treatment is, believe in its power.

Guidelines for Creating Healing Imagery

These seven steps may assist you in visualizing images of self-healing. Do a drawing on a large paper to illustrate the concepts below. Repeat your drawing daily to improve on the previous drawing.

1) Portray the cancer cells as being few in number, small in size, weak in strength, and lacking vividness.

2) Portray the white blood cells as being vivid, very active, strong and powerful, large and abundant, and overwhelming the cancer cells. Believe more in the potency of your body's ability to heal than in the disease process, and understand that nothing is fixed — it is a process than can go either way.

3) Portray the naturopathic and medical treatments with vividness and effectiveness.

4) Choose strong, powerful, active imagery that is well integrated yet personal.

5) Practice the imagery frequently, at least twice daily. Keep drawing, over and over, until it's as powerful as it can be for a healing response. Draw so that you believe it.

6) Visualize that your body's healthy cells are easily able to repair any slight damage the treatment might cause; that the dead cancer cells are flushed from the body easily and completely; and that at the end of the imagery, you are healthy and cancer-free.

7) See yourself accomplishing your goals and fulfilling your life's purpose — relate to your future rather than your past. Explore what your ideal future might be and shift your life in that direction so that your immune system responds with you. Draw one of your long term goals that you are moving towards achieving.

FACT

What we believe and imagine about our bodies has an incredible bearing on how we deal with an illness. Our minds create the most powerful drugs during the healing process. We can believe in our body's innate capacity to heal. We can familiarize ourselves with our immune system and visualize its components doing their jobs efficiently and perfectly.

FACT

A loss or grief from childhood that has never quite been healed or is reawakened by another loss in adulthood (such as the death of a loved one or loss of a relationship) can increase the likelihood of cancer.[3] Usually this second loss occurs one to five years before the diagnosis of cancer.

wanted to do for herself may appear selfish and different to those who have known her previously.

Take a minute to think about this for yourself. What would your new life script look like if you could rewrite the character in the play? How would you be different? How would you act differently to those around you? Write a few lines on how your character would be different on a separate piece of paper. We do not have to have an illness to do this. Do it now. Life is short for all of us.

Living with Joy and Purpose

The feeling of joy and the sense of having a purpose in life are dependent upon our emotional and spiritual well-being, our prevailing attitudes, development of our potential, sustaining relationships, who we are in a state of 'being', and what we 'do' in life. A lasting sense of joy and purpose comes from inner direction rather than from outside expectations. It is the voice inside of us linked to our intuition and to the universal energy that guides us to living our destiny.

Destiny is the path our life takes when we relate to our soul and listen to and obey our intuitive callings. Our soul is in the driver's seat. Fate is what happens to us when the soul is in the back seat and we let other people, parental expectations, societal norms, or 'shoulds' guide our lives. Disease sometimes manifests when we do the latter, as it can be the intelligence of the body-mind communicating to us that all is not well in the way we are living our lives. There may be some part of ourselves that we are not listening to or honoring, some aspect of unlived life. The psyche wants wholeness, integration of polarities and opposites, wants to embrace all parts of us.

Coping with Death and Disease

Still, death and disease can happen when we are living our lives fully. Why one woman should become ill and another may not is partially out of our control. We do not know what larger purpose is at work in the unfolding of our lives and in our dying. I believe that there is a time when each of us is slated to die and lessons we are meant to learn through our living and dying. The disease process can sometimes teach us those lessons more quickly. I also think that we have the capacity to change the time of our death by how we live our lives and how we respond to what is handed to us. Though the 'script' is there, we can rewrite it.

Clearly, breast cancer has many contributing causes. You did not cause your disease, nor are you responsible for curing it. If you have breast cancer, do not blame yourself. There are many causative factors that place all women at risk. However, if you orient your living to finding meaning, purpose, and joy, your immune system will respond positively to these cues and will help to protect you from breast cancer or to recover from it more quickly.

Our Unique Ways of Being in the World

In his book *Cancer as a Turning Point*, Dr Lawrence LeShan, a psychologist who has worked with cancer patients for over 35 years, claims that cancer in his patients goes into remission roughly 50% of the time. When he had his clients review their past and try to address what was wrong with them using Freudian and psychoanalytic techniques, they did not get better; but when he began to encourage patients to explore avenues for bringing meaning, fulfillment, and joy into their lives, they often became well.[4]

Dr LeShan noticed that in the majority of his clients, there had been a loss of hope in ever achieving a meaningful and satisfying way of living previous to discovering first signs of the cancer. He helped each client find her unique ways of being in the world and attempted to match these to a lifestyle and form of work which best suited her nature. One case he cites is 'Ethel', a woman with metastatic breast cancer who had been told that there was nothing else that could be done medically for her. She consulted a psychiatrist and described herself, her experiences, and how for her whole life she had longed to travel aboard an ocean liner and see the world, but her life situation had prevented her from doing so. The best memories in her life were when she was newly married and working as a saleswoman in an exclusive clothing store in Chicago. She had grown children now who lived on the other side of the United States.

The psychiatrist suggested to her that since her husband was dead and her children no longer needed her, there was nothing to hold her back now from taking a trip on an ocean liner. Her oncologists had told her that she had but two months to live. Ethel took all her money and invested it in a first-class cabin on the Queen Mary for a world cruise. Four months later she angrily stormed into her psychiatrist's office and complained that she had spent all her money and was still alive! The psychiatrist was able to get her a job in a boutique on another ship. She

PREVENTION
Live your life being aware of your death, so that you deepen relationships, experience life fully, achieve and accomplish your goals, and develop your talents and gifts.

PREVENTION
Strive to live a life in alignment with your true nature, where your passion and joy are kindled and you use your talents and gifts.

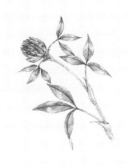

Activating Your Capacity to Heal

In addition to detoxification, eating a healthy diet, using herbal remedies and key nutritional supplements, we can assist our immune systems through techniques of visualization and imagery. Draw an outline of your body (full-size is best) showing the components of your immune system as you work through this exercise.

The Thymus Gland

Your thymus gland sits behind your upper sternum and is the commander-in-chief for many of your white blood cells, training them and telling them what to do. (Can you tell yourself what to do?) Tap the upper part of your sternum (which stimulates the thymus) as you repeat these phrases out loud, three times each:

'I am found behind your upper sternum, close to your heart. I am made stronger by your love.'

'I call white blood cells from the bone marrow to me. I train them to co-operate and perform specific jobs. I send them out into the blood to patrol the body.'

'I respond well to feelings of joy, hope, prayer and self-love. I need to feel supported.'

'I need you to be relaxed for me to function well.'

'I am strengthened by coordinated arm and leg movements on alternate sides (swimming, marching, yoga), tapping on the sternum, and brain hemisphere balancing.'

'I am nourished by vitamins A, C, E, B complex, B6, folic acid, the carotenes, selenium, zinc, melatonin, thymus extract, coenzyme Q10, probiotics, digestive enzymes, burdock root, echinacea, goldenseal, European mistletoe, poke root, wild indigo root, amla, astragalus, and ganoderma.'

The Spleen

Your spleen is located in the upper left part of the abdomen, beneath the diaphragm and behind your stomach. Tap the outer part of your body over your spleen as you repeat the following phrases out loud, three times each:

'I am found beneath your diaphragm and behind your stomach, and am the size of your fist.'

'I am packed full of powerful, intelligent lymphocytes.'

'The macrophages on duty in me identify and destroy all bacteria, viruses, and toxins as they circulate in the blood through me.'

'I am an amazing filter for debris in the blood.'

'I am nourished by burdock root, goldenseal, and echinacea.'

The Liver

Place your hand over your liver on the right side of your body beneath the rib cage as you repeat the following phrases out loud, three times each:

'I am a magnificent factory for manufacturing lymphatic fluid.'

'I am able to detoxify whatever comes my way.'

White Blood Cells
Macrophage

Open and close your hands in front of you as though you are a macrophage engulfing and destroying foreign particles. Repeat the following phrases out loud, three times each as you continue the arm movement:

'I am able to attack, engulf, and digest invaders in the blood.'

'I recognize what doesn't belong in this body; I engulf, digest, and inactivate anything that is harmful to me.'

'I like to hang out in the spleen, liver, lungs, lining of the intestines, lymph nodes, nervous system, bone marrow, and connective tissue.'

'I call on helper T-cells to come to the infection site.'
'I am made more vigorous by shitake and maitake mushrooms, echinacea, burdock, zinc, European mistletoe, and goldenseal.'

Helper T-Cell
Move your arms as though you are beckoning helpers to come to your aid and repeat the following phrases out loud, three times each:
'I am well trained in the thymus gland.'
'I respond quickly to the call of duty.'
'I signal the other cells of the immune system to come and help when we need to defend this body.'
'My numbers are increased by vitamin B6, zinc, and alpha lipoic acid.'

Killer T-Cell
Move your arms and hands as though you are shooting or targeting foreign organisms or cancer cells as you repeat the following phrases out loud, three times each:
'I recognize what needs to be destroyed and I destroy it.'
'I protect the life of this body.'
'Shitake and Turkey tail mushrooms make me a stronger warrior, as does MGN-3. So does the mistletoe preparation called Iscador and the mineral manganese.'

B-Cell
Punch out with alternate closed fists as though you are knocking down any enemies while you repeat the following phrases out loud, three times each:
'I can manufacture substances that make my enemies harmless.'
'I recognize my enemies and can defend myself against them.'
'I recognize what is harmful to me and can defend myself from it.'
'I quickly move to protect this body from what is harmful to me.'
'My home is in the spleen and lymph nodes, but I travel wherever I'm needed.'
'I have a helper who signals me to act.'

Suppressor T-Cell
Use your hands to make the 'time out' hand gesture with the left hand flat, palm down, and the right fingers perpendicular touching it underneath to form the letter 'T'. Repeat the following phrases out loud, three times each:
'I know when to stop attacking.'
'Things are safe now; I can be less aggressive at this time.'
(If you have cancer, you want to activate your Helper T-cells and Killer T-cells and decrease the activity of your Suppressor T-cells).

Memory Cell
Make circles with the fingers of each hand and place them around your eyes, as though you are looking through binoculars. As you look around you, repeat the following phrases out loud, three times each:
'I recognize you from before and know how to deal with you.'
'I will be around for a long time, watching for anything that is a threat to the life of this body.'
'I will protect you for life.'

PREVENTION
Build your 'meaning bank' by investing meaning daily into what you do and what you experience. Find meaning in the attitude you take to suffering or to illness. Ask of every situation that's given to you what you can learn from it to help you grow emotionally and spiritually.

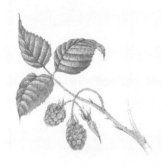

loved the work and found it completely fulfilling. Over the years, the breast cancer shrank to half its original size with no further treatment. She kept in contact with her psychiatrist until he died eight years later.[5]

What did Ethel do to generate self-healing? She rekindled and acted out a life-long dream. She let go of the mental obstacles that had previously thwarted the realization of that dream. She found a situation in life where she felt happy. She put everything on the line for herself. She made a commitment to her own happiness and her immune system responded.

When we recover our hope for living a satisfying and meaningful life, we strengthen our defenses against cancer as our body and mind respond to our spiritual commitment to live. By finding our own unique and joyous ways of being in the world, breast cancer will be less likely to find us.

Searching for Meaning

In his book *Man's Search for Meaning*, Viktor Frankl writes about the ways in which we derive meaning from life. Achievement is something we 'do' in the external world, while experience shapes who we 'are' internally. Meaning comes from both areas. For our well-being, what we expect from life is not as important as how we respond to life's expectations of us. Life is the teacher, continually presenting us with tests, choices, and opportunities. Daily and hourly we are being questioned by life and our answer can consist in right action and right conduct. Each of us is given tasks to fulfill, a piece to play on the world stage, and it is our responsibility to find our personal path that is in step with the grand scheme of things. Frankl called his method of responding to the world 'logotherapy' and wrote that we could discover the meaning in life in three different ways.

Meaning through Doing

The first way to find meaning is through creating a work or doing a deed. This includes meaningful work or a career, any artistic expression, as well as the day-to-day actions of our lives — greeting a friend, smiling at a stranger, writing a letter, making a charitable donation, doing volunteer work, buying organic food, planting a garden etc. For each of us these deeds will be different. We can bring meaning into the daily actions of our lives.

Meaning through Experience

The second way to gather meaning from life is by experiencing something or encountering someone. We may experience goodness, truth, beauty, nature, or culture.

To experience goodness, we can spend time with 'good' people and visit places where goodness is exemplified, such as in volunteer organizations, spiritual retreats, or healing centers. We can experience truth through studying the works of spiritual giants of whatever faith we find appealing. We can recognize beauty in the human body, a rose garden, faces of children, a well-made machine, or a decorated home. When we surround ourselves with beauty, we feed ourselves meaning.

Expanding Your Joy

Joyful experiences and play help us to live fully and renew our energy and creativity. When we connect to the miracle of each breath, we can bring joy into everyday moments. As women, we often sacrifice our personal joys for the needs of our families or career. It is valuable to put yourself first sometimes. Create balance between your inner life, family life, and career. This exercise will help you to access the states of 'being' and 'doing' that bring you the most joy.

1) In the first column, make a list of the 'being' states that have brought you joy in the past or experiences that are possible for you in the near future. These will include your favorite forms of play and relaxation as well as the ways you connect to your inner self or soul. In the second column, recall the 'doing' states that have brought you joy and fulfillment or things you have always wanted to do but have put off. Think back to recall any aborted dreams or forgotten desires.

For example, some 'being' states might include watching a sunset, having a bubble bath, or listening to a favorite piece of music. 'Doing' states could include horseback riding, teaching a skill, hosting a party, making pottery, traveling to the Galapagos, sky-diving, or swimming. Joy can also be an inner state that we bring to all our interactions. Because we feel joy, we can perform small acts of devotion or service, such as reading to a child, shoveling snow for a neighbor, or wishing someone a happy birthday.

2) If your list is short, then imagine what might bring you joy. What are the things you have watched others do that you have thought you would like to try? When you have exhausted your list, write beside each entry how often you would like this experience. Make it a priority to manifest at least three of these experiences each month and set dates for activities that need some planning, such as a vacation. If you are in a group, share your list with other women.

Joyful 'Being States' (more passive)	Joyful 'Doing States' (more active)
1.	1.
2.	2.
3.	3.
4.	4.
5.	5.
6.	6.
7.	7.
8.	8.
9.	9.
10.	10.

Nature is there for us to experience meaning. Running on the beach, walking in the woods, planting a garden, and travel to scenic places renews us spiritually. We can look for our own sacred spots in nature where we feel rooted and joyous. Culture also provides a source of meaning for many. Music, dance, art, theater — each of these has the potential to deepen our connection to our spiritual natures.

Of all interactions, it is loving encounters that bring us the most meaning. When we love another, we help them to actualize their potential, and when we are loved, we more easily realize our own potential. If we are feeling unloved, then we can make ourselves

FACT
If suffering is unavoidable, through our journey into the dark reaches of the soul, we can sometimes pass to the other side having gained in compassion, acceptance, tolerance, and wisdom. Illness is a great yet difficult teacher.

beacons of love and find people, plants, or animals that need our love. In giving it, we will receive it back. There are always organizations that need volunteers and plants and animals that need taking care of.

Meaning through Suffering

The third way we can experience meaning, according to Victor Frankl, is by 'the attitude we take towards unavoidable suffering.' When we suffer, we are challenged to change ourselves, and if the suffering is unavoidable, we can triumph in the way we bear it provided that we find meaning in it. Suffering can be the hero's path, although it challenges us physically, emotionally, and spiritually. If suffering is avoidable, then we should remove its cause, whether it be physical, psychological, or political.

The illuminating qualities that illness can bring us might never have been gained if we were able to cure our sicknesses instantly. Many of us call suffering into our lives so that we can help others. Once we have felt pain, we sense others' pain. We are then more able to extend our hearts and minds in compassionate service.

Why Am I Here?

In order to answer the question 'Why am I here?' we need to appreciate our unique qualities, gifts, talents, and capabilities. Think about what these are in you. What are the unique qualities that you perceive in yourself and the positive qualities that others have recognized? These might include qualities of optimism, insight, reliability, compassion, leadership, creativity, organizational ability, patience, assertiveness, sensitivity, grace, etc. Search for the hidden qualities that may lie buried in you that perhaps others don't see or you have not yet revealed to the world. Include those in your list, too. These may include such things as being forthright, adventurous, outrageous, wise, risk-taking, courageous.

'Why Am I Here' Exercise

List your gifts, talents, and capabilities and ways in which you can develop them to increase your joy and to seed your future — whether it's the next 50 years or a future life.

Qualities	Gifts, Talents, Capabilities	Passions, Interests, Causes
1.	1.	1.
2.	2.	2.
3.	3.	3.
4.	4.	4.
5.	5.	5.
6.	6.	6.
7.	7.	7.
8.	8.	8.
9.	9.	9.
10.	10.	10.

We all have unique gifts, talents, and capabilities. What were the gifts you came into the world with, have developed along the way or have wanted to develop? What are the talents you have not explored but which are calling you? What are the ways in which your creative energy expresses itself or has expressed itself in the past? Is it through writing, drawing, painting, acting, pottery, dance, cooking, dressmaking, athletic ability, music, weaving, gardening, carving — it is important to find your avenues of self-expression and nurture them.

Rudolph Steiner believed that as we prepare to die, we should choose the seeds we want to develop for our next life. We may never master a particular skill or talent in this life, but the seeds we plant will make it easier for them to germinate the next time around.

7 Steps for Finding Purpose

These seven steps will help you in your search for meaning and purpose in life.

1) Acknowledge that you have a spiritual self. People have called this the soul, inner guide, inner voice, Holy Spirit, higher self, etc. This aspect of us is divine, not bound by time or space, and is linked to a universal energy or universal mind. It is the God within linked to the God everywhere. It is not concerned with material possessions, success, or what others think. Even though you may not experience this aspect of yourself often, it is important to acknowledge its presence as a starting point. Close your eyes and take a minute now to link with your spiritual self.

2) Create a relationship with your spiritual self. As you create relationships with others through communication and time spent together, you can create a relationship between the mind and the soul. There are many forms that this can take, but essentially it is a daily spiritual practice. It is a regular setting aside of time to acknowledge and be with your spiritual self, a time of inner listening. It may be accomplished through one or more of the following practices: yoga and meditation; dreamwork; journal writing; creative activity such as drawing, painting, sculpture, music, poetry, dance; prayer and contemplation; service; and time spent in nature. As you acknowledge the soul's presence through a spiritual practice, you more easily recognize its voice and what it (or God) wants from you in the world. Take a moment to reflect upon what kind of spiritual practice best suits you and how you can establish it as a priority in your life. Make a commitment to explore alternatives or begin a regular spiritual practice.

3) Pay attention and actively listen to the soul's calling. This is synonymous with listening to God's will. It is the voice of intuition that gently urges you to see situations clearly and to act in certain ways. It opens you up to a state of 'being' in the fullness of the moment, experiencing love within the transitory nature of life, and feeling the interconnectedness of everything. It asks you to act in the world, to do what you are most suited for, and to contribute to the improvement of the planet and the human condition. It is the future pulling you to your potential. On some level, that potential is already manifest, only separated from you by time and space. You can answer the soul's calling, by asking yourself the following questions: Who am I? Why am I here? What did I come here to do? What is my passion? What is the potential in me that yearns for fruition? What did I come here to learn? What did I come here to heal? Who did I come here to love? What did I come here to express? What did I come here to teach? What causes did I come here to serve? Who did I come here to be? What brings me the greatest joy? What can I do that reflects my beliefs and values? In the following exercises we will explore the answers to these questions.

4) Agree to what is being asked of you. This is often painful as the ego allows the soul to be in the driver's seat. Sacrifice is required. Taking risks and trusting the process of change is also often necessary. Like a snake shedding its skin, you are asked to release old belief systems that limit your growth and expanding identity. The old persona, the old clothes, don't fit anymore. Faith must also be your companion through this process — faith in yourself, faith in a higher power or God.

5) Obey the guidance given to you from within, to act on the stirrings of the soul, moment by moment, leap by leap. Illness sometimes pushes us more quickly to do this or gives us permission to pursue a direction we may not have taken otherwise. This path may not be easy, as it can demand constant surrender of the ego. It may be terrifying to obey the inner voice. You may feel that you are not worthy or up to the task and ask, 'Why me?' You need consistency, commitment and courage to carry it out. You may need support and validation from at least one other person. Find that person.

6) Realize what must die or be transformed in your life for the soul to be affirmed. What do you need to say 'No' to in order to live a purposeful life that is in harmony with who you really are? If you are going to embrace a new way of living, then you must let go of parts of your old life that drain your energy, that reinforce negativity, or that no longer serve you. Sometimes you must let go of a relationship, shift careers, reassess friendships, give up comfort or wealth, and say 'no' to social engagements or responsibilities that you shouldered in the past. You can say 'no' to that part of you that reacts as a victim or is overly concerned with what others think. You can transform your anger into love and forgiveness.

7) Be fully present in your activity, acknowledging the unseen hands that help you and the opportunities and soul responsibilities that come your way at appropriate times. You can walk with an attitude of gratitude through life and welcome the joys and hardships of each day. Accept what comes your way and meet it head on. Every experience is an opportunity to trust in something larger than yourself. Release your resistance to the reality you've been handed and embrace the process of coming to terms with your life, or your death. You can release your need for control and acknowledge the mystery of living. You can act with commitment and integrity but surrender the outcome of your actions to a higher power or God.

Another way of understanding 'Why am I here?' is to recognize where your passion lies. What do you feel very strongly about that you would love to give your energy to? Think about your past and about when life drew the most from you, when you felt as though what you were doing really mattered, either for yourself, for others or the planet. Look for the things you love more than your own comfort or convenience, the things you could die for because you believe in them so strongly. Or what have you always wanted to explore but have been unable to so far?

Healing Dreams

For over 1000 years, the Greeks believed that dreams were an integral component in healing. This healing tradition began with Asclepius, who was born in the thirteenth century B.C., who legend says died when he was struck by lightning sent by Zeus, and who became the Greek god of medicine. His symbol was the snake we still see used in many medical insignia. Not only did Asclepius cure the sick, but also on occasion he brought the dead back to life. He established over 300 temples in Greece, usually in a country setting near sacred springs and rocks with crevices into the earth, presided over by priests who were also physicians. Snakes were commonly present in the temples and were considered to be the incarnation of Asclepius.

Healing was seen as a sacred tradition, and the physician-priests were required to take a sacred oath that evolved into what we now call the Hippocratic Oath. Patients came to sleep in the temple to be treated with herbs, surgery, exercise, hydrotherapy, and the laying on of hands — and to receive a healing dream. The patient would do a

Meaning Mandala Worksheet

Mandalas have been used in all cultures as symbols of the self, as meditation tools, and as expressions of healing and integration.

In this exercise you will make a 'meaning mandala' that will help you to define where you derive meaning from your life and propel you to manifest that meaning. It will remind you of your soul's purpose here and how to live that purpose. It will help to integrate the divergent directions in your life and bring you stability when you lose your compass or your anchor. As you relate to your meaning mandala, your body will mobilize its ability to heal.

1) Using this diagram as a model, redraw it on a large piece of paper, at least 24 inches by 36 inches (the bigger the better).

2) At the end of the spaces between two radiating lines at the outer edge of the largest circle, write words or phrases that answer the questions around the diagram. Between the radiating spokes list the progression of actions or experiences that would enhance or develop the meaning at the outer edge of the circle. These might include qualities to develop within yourself, tasks to do, other people to involve, phone calls to make, money to save, courses to enroll in, practice time, etc.

3) Place this drawing on the wall where you can see it regularly to remind yourself of all you have to live for. Focus on the drawing as you do your rebounding exercises. Let it speak to you and remind you of the next step in manifesting your potential.

4) In time, as you begin to actualize the meaning and purpose of your life, use colored markers to fill in the spaces from the center outward. Use many colors and make the mandala vibrant with life. For every step you take to experience meaning, purpose, and joy, acknowledge it by filling in an area around the section associated with it.

5) To make the mandala more powerful, draw images around the outer circle that represent your goals or fulfilled self. You can also cut up magazines to make a collage with images that remind you of your purpose.

Make your mandala uniquely your own, as your life is. Your body needs to know that you are serious about living for it to co-operate with you in healing. Trust in the future that's calling you.

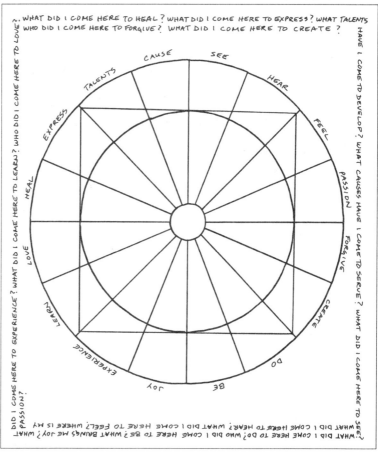

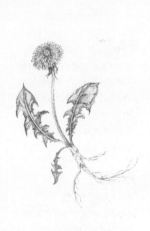

cleansing fast and don white clothing. In the evening, she would make an offering at an altar, while the priest read a prayer on her behalf. She was told that she would be visited by Asclepius through the night in a dream and perhaps be healed. In the morning, the priest interpreted the patient's dream and told her what treatment should be carried out in response to the dream. If she was healed, she made another offering and went home. If not, she could stay longer.

Many patients inscribed their healing stories on stone tablets around the temple. Here is one story:

A man came to the temple with paralyzed fingers, skeptical of the cures he read on the inscriptions around him. He slept and dreamed that as he was playing dice under the temple, Asclepius came and stepped on his fingers, stretching them out. He then asked the man if he still disbelieved. When the man said 'No', Asclepius said that if he trusted in the future, he would be healed. When the man awoke his fingers were no longer paralyzed.[7]

In my practice I have also encountered women who have experienced healing dreams. 'Lisa' came to me for follow-up care after traditional breast cancer treatment several years earlier. A cat scan and X-rays suggested that the cancer had metastasized to one of her ribs, though the bone biopsy was negative. Her doctors told her that they believed it to be a metastasis, but because of the lack of confirmation from the biopsy, they would not treat it. It left her feel-

Invoking a Healing Dream

It is possible to invoke a healing dream using the Asclepian tradition as a model. Here are the steps you can use:

1) Decide to whom or what you will direct your prayer.

2) Be conscious through the day of creating an air of sanctity in your surroundings and in your self. You can do this by cleaning your living space, playing devotional or meditative music, fasting or eating very pure foods, bathing with the intent to purify body and mind, and perhaps practicing yoga, meditation, or another purification practice. Through the whole day embody an attitude of quiet reverence in preparation for your healing dream. Let your home and your body become your temple or choose an outdoor location to receive the earth's healing energies.

3) Create a sacred spot inside or outside where you can establish an altar and make an offering. The location can be a place you revisit as needed. You can also visit or make a pilgrimage to an altar in an established place, such as a church, temple, synagogue, or healing shrine. The more frequently you visit the altar, the easier it will feel and the more it will work for you. We energize sacred spots with our devotion.

4) Place an offering at the altar, such as money, fruit, flowers, or time given in service to others.

5) Ask for a healing dream that will guide you in your journey to wellness or ask that you be healed. Often the less specific you are the better — leave it up to God or your unconscious to figure out how to heal you rather than trying to control the process.

6) Keep a paper and pencil beside your bed and tell your unconscious before you sleep that you are ready to receive a healing dream. If you receive a dream, write it down.

7) Reflect on your dream until you can discern its meaning or get help from someone skilled in dream interpretation, such as a Jungian analyst. A good book to help with dream analysis is *Inner Work* by Robert Johnson.[9]

8) Make another offering in the morning as thanks.

9) If you don't receive a dream, continue the process until you do. Be patient. You will eventually.

ing afraid and in limbo, not sure whether she was going to live or die. She had the following dream:

I was standing in a large 3-story house on the edge of a cliff, something like the Scarborough Bluffs. The house was dilapidated and was crumbling even as I stood in it. It was about to fall into the ocean, as was I. Just then a hand appeared and pulled me out of the house as it tumbled over the cliff. I was safe.

I told Lisa that I felt it to be a positive dream because she didn't fall over the cliff; an outstretched hand saved her. She could heal. Because of the inconclusive diagnosis, she had only her intuition to rely on and felt 'in her bones' that she was not going to die. Though the next few months were full of confusion, at different times she experienced distinct periods of elation when she felt connected to a source much greater than herself. During those months, I reminded her of her dream. Another CAT scan in three months showed that the lesion remained the same and there were no further metastases. In six months it had shrunk considerably.

The Power of Prayer

As you discover your reasons for living, you can reinforce your belief that a new life is possible and that you deserve it. Prayer is one of the tools that can strengthen your belief or faith. Health practitioners, family, and friends will either add to your faith (consciously or unconsciously) or diminish it. Prayer is an innate faculty of humans, existing in all cultures in a variety of forms. It reminds us that we are spiritual beings first, living a human life.[10]

Though our physical bodies are bound by time and space, our souls are not. Through prayer we connect to a higher source of power or energy. We don't have to do it all ourselves; we can draw on the unlimited power of the creator. We can gain access to a spiritual dimension to come to our aid. We are not alone. We call it God, the Infinite, or any name from the many world religions.

Prayer and visualization are inherently different. When we visualize, we consciously attempt to control an outcome in our body or in our life. It is accomplished through focused concentration, intention, and repetition. We attempt to fix ourselves or create the reality we want. When we pray we give up control. We surrender. We entreat a power greater than our own to help us. We admit that we need help; we can't fix the part of us that is broken. We are vulnerable. Though they are different, they are not mutually exclusive.

Prayer and meditation are complementary practices that each have a place in a healing program. I once attended an imagery workshop in Toronto with Jeanne Achterberg and Frank Lawless. Jeanne said that she noticed that the AIDS patients who did the best were the ones who were actively engaging the warrior archetype to be victorious over their disease but had given up trying to influence the outcome. In other words, do the best you can and leave the rest up to God. Visualization is 'doing'; prayer is 'leaving the rest up to God'. We need both. Whatever the outcome, we did the best we could. We are not responsible for the outcome. God is in charge.

FACT
At least some of the time prayer works to reverse diseases of all kinds. Spontaneous regression of cancer is possible but not predictable.

FACT
Spiritual growth is not necessarily proportional to an improvement in physical health. Poor physical health, however, is often the gate through which we pass to explore our spirituality.

FACT
People who are true to themselves and honor the experiences that come from the depths of their being are sometimes graced with a miraculous cure. They can but do not always have the following traits in common. They use surgery, medication, complementary medicine, and any other healing modalities that may be helpful. They do not desperately seek a miracle and are not determined to be healed of their disease. Rather, they believe that God's will is being done, no matter what the outcome. They live with gratitude for their lives despite their disease. They focus on 'being' and live fully in the present rather than getting caught up in 'doing'. They have a fighting spirit yet a capacity to surrender.

My Prayer of Intercession for You

May you be guided and protected on your healing journey. May we all be blessed in our efforts to heal ourselves, each other, and the Earth.

FACT

Saint Peregrine is the patron saint for spontaneous regression of cancer in the Christian tradition. While a young priest, he developed cancer in his leg and was scheduled for amputation. He prayed earnestly the night before surgery and dreamed he was cured. When he awoke, he was surprised to find that his dream had come true. In 1345 he died at the ripe age of 80, without any recurrence of cancer. He lived in service of those people afflicted with cancer, as many breast cancer survivors do today.[11]

A Gateway to the Spirit

Prayer heals us spiritually. We turn to prayer in times of crisis or illness. It helps us psychologically through difficult times, though it may not outwardly change a particularly situation or reverse disease. If you are ill and prayer does not reverse your illness, even though you are doing the best you can through allopathic and complementary medicine and psychological change, you can consider the following.

Illness can be a path of purification for the mind, body, and spirit. Sickness is part of the natural order on earth. Plants and animals get sick and die, as we do. Perhaps the purpose of our lives is to link to the totality and divinity within ourselves and all around us. The length of your life is not as important as how fully you receive your soul and how well you live in accordance with your true nature and your values. If the soul is infinite, then an opportunity may exist for it somewhere else to express itself, perhaps through reincarnation or through another form. Who are we to know when or where that opportunity lies? Many things are beyond our control. That is as it should be.

Reversing disease is not the ultimate goal. We are obliged to do all we can to live as fully as possible and to purify and heal as deeply as possible and then surrender the outcome of our efforts. Our soul never dies. Physical death can come sweetly as an exit point when we have finished our work here. It heralds a new beginning. For those of you who have cancer, there is no formula that will result in spontaneous healing. You must create your own path, reclaim your authentic life. You may or may not be 'cured' but your living will be more vital.

Types of Prayer

Several types of prayer are used in different religious traditions. They include 'petition', when we ask for something for ourselves; 'intercession', when we ask for something for others; 'confession', when we ask for forgiveness for a wrongdoing; 'invocation', when we call on the presence of God; 'thanksgiving', when we express gratitude for what we have received; and 'submission', when we accept God's will for us and surrender our personal will.

Patrons of Prayer

'Whom do I pray to?' you may ask. You can pray to the particular deities, saints, enlightened beings, or teachers associated with a spiritual tradition. You can pray to a divine spirit or energy that is all pervading, with no particular face. You can pray to the feminine creative power of the universe, known as Adi Shakti in India, or to the Virgin Mary in Christianity. You can pray to Jesus, Buddha, or Krishna. You can pray to one of the Greek goddesses, such as Athena. You can pray to the Greek healing God, Asclepius, or to Guru Ram Das, a healing divinity in the Sikh tradition.[12]

Go to the library and research world religions or talk to religious people if none of them seem right. We all have links to teachers and saints. It's up to us to find out who they are, recognize and accept them. But for now, just pray. Make the connection in your heart to something larger and more powerful than yourself. Over time, let there be intimacy between you and your spiritual source, and talk regularly to it as you would talk to a close friend who is a good listener. Remember the first law in physics, 'for every action there is an equal and opposite reaction.' There will be a response to your prayer, though it may not be what or when you expect it.

Your Personal Prayer

Each of the spiritual traditions has a large body of prayers to choose from and to recite. If you have a religious heritage, you might begin to search for your personal prayer in some of these religious books or in the writings of the saintly persons associated with your tradition. Find a few prayers, read them out loud, and notice how they make you feel. Change the wording if necessary.

With practice, prayer can replace worry and fear. Use it when you feel overwhelmed with either of these emotions.

PREVENTION
Design your own prayer or use a traditional prayer upon rising each morning and before bed. When you find yourself feeling a loss of hope, worry or fear, use prayer as a centering device.

How to Pray

We all will find different ways to pray as we listen to the longing of our soul and follow its directives. If you feel a little inept entering the world of prayer, here are a few suggestions to get you started.

1) Create a Time and Space for Prayer: As religious groups establish places of worship and set times for prayer, so too we can do this in our own homes. Find an area in your living space which you can designate as your place to pray. Claim your space with a blanket, pillow, or sheepskin that you can sit on for prayer. Over time you will associate this object with prayer and it will become easier to do — it may also be something to take with you when you travel. Create an altar if you like. Find some symbols that are meaningful to you and decorate the area with them. You might use religious pictures, natural objects such as flowers and shells, drawings or photographs. You want the images to be uplifting and transcendent so that they will help put you into a prayerful state. Change the symbols occasionally to create an ongoing relationship with your prayer space.

Establish a regular time for prayer. Typically this is in the morning on awakening or in the evening before bed, but it can be any time. If you pray at the same time daily, you establish a habit in your psyche that makes it easier to sustain. Be consistent, even when it's difficult. Like any discipline, it requires practice. Think of it as exercising your spiritual muscle — spirit-building, rather than body-building.

2) Begin with a Gesture: Initiate your prayer time with a gesture. Whatever feels natural to you — you can touch your forehead to a sacred object, bow or genuflect, put your palms flat together at your heart center, or simply close your eyes. This gesture becomes a signal for your body and mind to enter into a prayerful state.

3) Decide on a Type of Prayer: Decide which of the six types of prayer you will use at this time. Will it be a prayer for yourself, a prayer for another, a prayer of thanksgiving, a request for forgiveness, a call for God's presence, or a prayer for the ability to submit to divine will?

Center yourself by focusing your attention on your breath rather than any distracting thoughts. Bring your awareness to the heart center, between the breasts, and adopt an attitude of reverence and devotion as though you are in the presence of a great spiritual being or power. Feel compassion, receptivity, and surrender to a higher will. Give up control.

4) Begin Your Prayer: Your prayer may be a feeling state without words that you maintain for a period of time. It may be a formal prayer that you recite one or more times until you feel finished. You might keep a little notebook in your prayer space and let your prayer come out as written thoughts or as letters or drawings to God. Find what works for you.

5) Finish with Thanks: Finish your prayer with a moment of gratitude for having had the opportunity to pray. Acknowledge yourself as a spiritual being living a human life.

Summary

During an illness, we often need help to generate a healing response. A health practitioner can assist by creating a safe and relaxed environment, providing an opportunity for you to feel deeply, and to get in touch with emotions which may have gone unnoticed far too long, resulting in disease. You can gently be coaxed into the future that is calling you and there realize the full meaning of your life. You can also utilize spiritual practices to attune to your innermost self and learn to walk with faith as your companion.

Many people sense that their disease is a 'wake-up call'. What if we were to wake up to our psychological and spiritual needs and embark on a path of purification before a disease summoned us?

Here are some further guidelines for you to generate a healing response.

1) Learn to watch your thought processes. Identify with healing imagery and use it to replace self-destructive thoughts. Explore disturbing thoughts to understand their source, the need that lies beneath them, and ways to transform them. Remind yourself of the following:
   i)   illness is not a form of punishment — you are not guilty;
   ii)   others have recovered from the same illness;
   iii) your symptoms are a messenger & can be a catalyst for change;
   iv)   you have an innate capacity to heal;
   v)   the body is in a constant state of change — nothing is fixed — all is process.

2) Use meditation tools such as mantras, witnessing thoughts and feelings, and attention to the breath to disengage from the temporary reality created by your thoughts.

3) Use sensory stimuli to create healing responses. For example, when you turn on a water faucet, visualize any toxins, illness, or cancer cells being flushed out of your body; when you walk outside allow the wind to blow out any cancer cells; when you hear music direct it to breaking up any tumors, etc. Let these sensory experiences become a celebration of your body's self-healing ability. Make a list of all the ways you can use sensory stimuli to generate healing.

4) Use particular images that have power and significance for you. Find your totems — a rock, a tree, a piece of music, an animal — whatever contains healing power for you. Look for these in your dreams, honor them in your life. Place these images around you to remind you of healing. Believe in the power of nature to heal or in a spiritual force or deity. Identify with and pray to that higher power regularly, believing that it will heal you. Let a healing animal, person, or deity come to you in a state of relaxation and absorb the power of that animal or deity, letting it fight for you even as you sleep. Make a list of images that have power and significance for you.

5) Use meditation, imagery, prayer, and visualization regularly, two to five times daily. Enter a relaxed state beforehand. This usually takes a minimum of 11 minutes.

6) Remind yourself that the body-mind is in a constant state of change. If your mental state can change, so can the physical.

CHAPTER TEN

Breast Disease Treatments

CONTENTS

EXERCISES, CHARTS, CHECK LISTS & WORKSHEETS

Most women newly diagnosed with breast cancer come to see me for naturopathic support to help them through their conventional treatments of surgery, chemotherapy and radiation. Few women forego these recommended treatments to rely solely on natural therapies for their recovery. Although it is possible to coax breast cancer into retreat using naturopathic therapies alone, it is not predictable. It is also an immense task. Radical shifts in the psyche, specialized diets, lifestyle changes, detoxification regimens, and the use of numerous nutritional and herbal supplements are necessary to reverse breast cancer naturally. This undertaking is probably best done in a supervised setting, in a comprehensive medical clinic specializing in the natural treatment of cancer, where everyday stresses are removed, where food is prepared for you, and where progress can be monitored with very specific testing. Some clinics use additional treatments like ozone therapy, hyperthermia, and intravenous solutions that provide further benefit. See the 'Resources Directory' in the back of the book for several reputable international clinics.

It is my great hope that in the near future we will know more precisely what combination of natural therapies and healing practices we can consistently rely on to reverse breast cancer in women. I have outlined many of them in this book, but we are not there yet. There have been no large-scale studies of women who used a specific protocol of natural therapies for breast cancer to compare their long-term outcome to other women who used chemotherapy and radiation. The integration of natural therapies with conventional treatment is an evolving science.

Assessing Treatment Methods

While it is not my role to analyze the benefits or risks of chemo and radiation, I think we need to 'individualize' treatment more when recommending these harsh therapies. Women should clearly evaluate the long-term effects of chemotherapy and radiation before they begin, weighing those effects against the statistical benefit these treatments might give them for their specific situation. Often the reduction in mortality for either chemotherapy or radiation is limited.

Women with small, contained tumors are commonly over treated, and it is in these cases that we may draw on the use of natural therapies after surgery to prevent a recurrence, rather than use harsh treatments. Otherwise, natural therapies can be used before, during, and after surgery, chemotherapy, and radiation treatments to decrease side effects and improve outcomes. Because breast cancer is a chronic disease with the possibility of recurrence at any time, the strength of natural therapies at present lies in promoting long-term wellness after conventional medical treatment is completed.

Surgery Support

When to Schedule Your Surgery

If you are pre-menopausal, schedule your breast surgery during the latter half of your menstrual cycle when progesterone levels are highest.

Pre-Surgery Preparations

Consider the following strategies to prepare for surgery:[3]

1) Take time in the weeks leading up to surgery to eat well, with plenty of fruits and vegetables, to decrease your stress levels, to exercise and to relax.

2) Utilize a daily visualization practice to rehearse a positive experience during surgery, modifying the visualization script below to suit your temperament and situation. Read the script into a tape recorder, and listen to it daily. (You may also order a tape using the order form at the back of the book).

3) Create a ritual to transform your surgery into a more meaningful experience. If you are having a lumpectomy or a breast removed, ask yourself what else you can let go of at the same time. Can you use the surgery to release an old hurt, or conflict, or a piece of your past that no longer serves you? Write a poem or song, make a drawing or sculpture, talk to a friend or therapist, or create a ceremony to mourn and honor the loss of your breast (or part of it).

Similarly, if you are having breast reconstruction, make it a richer experience by exploring what else you can bring into your life at this time. How can surgery be a turning point for you in a journey to a more fulfilling future? What commitment can you make to yourself to mark the surgical event? Yes, breast surgery is a traumatic event, but our interpretation of it,

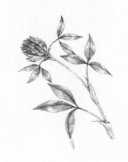

how we choose to react to it, will make all the difference.

4) Do not take the following supplements during the week before surgery, other than in amounts found in a multivitamin, as high amounts may thin the blood and cause increased bleeding: vitamin E, vitamin C, gingko, feverfew, garlic, ginger, Asian ginseng and conventional blood thinners.

5) There are other supplements you can use before surgery to heal faster. Use these during the 10 days prior to surgery: Zinc Picolinate: 30 mg 2 x per day between meals. Vitamin A: 20,000 IU 2 x per day. Beta carotene: 30,000 IU 2 x per day. Vitamin B Complex: 1 daily. Use immediately before surgery the following homeopathic remedies: Arnica 30 CH: 3 pellets. Calendula 30CH: 3 pellets, dissolved under the tongue. Traumeel drops (Heel): 10 drops.

6) Arrange for someone to cook for you for a few days after surgery or cook and freeze dishes in advance, so you are more able to focus on healing.

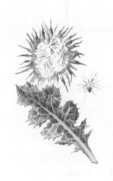

Healing After Surgery

Use immediately following surgery these supplements and homeopathic remedies:

N-acetyl cysteine: 500 mg 2 x daily for 5 days (to eliminate the anaesthetic).

Milk Thistle tincture: 30 drops 3 x daily (to protect the liver).

Curcumin and Bromelain: 500 mg of each 3 x daily between meals (to decrease swelling).

Proteolytic Digestive Enzyme (i.e. Wobenzyme): 2-5 capsules 2 x daily between meals (to decrease swelling and pain).

Vitamin C with bioflavonoids: 2 grams 3 x daily (to promote healing).

Vitamin E: 400 IU 2 x daily (also apply vitamin E directly on the incision).

Vitamin A: 20,000 IU 2 x per daily.

Beta carotene: 30,000 IU 2 x per daily.

Vitamin B complex: 1 tablet daily.

Zinc picolinate: 30 mg 2 x daily (to improve wound healing).

Fish Oil capsules: 2000 mg daily.

Arnica 30 CH: 3 pellets 3 x daily, for 1 week (to reduce bruising).

Calendula 30 CH: 3 pellets, once daily for 1 month (to prevent scarring).

Traumeel drops: 10 drops 3 x daily for 1 week (to reduce bruising).

To speed up the healing around the incision, you can use salves that contain vitamin E, zinc, calendula, comfrey and/or St. John's wort over the wound.

Dealing with Lymphedema

Lymphedema may occur after surgery and/or radiation has damaged or removed the lymph nodes in the underarm area. Anyone who has undergone a mastectomy or lumpectomy with axillary node dissection is at risk for developing lymphedema in the arm on the affected side. It can occur immediately after surgery, within a few months, or even 10 years or more after cancer therapy, and may occur gradually or suddenly. Swelling of the arm occurs due to an abnormal accumulation of lymph and its inability to flow back into the circulatory system. The condition may be accompanied by a feeling of heaviness, discomfort or pain in the arm, repeated infections, and thickening of the skin.

Lymphedema is best treated by someone trained in manual lymphatic drainage and combined decongestive therapy, usually a massage therapist or physiotherapist. Combined decongestive therapy includes manual lymphatic drainage, a gentle type of massage that works with improving the flow of the lymph; compression therapy, which includes compression garments or bandaging of the affected limb; education in self-massage; exercise; and skin care techniques.

The Hoxsey Formula, Essiac, Floressence, or the Healthy Breast Formula will also help to ease lymphedema. Certain homeopathic products have proven themselves over the years to help many patients with lymphatic congestion, including Lymphdiaral cream or drops from Pascoe, a German company, and Lymphomyosot, made by Heel.

Visualization Script for Surgery

If you have been diagnosed with or treated for breast cancer, you can follow this script as is or adjust it to better suit your particular needs and personality. Rehearse it one or more times daily as you are preparing for surgery or use it during your recovery.

1) Create a sacred space for yourself by changing your environment in such a way to set the stage for healing. This time is for you and your healing process. Ensure that you won't be disturbed. You might want to light a candle or incense, use a special blanket to cover yourself, or arrange flowers in the room. (Long Pause)

2) Begin sitting or lying down in a comfortable position. Support your neck and back with pillows if needed. Close your eyes. Give yourself permission to be still and to focus on relaxation and healing for at least twenty minutes. Open to a greater energy than yourself and invite it into your life. Imagine you can feel a healing presence in the room with you. Visualize a powerful healing force assisting you now. Receive the presence of your higher self and spiritual guides and ask them to help you through this healing journey. Become aware of your breathing, in and out through your nose, and notice the breath becoming slower and deeper. Experience your abdomen rising gently as you inhale and falling softly as you exhale. Feel your breathing for a few long, deep breaths. Inhale… Exhale… Inhale… Exhale…. (Medium Pause) Listen to the sound of the breath as though you are listening to the sound of the ocean waves coming in — and going out. (Medium Pause) Inhale the smell of a pine forest and allow that scent to fill you with rejuvenating and healing energy. With each exhale notice more tension being released. Take a few very slow, long deep breaths to enjoy this fully. Each breath brings more relaxation than the one before it. (Medium Pause) Notice where you feel numbness, pain or discomfort in your body and breathe into those areas.

3) Feel more relaxed now, more relaxed with each breath. Give yourself permission to ignore all sounds in your environment and choose not to interact with thoughts that come to mind. As you breathe in, imagine a cleansing and peaceful warmth filling your body. Feel it spread from your head and neck down through the shoulders, chest and arms, to your back, abdomen, and pelvis, then down through your legs and feet as though you are a plant drinking in energy from the sun. Take your awareness to your feet and let any tightness and tension dissolve. Notice the muscles feeling loose and smooth and warm as though they have just been given a gentle massage. Relax your lower legs and let the muscles soften. Breathe relaxation into your knees and thighs. Notice them becoming warm and relaxed, as though being bathed by rays of light. Become aware of your hips, buttocks, and pelvic area. Allow the breath to circulate there like a gentle wind, bringing warmth and relaxation with it. Relax your hips and pelvis. Let go of any tension you experience there. Breathing slowly and deeply, be aware of the muscles in the abdomen and release any tightness or anxiety you find there. Watch it dissolve. Feel the muscles in your back, allowing them to relax and let go. Imagine you are lying on warm sand and release tension from your back into the earth. As you breathe fully and deeply, let go of any tightness or tension stored in your chest. (Pause)

4) Direct healing and relaxation to the area of your breasts. Pick a healing color and let this color completely fill and wash through the breast area. Feel it cleansing the area, bringing renewed vitality. Notice the feelings you have associated with your breasts. Watch and listen to those feelings, acknowledge them, and then release them. (Pause)

5) Imagine a nurturing female presence beside you. It may be someone in your life now, someone you have known in the past, or an energy that you invoke. (Medium to Long Pause) She brings grace into your life. She fills you with courage, acceptance and love. She brings healing to the area of your breasts. (Pause) She can respond at any time to your questions. The response may be in the form

of words you hear internally, a feeling in your body, or an image. It may also come in a dream or an incident in your life. If you have a question for her, ask now — and be open to her response. (Long Pause) She reminds you of your own needs and when it is time for you to take care of yourself. She is available to you in your daily life. You have only to ask for her and listen to her response.

6) Now move your attention from the breast area, maintaining a long, deep breath, to your shoulders. Imagine healing hands massaging the shoulders as you allow tension to melt away. Let them become like soft wax. Allow relaxation to spread down your arms and to your hands. Let any stiffness or tightness be released. Open and close your fingers a few times and release constriction from your body and mind the way a butterfly releases itself from a cocoon. Open your mouth slightly and relax the muscles in your jaw. Relax your lips. Relax your cheeks, eyes, and eyebrows. Send the breath to your eyes as you feel them relax. Enable your eyes to see new choices available to you in your life. As you continue to breathe very slowly and deeply through your nose, become aware of your forehead and scalp. Allow them to relax and feel warm. Let any tension be released.

7) Now become aware of your whole body. If you notice pain, tension, or fear in any part of your body, send the breath there to soothe it. Inhale deeply… Exhale… Inhale… Exhale… With each breath, send your healing color through the entire body, washing it clean. Let that color permeate every cell, as though each cell receives pure air. Allow your mind to become very open, centered, and still. (Long pause)

8) Imagine a feeling of complete harmony, safety, and empowerment within yourself. Know that your body is a miracle and is in a state of constant change, responding to the myriad of messages it receives moment by moment. Your body is able to shift as your mind shifts. This body is your vehicle in this lifetime, and is meant to be used by you for a unique purpose, for your own life story. It has built-in mechanisms that protect it and heal it from illness, including cancer. You have millions of white blood cells, many of them targeted for healing cancer, active right now within your body. These cells are powerful allies. They help to protect your body from all diseases. As you imagine them, enliven them with an image that is fitting. It may be an archetypal religious figure or goddess, a historical person of power, an angel, an animal, or other image. Choose an image that has significance for you, that you can believe in, and that is vivid and powerful, as your white blood cells are. Feel and visualize that your white blood cells are fueled by the energy of this image. Internalize your image and let it feed the white blood cells. For example, you may imagine that the spirit of Joan of Arc is commanding your white blood cells into action, or that they are potent rocket ships set on a particular course and mission to destroy any loose cancer cells. You might use the image of a team of expert gardeners consciously and consistently weeding any unhealthy cells, or a pack of wolves ever on the alert for stray cancer cells. You might utilize the precision of an army of archers shooting arrows at cells that have become harmful to you, or you might lull your cancer cells to sleep and inactivity with beautiful music. Take a moment to let an image become clear in your mind. Be sure that it is an image that you are comfortable with, and that fits your belief system. (Pause)

9) See your white blood cells as your helpers. There are millions of them to protect you, many more of them than there are cancer cells. The white blood cells are large, vivid, and clear in your mind. Give them energy. Imagine these being formed in the bone marrow, traveling to the thymus gland in the sternum where they are become potent, intelligent, determined, energized, and assigned specific tasks. Let them flow purposefully from there to the rest of the body. They are able to identify and attack or inactivate any invaders in the body. They are controlled by a center in your brain. Feel their sense of direction and purpose in your mind, patrolling, engulfing, and eliminating any stray cancer cells. Send the white blood cells into the breast area, keeping it healthy. Feel their courage and collaboration as they swiftly identify toxins, viruses, bacteria, and cancer cells, then

execute a marvelous attack on whatever is harmful to you and your breasts. They are a fantastic clean up crew, protecting every millimeter of your breasts and body. They are determined to defend you to live your life to accomplish your soul's purpose. The more relaxed you are, the more powerful and capable they are of protecting you. (Long Pause)

10) Take some time to imagine whatever treatments you are using working effectively in your body. If you are taking anything to strengthen your immune system, see and feel it activating and energizing your white blood cells with a spark of life, making them brighter and more alive. Picture and hear your white blood cells responding enthusiastically to the boost that you are giving them. Listen to their sound. Visualize any anti-cancer drugs or therapies going directly to the cancer cells and shrinking them hourly, until you are free of disease. See the medication affecting only the unhealthy cells, protecting what is healthy. See and feel the treatment interacting in a positive way with the rest of the body. Experience the treatment assisting your return to health and helping you to maintain perfect health. See, feel, and hear the body's debris being eliminated like a great river flushing through you. The liver effectively breaks down toxins, while the colon, kidneys, and skin are able to eliminate them.

11) As you finish, feel that your body is more relaxed, your defences against disease are stronger, and you are more able to participate in your medical treatment. You are resistant to cancer, immune to it. Visualize yourself as billions of molecules being able to shift and move and connect to the web of life. Feel your connection to your surroundings, to an inner guiding force, to the living beings around you, and to your future. Stay with this feeling and know that you have skills and inner resources to cope with whatever comes your way. Imagine yourself in a state of perfect balance — mental, emotional, physical, and spiritual. Experience these working together. Congratulate yourself for having allowed time for healing and quiet reflection. As you begin to stretch, become more alert to your surroundings and at your own pace, go back to your daily living.

Botanical Surgery

At times, women may have a secondary tumor that is inoperable because of its location, or surgery is not recommended because the cancer has already spread to the liver or lungs. Some women refuse surgery for reasons of their own. In these cases, removal of cancerous tissue can be accomplished with the use of herbal salves, or botanical surgery.

Native Americans commonly used poultices of roasted red onion and bloodroot or goldenseal to destroy and remove tumors. Some of these practices were adopted by European medical doctors in the 18th century, and Ingrid Naiman has revived this tradition with the publication of her book, *Cancer Salves: A Botanical Approach to Treatment.*[4] Please read her book before using any of the following treatments, so that you know what to expect, or link to her web site at www.cancer-salves.com.

The advantages of using the salves are that there is commonly next to no bleeding, there is very little scarring, and there is less trauma to the patient. Tumors can be removed using this method within 5-21 days, although it may take many months for the process to be completed. The disadvantages are that it is messy, it hurts, the duration of use is unpredictable, it is time consuming as dressings are changed daily, and there is no guarantee what the outcome will be.

Having used the salves on several patients, I have the utmost respect for the power of the herbs and consider their ability to remove cancerous tumors one of the most miraculous things I have ever seen.

However, do not attempt to use the salves on your own. Find someone with experience to supervise you. Do not use more than 2000 mg of vitamin C or 400 IU of vitamin E while using the salves, as increased bleeding may result.

Cancer Salve Recipes

Here are recipes for 2 commonly used salves.

Black Salve Formula

Preparation: Put the zinc chloride in an uncovered glass bowl and add enough distilled water to liquefy. Grind the herbs, keeping the temperature below 100°F. Add the herbs to the zinc chloride and stir with a wooden utensil until it is the consistency of toothpaste. Heat the mixture at 100°F overnight in a yogurt maker or kefir maker. Place in a dark glass jar.

Application: Using a wooden utensil, apply a dime sized patch once daily to the affected area, covering with gauze, plastic and surgical tape to retain moisture. Use cautiously, as it can irritate the skin. This paste will cause pain to the breast during the first several days of application. Never use a metal spoon or utensil with the zinc chloride. Read Ingrid Naiman's book, *Cancer Salves*, before you begin.

Ingredients
25% Bloodroot
25% Galangal (chopped at low heat using a mortar and pestle or food processor)
25% Slippery elm powder
25% Zinc chloride
Distilled water

Goldenseal Salve

Preparation: Place the powdered herbs in a glass bowl. Add 1 drop of calendula CO2 concentrate and enough apricot kernel seed oil to make a thick paste and stir with a tongue depressor or wooden spoon until all ingredients are well blended. Heat the mixture at 100°F overnight in a yogurt maker or kefir maker. Place in a dark glass jar.

Ingredients
5 oz. goldenseal
4 oz. turmeric
3 oz. white willow bark
1 drop of calendula CO2 concentrate
apricot kernel seed oil

Materials Checklist for Dressings and Salve Application

You will need the following materials when applying cancer salves.

1) Kendall Tendersorb ABD pads to be used around the wound to address leakage.
2) Tegaderm transparent dressing to be applied over the salve area and surrounding skin (Less ideal alternative is an Op-Site dressing).
3) Wooden tongue depressors used to apply the paste. Never touch the tongue depressor to the skin and then insert it into the jar of paste. Use a new tongue depressor rather than contaminating the batch.
4) Mefix soft elastic, self adhesive fabric tape, used to tape around the dressing.
5) Latex gloves, always to be worn by the person doing the dressing.
6) Gauze sponges to absorb moisture.
7) 3% hydrogen peroxide and a spray bottle, used to clean the site before salve application.
8) Plastic kidney tray to collect the debris while spraying. Hold it against the chest while the patient sits.
9) Scissors.
10) Goldenseal and bloodroot pastes.

Application: This formula acts more slowly than the Black Salve formula above, but does not cause pain. Zinc chloride can be added to make it a more aggressive formula. If the pain is too intense from the black salve, this formula can be used intermittently with it. Read Ingrid Naiman's book, *Cancer Salves*, before you begin a salve treatment.

Chemotherapy Support

Many strategies can help you through the difficult days of chemo, such as exercise, visualization, yoga, meditation, healthy food, nutritional supplements, and careful use of antioxidants. Reiki, massage, and acupuncture help to relieve feelings of fatigue and other side effects of chemo. Set up a support network of friends or professional healers before the chemo begins who can be there for you when you need them, or join an existing breast cancer support group.

Exercise

If you are going through chemotherapy, a moderate exercise program, such as walking 30 minutes three times a week will help to alleviate fatigue, improve your cardiovascular fitness, relieve stress, and maintain a positive body image.[5,6,7] Think about what type of exercise program will suit you best during the coming months, and schedule it at least three times weekly.

Food

Chemotherapy treatment decreases appetite in many women, so have on hand some healthy foods you really love to tempt you. Foods that are simple to make, easy to digest, and nourishing are best, like your favorite soups and smoothies. Eat as soon as you are hungry to reduce nausea. Support your immune system with shitake mushrooms, onions, garlic, fresh vegetable juices, tomato dishes, and cooked orange vegetables. Avoid grapefruit throughout chemo, as it may alter the way your liver breaks down the drugs.

Nausea

Ginger tea or ginger capsules can help relieve nausea but should be used cautiously in patients who have low platelets because ginger can inhibit blood clotting. Chemotherapy also has an anti-clotting effect, and the two used together may thin the blood to levels that are too low in patients whose platelets are reduced (60,000 or less), possibly causing hemorrhaging.[8]

The acupuncture point P6, found three finger widths (about two inches) above the center of the wrist crease on the underside of the arm, relieves nausea when stimulated daily with a needle or magnet, or simple finger pressure. Several studies demonstrate the effectiveness of acupuncture at reducing nausea from chemotherapy.[9,10,11] Anti-nausea wristbands are available that stimulate this point with a magnet.

FACT

Nausea from chemotherapy can be counteracted with ginger, the Chinese medicinal mushroom called hoelen (fu ling), and the underground stem of pinellia. Collectively, these three herbs will reduce nausea, vomiting, and diarrhea. Catnip, peppermint, chamomile, and red raspberry can be used as alternatives to relieve nausea.

FACT

A good quality acidophilus supplement taken once or twice daily is helpful in maintaining healthy gut flora and preventing diarrhea and yeast infections caused by antibiotics or lowered immunity. Fish oil at 2000 mg daily also helps to lessen diarrhea and control inflammation.

Protecting the Lining of the Mouth and Gastro-Intestinal Tract

L-Glutamine is an amino acid found in protein that will help to prevent mouth sores and digestive upset caused by 5FU or methotrexate.[12] It should be taken for 3 days before and during chemo treatments. As the chemotherapy works on disrupting cell division in cancer cells, it also damages the cells lining the digestive tract, because they have a faster turnover rate than most other body cells. When 4 grams of L-glutamine are used twice daily in a mouthwash that is swished and swallowed, both mouth sores and diarrhea are significantly reduced.[13,14] Vitamin E oil applied directly twice daily to mouth sores will shorten their duration.[15]

Low White Blood Cell Count

Chemotherapy and radiation can cause leukopenia, or suppression of your white blood cells, leading to lowered immunity and risk of infection. Many natural substances can be used to either prevent this from occurring or to increase the white blood cell count.

Chinese herbs that sustain the white blood cells and are safe to take during chemo are astragalus, codonopsis, ligustrum, millettia, salvia miltorrhizae, white atractylodes, lycii fruit, salix root, and royal jelly.[17] Schizandra also improves immunity but it has a strong effect on Phase 1 detoxification in the liver and may decrease the effectiveness of chemo. To be safe, use it in only very small quantities or not at all. The following three formulas have many of these herbs present in them and are recommended specifically during chemo: Astragalus and Ligustrum Formula, manufactured by Golden Flower Chinese Herbs; Millettia 9, from Seven Forests; and Astragalus 10+, also from Seven Forests. See the 'Resources Directory' for sources of these herbs.

Should your white blood cell count drop so low that you are at risk of infection, pau d'arco and echinacea can be added to increase resistance and may be a better choice than antibiotics.

Mushrooms that have a restorative effect on your immune system include ganoderma (reishi mushroom), maitake, shitake, and coriolus. Maitake D-Fraction and MGN-3 can also be considered. I generally recommend both a blend of immune enhancing Chinese herbs as well as a combination of medicinal mushrooms to women going through chemotherapy.

If your white blood cell count is chronically low, consider acupuncture treatments to elevate it.

What to Take for Anemia and Low Platelets During Chemotherapy Treatments

Chemotherapeutic agents can injure the bone marrow's capability to produce white blood cells, red blood cells and platelets. Low platelets will increase your risk of excess bleeding, as they are necessary for blood clotting.

To counter anemia, or a low red blood cell count, the herb yellow dock can be used in tincture form, at a dosage of 5-20 drops daily.

FACT
Several studies have shown that acupuncture is effective in increasing low white blood cell counts in patients undergoing chemotherapy.[16]

PREVENTION
To elevate white blood cell count, use the protective minerals, zinc and selenium. Helpful vitamins are A, B6, B12, C, and E. Weekly intramuscular injections of 1000 mcg B12 throughout chemo has been found by some naturopaths to elevate white blood cell count and help with fatigue.[16]

FACT
Goldenseal, a North American herb, will both elevate white blood cell count and decrease the risk of infection because of its antibiotic effect. It should be used for only 3 weeks at a time, followed by a one-week break.

FACT
In one study of 48 patients with chronic leukopenia, acupuncture resulted in an increased white blood cell count in over 90% of the patients.[18] A second study of 121 patients undergoing chemotherapy demonstrated a significant increase in white blood cell counts after 5 days of daily acupuncture.[19]

FACT
Platelets can be increased with concurrent use of the pineal hormone, melatonin, during chemotherapy.

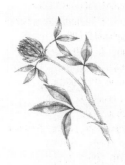

The herbal iron tonic, Floravit, may also be used. Because iron is used by cancer cells to divide, supplementation with iron tonics should only be used when there is a demonstrated deficiency, or it may promote tumor growth.

The classic Chinese medicine, Shih Chuan Da Bu Wan, tonifies blood and energy and improve anemia. One of the herbs contained in it is Angelica, which strengthens the spleen and increases the red blood cell count. A Chinese herb used for restoring both the red and the white blood cell count is millettia, present in Millettia 9, from Seven Forests. Dietary blood builders include pumpkin seeds, oatmeal, dried apricots, beets, nettle, kale, and seaweeds.

Melatonin is likely to improve the overall outcome of chemotherapy. In one study, 250 patients with metastatic solid tumors were randomized into chemotherapy with and without melatonin. The one-year survival rate was significantly higher for patients treated with chemotherapy plus melatonin — 38% as opposed to 23% for those treated with chemotherapy alone.[20]

How to Combat Fatigue During Chemotherapy and Radiation

Fatigue is a common symptom in women undergoing chemotherapy or radiation. To combat fatigue, consider using nettle tea, an ounce a day of fresh wheat grass juice, Siberian ginseng (30 drops, 3 x daily), astragalus in tea or tincture form, or the formula Astragalus 10+(Seven Forests) or Astragalus and Ligustrum Formula (Golden Flower Chinese Herbs).

Peripheral Neuropathy

Cumulative treatments with the chemotherapy drugs Taxol and Taxotere can cause a reversible pins and needles sensation in the hands and feet, known as peripheral neuropathy. Natural therapies to prevent or reverse this include weekly intramuscular injections of vitamin B12, regular acupuncture treatments, or the use of the nerve-regenerating herbs, Gastrodia root and Eucommia bark.[22]

Cognitive Function

Chemotherapy affects the cognitive function of some women, with decreases in the speed of taking in information, visual memory, motor function, mental flexibility, and difficulty in concentration.[23] Antioxidants taken during chemo, along with fish oil capsules, will help to decrease these effects. The homeopathic tissue salt Kali phos 6X and the homeopathic formula Acidum phosphoricum plex (Unda) are remedies I have used successfully with patients to improve cognitive function.

Protecting Your Heart

Doxorubicin (also known as Adriamycin) is toxic to the heart; patients treated with it may experience heart failure in later years. Coenzyme Q10 has been shown to reduce the degree of chronic heart damage caused by doxorubicin without interfering with its efficacy.[24,25,26,27] Vitamin E protects from the acute but not the chronic heart toxicity of doxorubicin. If this drug is part of your chemotherapy regimen, protect your heart by using 400 mg coenzyme Q10 and 800 IU natural source vitamin E throughout your chemo.

Other Supporting Supplements

Other supplements that one can safely take during chemotherapy are vitamin B6, inositol, IP6, kelp, chromium, modified citrus pectin, and fish oil capsules.

Fish oils contain long-chain omega 3 fatty acids, which have been shown to inhibit the growth of human breast cancer cells.[28] Fish oils may help to deliver chemotherapy drugs across tumor cell membranes. In one study, mice were given doxorubicin for their cancer in addition to either 3% fish oil concentrates or 5% corn oil. Tumor-growth rates were significantly decreased in the fish oil group compared to corn oil, and the fish oil did not increase the toxicity of doxorubicin to the host mouse.[29] This was confirmed in a double-blind, randomized study of dogs on doxorubicin.[30] In another mouse experiment with cyclophosphamide, fish oil increased cyclophosphamide's therapeutic effect and decreased its toxicity.[31] When buying fish oil, check for purity. Brands that are reliably free of PCBs and dioxins include Eskimo 3, Thorne, Carlson's, Nordic Naturals and Nutrasea herring oil.

Using Antioxidants During Chemotherapy and Radiation

The rationale in favor of using antioxidants throughout chemotherapy and radiation is to protect healthy cells and the individual from the damaging effects of the treatments without decreasing their efficacy, and to reduce long-term side effects that may include injury to the heart and lungs, a decrease in cognitive function, chronic bone marrow suppression, and leukemia later in life.

Chemotherapy regimens for breast cancer typically consist of drug combinations using cyclophosphamide, methotrexate, 5FU, epirubicin, doxorubicin (adriamycin), taxol, and or taxotere.

Two naturopathic doctors, Davis W. Lamson, ND, and Matthew S. Brignall, ND, have carefully summarized the existing literature on antioxidant use in chemotherapy and radiation, and some of their findings are shown in the chart below. After reviewing 93 studies, there were only three instances where they found a particular antioxidant decreased the effectiveness of chemo or radiation in animals or humans. These three instances were: 1) N-acetyl cysteine reduced the effectiveness of doxorubicin in animal studies[32]; 2) beta carotene decreased the therapeutic effect of 5-fluorouracil (5FU) in fibrosarcoma[33]; and 3) tangeretin, a flavonoid found in tangerines, decreased the effectiveness of Tamoxifen.[34] The other 90 studies showed either no effect or decreased toxicity and/or increased therapeutic effect of combining antioxidants with chemo and/or radiation.[35]

FACT

Differing opinions exist in the naturopathic community as well as among oncologists about which supplements, particularly antioxidants, should be taken (or not taken) during chemotherapy and radiation treatments.

Recommended Safe for Chemotherapy

Vitamin C : 4000-8000 mg.
Vitamin E (natural source mixed tocopherols): 800 IU.
Vitamin A : 20,000 IU.
Vitamin B6 : 50 mg.
Vitamin B12 : 1000 mcg
Zinc picolinate : 50 mg.
Selenium : 200 mcg.
Chromium picolinate : 200 mcg.
Kelp tablets : 1000 mg.
CoQ10 : 300-400 mg.
Fish oil (combination of EPA and DHA): 2000-3000 mg.
Melatonin : 9-20 mg before bed.
Kali phos 6X : 3 pellets 3 x daily.
Herbal Blend: astragalus, codonopsis, ligustrum, millettia, salvia, white atractylodes, royal jelly, lycium.
Mushroom Blend: shitake, reishi, maitake, coriolus.

Do Not Use During Chemotherapy

Beta carotene
Curcumin
Grapefruit
St. John's Wort
Ellagic acid
Indole-3-carbinol
DIM

Cautionary Use

Milk Thistle, Quercetin, NAC, and Rosemary: do not use these 5 days before chemo or 1 week after chemo, but do use between these times.

Antioxidants in Cancer Therapy

Antioxidant	Radiation	Chemotherapy
Vitamin A	• increases survival time and decreases tumor size when administered with radiation in mice • improves response rate to radiation in humans	• does not interfere with methotrexate, cisplatin, etoposide, doxorubicin • protects the small intestine from damage due to methotrexate • use dosages between 15,000 – 50,000 IU/daily
Carotenoids	• improves its effectiveness	• in mice with breast carcinoma, beta-carotene enhanced the antitumor effect of cyclophosphamide[45] • in mice, beta-carotene (5-50 mg/kg) has been shown to reduce the genotoxicity of cyclophosphamide[46]. • beta carotene may interfere with the action of 5-fluorouracil.
Vitamin C	• increases the effectiveness of radiotherapy in humans and in mice	• in vitro studies with several tumor cell lines have shown vitamin C to enhance the cytotoxic activity of doxorubicin, paclitaxel, and 5-FU[47,48,49] • animal studies have shown that vitamin C at 500 mg/kg 43 and 1,000 mg/kg44 enhanced the chemotherapeutic effect of cyclophosphamide, 5-FU, and doxorubicin[50,51] • other studies found that vitamin C was without effect on the activity of doxorubicin when vitamin C was administered at 2 g/kg/day to mice or 835 mg/kg/day to guinea pigs[52] • simultaneous adminstration of vitamin K can increase the activity of vitamin C
Vitamin E	• increases the effectiveness of radiotherapy in mice when doses below 500 mg/kg are used (approximately 35,000 IU human dose) • more research needed	• vitamin E, in vitro, has been shown to enhance the cytotoxic effect of several anticancer drugs, including 5-fluorouracil (5-FU), doxorubicin/adriamycin, vincristine, dacarbazine, cisplatin, and tamoxifen[53,54,55,56] • in animal studies Vit E enhanced the anticancer effect of fluorouracil, although it had no apparent effect on the tumoricidal properties of doxorubicin[57,58] • in a human trial, 21 patients with metastatic breast cancer who were treated with 5-fluorouracil, doxorubicin, and cyclophosphamide were given vitamin E (2,000 IU/day), beginning seven days before and continuing throughout chemotherapy. Vit E did not prevent myelosuppression or alopecia, did not alter the incidence of nausea, vomiting, and stomatitis, and did not prevent chronic doxorubicin-induced

Antioxidant	Radiation	Chemotherapy
Vitamin E (cont'd)		cardiotoxicity. Vit E did not compromise the antitumor activity of the chemotherapy, based on the fact that it did not interfere with the cytotoxic effects of the drugs on bone marrow and hair follicles[59] • 20 patients (no controls) were treated with doxorubicin in combination with vincristine alone, 5-FU plus cyclophosphamide, cyclophosphamide alone, 5-FU alone, or cisplatin plus cyclophosphamide plus vitamin E (1,600IU/day po). The Vit E did not prevent alopecia from developing[60] • in addition to its activity as an antioxidant, vitamin E may enhance anticancer activity by inducing apoptosis through inhibition of protein tyrosine kinases (PTKs)[61]
Selenium	• low selenium may reduce the lethal dose of radiation. Selenium may therefore decrease the effectiveness of radiotherapy • until more research is available limit selenium intake to less than 400 mcg daily during radiotherapy	• reduces acute toxicity of doxorubicin on the heart[62] but does not protect from chronic toxicity. • decreases the toxic effect of cisplatin on the kidneys while improving its anti-tumor activity • increases white blood cell count when taken during chemo • may interfere with the effectiveness of the anti-tumor drug, bleomycin • no other evidence in humans suggests that selenium reduces the effectiveness of chemo
Coenzyme Q10	• may interfere with the effectiveness of radiotherapy if doses above 700 mg/day are used. • safe to use in doses of 100-400 mg/day	• in vitro, CoQ10 has been shown not to interfere with doxorubicin[63] • in mice, CoQ10 has been shown not to interfere with the antitumor activity of doxorubicin, and in rabbits CoQ10 did not change doxorubicin-induced bone marrow suppression[64,65] • animal studies showed that intravenous administration of 1, 10, or 15 mg/kg/day of CoQ10 prevented acute doxorubicin-induced cardiotoxicity[66] • in mice and rabbits, oral and i.v. administration of CoQ10 protected animals from chronic irreversible cardiomyopathy[67] • in a third human trial, there was a reduction in the degree of chronic doxorubicin-induced cardiotoxicity with CoQ10 administration[68] • reduces diarrhea and stomach irritation when used with doxorubicin

Antioxidant	Radiation	Chemotherapy
Flavonoids: Quercetin, Green Tea, Genistein	• flavonoids increase the sensitivity of cancer cells to radiation in vitro	• green tea, quercetin and genistein increase the concentration of doxorubicin in some resistant cell lines • quercetin inhibits topoisomerase II activity and is particuluarely good at inhibiting breast cancer cell growth in vitro. • in multidrug-resistant breast cancer cells, quercetin markedly enhanced the growth-inhibitory effects of doxorubicin, although it did not affect the cytotoxicity of doxorubicin in drug-sensitive cells [69,70] • soybeans reduce the damage of methotrexate to the intestine[71] • tamoxifen activity is decreased by tangeretin (from tangerines) in vivo and by genistein in vitro
N-acetylcysteine	• does not block the effectiveness of radiation	• animal and human studies show it partially protects against the cystitis caused by cyclophosphamide without reducing the drug's effectiveness[72] • one out of two animal studies showed NAC to reduce the effectiveness of doxorubicin, but this was not confirmed in human trials; therefore, caution is required before using NAC with doxorubicin
Glutathione	• is not thought to interfere with radiotherapy	• decreases toxicity and increases the anti-tumor effect of cisplatin[73] • caution is advised before using glutathione with alkylating agents such as cyclophosphamide. More research needed[74]
Melatonin	• increases the effectiveness of radiation and increases survival time when used with it • fewer side effects from radiotherapy when melatonin is used with it	• 20 mg/day of melatonin normalized platelet counts in breast cancer patients undergoing chemotherapy • increases survival time when used with tamoxifen, cisplatin, and etoposide • decreases weight loss during chemo • no evidence in humans suggests that it reduces the effectiveness of chemo

This chart merges the research of Lamson and Birdsall, published as "Antioxidants in Cancer Therapy; Their Actions and Interactions with Oncologic Therapies," *Alternative Medicine Review*, 1999;4(5):304-329, with additional research from the noted authors.

Discuss antioxidant use with your oncologist, naturopathic doctor, and other health care providers. Research the issue as much as possible so that you believe in the decision you make. I recommend that my patients use specific antioxidants throughout chemo and radiation, and that they avoid others. If you are caught between two different points of view, another alternative is to use antioxidants up until about five days before chemo starts, and then resume them again seven days after a chemo treatment. In this way the supplements will be unlikely to interfere with the action of the drugs but will still offer some protection.

Radiation Support

Radiation treatments may cause fatigue and inflammation and redness to the skin. Radiation can exacerbate lymphedema, injure the heart and lungs, leaving them vulnerable to future illness, decrease white blood cell count and immune health, and precipitate depression. Radiation treatments have a cumulative effect in damaging DNA, which may increase our life-long cancer risk. We can significantly decrease the possibility of these side effects with natural therapies.

FACT
While in theory antioxidants may protect cells, including cancer cells, from the toxic free radicals generated by chemotherapy and radiation, in practice most combinations of antioxidants have been shown to act synergistically to reduce tumors in humans, and when combined with chemotherapy and radiation, they increase survival time and reduce toxicity. The patient who takes antioxidants will usually have fewer short and long-term side effects from chemotherapy and radiation.

Recommended Supplements Checklist for Radiation Treatments

Continue as much of this regimen as you can manage for at least one month after radiation therapy has finished:

- ❑ Turmeric, 2 or more tsp daily or curcumin, 1000 mg 3x daily to substantially decrease the damaging effects of radiation.[40]
- ❑ Quercetin, 500 mg, 3 x daily, to improve the effectiveness of radiation.
- ❑ Sea vegetables, $\frac{1}{2}$ cup daily or 9 kelp tablets for their iodine and sodium alginate content.
- ❑ Yams, squash, carrots, Swiss chard or spinach daily for beta carotene, or a supplement containing Dunaliella algae, equalling 60 mg beta carotene daily.
- ❑ Cooked tomato sauce, $\frac{1}{2}$ cup daily during exposure for its lycopene content.[41]
- ❑ Foods or supplements high in calcium and potassium which aid in the excretion of radioactive particles.[42]
- ❑ Antioxidant supplements containing vitamin C (8000 mg calcium ascorbate), E (200 IU), A (20,000 IU), Coenzyme Q10 (100 mg), zinc (50 mg), and grape seed extract (100 mg) to quench free radicals.
- ❑ Melatonin, 9-20 mg before bed.
- ❑ Flax oil (unheated), 2 tbsp daily, to protect cell membranes or 3 uncontaminated fish oil capsules daily.
- ❑ Vitamin B3 or niacin (300 mg), B12, and B complex to help to repair DNA damage.[43]
- ❑ Green tea daily to remove radioactive isotopes and protect from cancer.
- ❑ Reishi, maitake, coriolus and shitake mushroom blend to sustain immune health.
- ❑ Astragalus, codonopsis, ligustrum, millettia, salvia, white atractylodes, royal jelly, Siberian ginseng, lycium herbal blend for strong immunity and to combat fatigue.
- ❑ A high fiber diet, 40 grams daily, to deter absorption of radiation and improve its excretion.
- ❑ Foods from the brassica family daily, kale, cabbage, broccoli, cauliflower etc.
- ❑ Miso soup a few times a week.
- ❑ Dried beans, lentils or tofu daily in the diet.
- ❑ Avoid manganese, copper and iron during radiation as they interact with vitamin C to form free radicals.
- ❑ Consult a homeopath. — Some of the remedies used for radiation exposure include Calc- fl., Rad-brom., Rad-iod., X-rays, Fl-ac., Cad-iod., Cad-sulph., Bell., Phos-ac., Rhus-ven., Cobaltum.[44]

Phytochemotherapy for Life

Cell division, known as mitosis, occurs in several carefully engineered sequential steps or phases. In cancer cells the normal mechanisms for DNA repair and programmed cell death are disturbed, so that cancer cells record mistakes in their DNA. We can use specific plant chemicals to intercept phases of the cell cycle, helping to stall cell division in cancer cells. You can think of this as 'phytochemotherapy', and use it to discourage breast cancer cell division for the rest of your life. A combination of phytochemicals used for various phases of the cell cycle will help to put breast cancer cells to sleep.

The phases of the cell cycle and the plant chemicals that modify them are shown below. For maximum benefit, a combination of all of the phytochemical bearing substances listed can be taken throughout the day. See Chapters 6 and 8 for dosages of phytochemicals.

1) 'G0' Phase: Most cells are resting in this phase until they receive a signal to divide.

2) 'G1' Phase: This is the most variable phase of cell division that determines the length of the cell cycle. This phase can be almost instantaneous or last up to 9 hours. Aggressive cancers tend to have a short G1 phase. In G1, cells prepare themselves for entry into the more active S phase, and wait for cues from inside or outside the cell to signal them to proceed. Phytochemicals that help to keep cells in G1 include allicin (garlic),[80] docosohexanoic acid (fish oil),[81] ellagic acid (red raspberry),[82] IP6 and inositol (beans and bran),[83] indole-3-carbinol (brassicas),[84] quercetin (onions), perillyl alcohol (essential oils of palmarosa, lavender; cherries),[85] D-limonene (essential oils of lemon, sweet orange, celery, lemongrass),[86] epigallocatechin (green tea).[87]

3) 'G1' Checkpoint: Before entering the S phase, cells are inspected by regulating genes that either signal their repair or destruction. The p53 gene should act here to destroy abnormal cells, but this gene is often damaged in cancer cells, allowing abnormal cells to make it through to the next phase. Substances that assist the normal function of p53 or help to repair damaged genes are niacin,[88] IP6, reishi mushroom,[89] and melatonin.[90,91]

4) 'S' Phase: During the S phase, cells reproduce their entire genetic material to make 2 sets of paired chromosomes. This phase lasts 6 hours. Phytochemicals that help to keep cells in the S phase include genistein (soy), quercetin, curcumin (turmeric),[92] perillyl alcohol and limonene.

5) 'G2' Phase: In this phase, lasting approximately 4 hours, the chromosomes arrange themselves in preparation for the final stage of cell division. We can help to arrest the cells in G2 with lycopene (tomatoes),[93] beta-sitosterol (black caraway and black cumin seeds, sage leaf),[94] docosohexanoic acid, perillyl alcohol,[95] curcumin (turmeric),[96] quercetin,[97] genistein,[98] and berberine (goldenseal, bloodroot, barberry, Coptis chinensis [Huang lian]).[99] At the end of G2, cells go through another inspection before proceeding.

6) 'M' Phase: This is when cell division is complete and 2 cells result from the original parent cell. We can help to halt this phase in breast cancer cells with allicin and curcumin.[100,101,102]

Niacin in particular is useful prior to and during radiation treatments. It is required to make the enzyme ADP ribose polymerase, used in DNA replication and repair.[36] When niacin is administered before radiation treatments, it increases its effectiveness, and will result in less damage to healthy cells.[37]

Brown seaweeds such as Kelp (Laminaria sp.), Sargassum, and Bladderwrack (Fucus vesiculosus) contain sodium alginate, which reduces the uptake of radioactive particles in bone by 80% when added to the diet.[38,39] During radiation therapy, make seaweeds a big part of your diet, consuming at least a ½ cup daily. Use nori with your rice, make an arame or hiziki and vegetable salad, add wakame to a miso soup, and mix them in with bean dishes.

Phytochemotherapy and the Breast Cancer Cell Cycle

TO ARREST CELLS IN 'M':
curcumin (turmeric)
allicin

TO STALL CELLS IN 'G2':
lycopene (tomatoes)
beta-sitosterol
docosohexanoic acid
perillyl alcohol
curcumin (turmeric)
quercetin
genistein
berberine (goldenseal, blood
root, barberry, Coptis
chinensis)

TO STALL CELLS IN 'G1':
allicin (garlic)
docosohexanoic acid (fish oil)
ellagic acid (red raspberry)
IP6 and inositol (beans, bran)
indole-3-carbinol, DIM
quercetin (onions, etc.)
perillyl alcohol (palmarosa,
lavender oils)
limonene (lemon essential oil)
epigallocatechin (green tea)

P53 CHECKPOINT:
IP6
reishi mushroom (ganoderma)
melatonin

TO STALL CELLS IN 'S':
genistein (soy)
quercetin
curcumin (turmeric)
perillyl alcohol
limonene

(cell cycle labels: M, G1, S, G2, DIVISION, 4 hrs, 9 hrs, 6 hrs)

Topical Treatments

Pure aloe vera gel and a topical cream called Unda 270 applied twice daily to the skin during radiation treatment can minimize damage to the tissue and decrease burning. Essential oils can be used during radiation to protect from radiation burns. Niaouli oil and tea tree oil can be applied prior to treatment to accomplish this, while lavender with St. John's wort oil can be used after radiation treatments are completed to stimulate rapid healing.

Managing Side Effects

What to Use with Tamoxifen

To decrease the side effects of Tamoxifen, we want to decrease blood viscosity; protect the liver; improve thyroid nutrition; increase antioxidant intake to protect from cancer; and manage hot flashes.

1) To decrease blood viscosity: curcumin 1500 mg , quercetin 1000 mg, bromelain 600 mg, proteolytic enzymes between meals, vitamin E 800 IU, fish oil 3000 mg.
2) To protect the liver: milk thistle 300 mg standardized extract, rosemary.
3) To provide iodine for the thyroid: kelp tablets, 3 daily.
4) To increase anti-oxidant intake: vitamins C, E, beta carotene, zinc, selenium, alpha lipoic acid.
5) To manage hot flashes: black cohosh and the Chinese herbal formula Chih Pai Pa Wei Wan 8 pellets, 3 x daily, and freshly ground flaxseed, 2-4 tbsp daily.

Both melatonin and indole-3-carbinol have been found in laboratory studies to assist Tamoxifen in reducing breast cancer recurrence without interfering with its effectiveness.[75,76]

Hot Flashes

I commonly recommend for hot flashes vitamin E mixed tocopherols 800 IU, black cohosh 500 mg, Chih Pai Pa Wei Wan 8 pellets 3x daily or an equivalent formula, freshly ground flaxseeds 2-4 tbsp, daily practice of relaxation or meditation, and a high potency vitamin B complex. Acupuncture and/or specific homeopathic remedies can also reduce hot flashes.

Vaginal Dryness

Vaginal dryness can be eased by lubricating with cold pressed almond oil with added vitamin E, using black cohosh 500 mg daily, and considering the use of estriol cream applied topically to the vagina at a dose of 0.5 mg twice weekly.[77]

Loss of Libido

Herbal treatments for loss of libido include a combination of saw palmetto and damiana, 30 drops of tincture 2 or 3 times daily of each. Acupuncture treatments and individualized homeopathic remedies may also be helpful.

Preventing Osteoporosis

Both chemotherapy, aromatase inhibitors, and removal of the ovaries make a woman with a breast cancer history more susceptible to osteoporosis. Maintaining an alkaline diet with many foods high in potassium will help to keep calcium in your bones, rather than causing it to be leached out to balance an overly acid condition. Other nutrients that improve calcium absorption are vitamin D, boron, manganese, and zinc.

Stimulating the stomach by using lemon in water before meals or 1 tbsp daily of apple cider vinegar will help produce adequate hydrochloric acid to absorb calcium. Ipriflavone is a synthetic isoflavone that has been shown to improve bone density in post-menopausal women, and in animal studies, inhibited growth of bone metastases related to breast cancer.[78,79]

Treating Other Breast Ailments

In addition to these adjunct treatments for cancer, other natural medicine therapies are recommended for specific breast ailments.

Premenstrual Breast Pain and Swelling

Experiment with B6 and magnesium for a few months to see if there is improvement in your breast swelling. Include more sea vegetables containing iodine in your diet. Decrease your consumption of fats to less than 15% of your total caloric intake, with the exception of flaxseed oil and extra virgin olive oil. Increase aerobic exercise to four hours weekly and develop a regular relaxation or meditation practice.

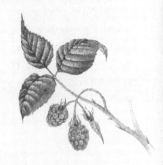

Other therapies that are effective are the Chinese patent formula Xiao Yao Wan, which circulates the liver energy;[103] the Hoxsey Formula, a lymphatic cleanser; a balanced ratio of Omega 3 and Omega 6 essential fatty acids; and vitamin E. In many women, the homeopathic remedy Folliculinum 9CH, taken on days seven and 21, relieves breast swelling by stimulating progesterone production.[104] Increasing progesterone through the use of herbs like chaste tree berry or by using a natural progesterone cream is also effective.

Supplements and Dosages
    Vitamin B6: 50 mg 3 x daily with meals as well as a B complex.
    Magnesium: 150 mg 2 x daily with calcium, with meals.
    Xiao Yao Wan: 8 small pills 3 x daily between meals to assist liver function.
    Hoxsey Formula: 15-30 drops 3 x daily between meals starting 7 days after your period begins and stopping at the onset of your period. It can be toxic in high dosages and should not be used in pregnancy.
    Evening Primrose Oil: 2 g daily, combined with twice as much flaxseed oil; or balanced oil with 2:1 Omega 3: Omega 6 fatty acids.
    Vitamin E: 600 IU daily.
    Folliculinum: 9 CH—one dose on the seventh day and another on day 21 of the menstrual cycle; an extra one on day 14 if necessary.

Fibrocystic Breast Disease

Correct homeopathic treatment may help fibrocystic breast disease, as will Chinese herbal formulas. I usually start a patient on two or three of these therapies and add or subtract as symptoms call for it.

Supplements and Daily Dosages

   Vitamin E, mixed tocopherols: 600 IU.

   Beta Carotene: 25,000-40,000 IU.

   Kelp tablets and/or Iodine (in one of the following forms):

   a) aqueous molecular iodine: 0.07 to 0.09 mg per kg of body weight for 6 months.

   b) Lugol's Solution (sodium iodide): 5 to 10 drops.

   Evening Primrose Oil: 1500 mg plus 3000 mg flaxseed oil.

   Vitamin B6: 50 mg 3 x daily plus a B complex.

   Coenzyme Q10: 60-200 mg.

   Progesterone Cream (if indicated by low amounts in saliva): 2 oz per month or 15-20 mg.

   Xiao Yao Wan: 8 pills 3x daily; and/or

   Milk Thistle or Dandelion Tincture: 25 drops, 3 x daily for liver support.

   Turmeric, Soy and Rosemary: dietary use.

   Hoxsey Formula: 15-30 drops, 3 x daily starting 7 days after your period begins and continuing until the next period. (The Healthy Breast Formula may be used as a substitute).

   Folliculinum 9 CH: on day 7 and day 21 of the menstrual cycle; an extra one on day 14 if necessary.

Mastitis

Supplements and Dosages

   Vitamin C: 500 mg every 2 hours.

   Homeopathic Phytolacca 30K: 3 pellets hourly.

   Hoxsey Formula: 15 drops every 2 hours.

   Goldenseal/Echinacea Herbal Tincture: 15 drops every 2 hours.

Homeopathic Symptom Pictures and Remedies for Breast Care

Homeopathy is an art and a science that relies on the principle of 'like cures like'. A given substance, which in the crude form may cause a particular set of symptoms, can stimulate the body to heal when it is used in the diluted or 'potentized' form. Individual remedies are prescribed based on the totality of a person's symptoms, known as the 'symptom picture', which includes details about a particular illness, food preferences, emotional well-being, body temperature, and times of aggravation, among others.

What follows is a brief list of some homeopathic symptom pictures and remedies that have an affinity with the breasts. These can be prescribed for breast ailments and as an adjunct to standard breast cancer treatment.

A full homeopathic case-taking should occur before choosing a particular homeopathic remedy. Since it takes years of training and experience to be a good homeopath and to prescribe correctly, search for a qualified homeopathic or naturopathic medical professional to advise you.

Homeopathic Remedies Indicated for Breast Cancer

- Apis (Honeybee)
- Arsenicum album (Arsenic Trioxide)
- Asterias rubens (Red Starfish)
- Baryta iodata (Iodide of Baryta)
- Belladonna (Deadly Nightshade)
- Bromium (Bromine)
- Bufo (Toad Poison)
- Calcarea carbonica (Carbonate of Lime)
- Calcarea oxalata (Oxalate of Lime)
- Carbo animalis (Animal Charcoal)
- Chimaphila umbellata (Pipsissewa)
- Cistus canadensis (Rock Rose)
- Clematis (Virgin's Bower)
- Condurango (Condor Plant)
- Conium (Poison Hemlock)
- Graphites (Black Lead)
- Hepar sulphuris calcareum (Calcium Sulphide)
- Hydrastis canadensis (Goldenseal)
- Lachesis (Bushmaster Snake Poison)
- Lapis albus (Silico-fluoride of Calcium)
- Lycopodium (Club Moss)
- Mercurius (Quicksilver)
- Natrum muriaticum (Table Salt)
- Nitric Acid
- Phosphorus
- Phytolacca (Poke Root)
- Pulsatilla (Windflower)
- Scirrhinum
- Sepia (Cuttlefish Ink)
- Silicea (Silica)
- Tarentula cubana (Cuban Spider)

LEFT-SIDED AND RIGHT-SIDED REMEDIES

Many of these remedies are associated with the left or the right side:

LEFT-SIDED REMEDIES
Asterias rubens, Bromium, Calcarea oxalata, Carbo animalis, Clematis, Lachesis, Hydrastis canadensis

RIGHT-SIDED REMEDIES
Apis, Arsenicum album, Lycopodium, Phytolacca

Other remedies can be left- or right-sided, including Baryta iodata, Belladonna, Bufo, Calcarea carbonica, Chimaphila umbellata, Cistus canadensis, Conium, Graphites, Hepar sulph., Lapis albus, Mercurius, Natrum muriaticum, Nitric acid, Phosphorus, Phytolacca, Pulsatilla, Sepia, Silicea.

Summary

Breast diseases often occur on a continuum. If we treat fibrocystic and other breast conditions with natural therapies early on, we can improve breast health, possibly preventing breast cancer. If we use natural therapies along with conventional treatments of surgery, chemotherapy, and radiation, treatment outcomes are improved and healing occurs more quickly with fewer side effects. Certain plant nutrients, like ellagic acid, genistein, allicin, curcumin, and quercetin, help to stall cell division in cancer cells and can offer us some protection throughout our lives from breast cancer or its recurrence. Many of these are available in our foods, so we can plan our meals with healing nutrients in mind. With the knowledge gleaned from this chapter, you are better equipped to cope with breast cancer treatments and to plan a lifelong strategy that focuses on maintaining breast and whole body health.

CHAPTER ELEVEN

Working with
Healthcare
Professionals

CONTENTS

EXERCISES, CHARTS, CHECK LISTS & WORKSHEETS

*T*he success of any breast health program depends on an equal and active partnership between a woman and her healthcare practitioner. Natural therapies are not a quick fix — there will never be one 'cure' for breast cancer — but there are a great many healing practices and supplements that can work together to sustain health so that breast cancer will be unlikely to occur or may be coaxed to retreat. It is, after all, a systemic disease. Improving the function of the body systems — the lymphatic system, the immune system, the digestive system, the circulatory system, and detoxification systems — will decrease your susceptibility to breast cancer. If you are working with a healthcare practitioner such as a naturopath, you need to find someone you will feel comfortable working with over several years. It will take time to evaluate the areas of your physical and emotional health that need to be addressed, and it will take even more time for you to adapt to and sustain those changes. A skilled healthcare practitioner can guide and support you through the steps you need to take to recover your health.

Responsibilities of Patients

As breast care patients, you have a responsibility to yourself for your own well-being. The following resolutions may help you to stay on track.

1) Maintain regular visits with your health care practitioner (every 1-3 months).
2) Practice breast self-exam and breast mapping once monthly and notify your naturopathic doctor and your medical doctor of your findings.
3) Have your doctor perform a clinical breast exam with you every 6 months and follow-up with any recommended testing procedures as your finances allow.
4) Comply with your health care practitioner's recommendations and explain any side effects or financial difficulties that require you to alter your regimen.
5) Be an active participant in understanding the disease process and in taking the necessary steps to reverse it.
6) Complete and revise periodically the various worksheet exercises presented in this book and provide them to your health care professional.

Exercise and Worksheet Checklist

- ❑ Breast Health Balance Sheet (p. 29)
- ❑ Breast Map Worksheet (p. 44)
- ❑ BBT (Basal Body Temperature) Chart (p. 82)
- ❑ pH Balance Chart (p. 152)
- ❑ Weekly Diet Diary (p. 238)
- ❑ 14-Day Diet Routine Worksheet (p. 239)
- ❑ Daily Therapeutic Amounts of Vitamins and Minerals Chart (p. 261)
- ❑ Daily Supplement Schedule Worksheet (p. 264)
- ❑ Exploring Your Beliefs Exercise (p. 270)
- ❑ Letting Go Exercise (p. 271)
- ❑ Communication Style Worksheet (p. 274)
- ❑ Assertive Behavior Worksheet (p. 276)
- ❑ Meaning Mandala (p. 289)

PREVENTION
Use the following 'Breast Health Data Sheet' to summarize your breast history for your healthcare practitioner.

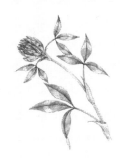

Breast Health Data Sheet

Complete this questionnaire, bringing it up-to-date at least once each year, and provide copies to your healthcare practitioners so that they can have clear records of what you have been doing and how you are responding.

Name:_____

Address:_____

Tel: _____ Fax: _____ E-mail: _____

Age: _____ Birthdate: m_____/d_____/y_____ Breast Exam Date: m_____/d_____/y_____

PERSONAL HISTORY

1. Age when periods began _____ Age when periods stopped _____

2. Length in days between menstrual cycles _____

3. Number of live births _____

4. Age at birth of first child _____

5. Total number of months spent breast-feeding _____

6. Number of bowel movements per day _____week _____

7. History of fibrocystic breast disease? ❑ yes ❑ no Other breast disease? _____When? _____

8. Dates of previous mammograms _____ Frequency _____

9. Family history of breast cancer? yes no Who, and at what age were they diagnosed?_____

10. Family history of ovarian, endometrial or prostate cancer? Who, and at what age?_____

11. Personal history of breast cancer? ❑ yes ❑ no

   If yes, complete the following:

12. Location of tumor ❑ L ❑ R _____ Size of tumor _____

13. Grade of tumor cells _____ Cancer stage 0 I II III IV Estrogen/progesterone receptor ❑ + or ❑ -

14. How many lymph nodes removed _____ # of positive nodes _____When? _____

15. Bone metastases? ❑ yes ❑ no If yes, where? _____ When? _____

   Other metastases? ❑ yes ❑ no If yes, where?_____ When diagnosed? _____

16. Current weight _____ Previous normal weight _____ Height_____

17. Any recurrence of breast cancer? ❑ yes ❑ no If yes, when and where?_____

HORMONE PROFILE AND PREDICTIVE TESTS

1. Saliva estrogen quotient Estrogen quotient = $\dfrac{\text{estriol}}{\text{estrone} + \text{estradiol}}$ Date tested _____

2. Ratio of C2 to C16 estrogen _____ Date tested _____

3. Saliva progesterone (days 20-23) _____ Date tested _____

4. TSH, T3, rT3, TPO Ab, Tg Ab _____ basal body temp: ❑ Norm ❑ Hi ❑ Lo Date tested _____

5. Melatonin level at 3:00 a.m. _____Date tested_____Testosterone _____ Date tested_____

6. IGF-1 in saliva_____Date tested _____Fasting insulin_____Date tested_____

7. Cortisol a.m. _____Cortisol p.m. _____ Date tested _____

8. AMAS test _____When? _____Thermography result _____ When?_____

9. Stool or blood glucuronidation rate _____

10. Tumor markers _____

11. pH of urine (2nd urine of the day) _____ pH saliva after breakfast _____

12. Monthly breast self exams? ❑ yes ❑ no Breast mapping? ❑ yes ❑ no Attach copy of breast map.

13. Other tests _____

_____

_____

PREVIOUS MEDICAL TREATMENTS FOR BREAST CANCER

1. Surgery ❑ yes ❑ no If yes, date(s) _____ lumpectomy mastectomy (circle one)

2. Tamoxifen ❑ yes ❑ no If yes, dates of use _____

3. Raloxifene ❑ yes ❑ no If yes, dates of use _____

4. Chemotherapy ❑ yes ❑ no If yes, names of medication and dates of treatment _____

_____

5. Radiation ❑ yes ❑ no If yes, when and number of treatments _____

_____

6. Other _____

Dates_____

PAST AND PRESENT RISK FACTORS

1. History of birth control pill use ❑ yes ❑ no   Age with use and for how long _____

2. History of estrogen/hormone replacement therapy ❑ yes ❑ no   Age began and for how long _____

Type of ERT/HRT_____

3. History of fertility drug use? ❑ yes ❑ no   How often _____

Attach a copy of your completed Breast Health Balance Sheet.

NATURAL MEDICINE TREATMENTS

1. Evening meditation practice ❑ yes ❑ no   When did you begin? _____

Type of practice and duration. _____

2. Rebounding/exercising ❑ yes ❑ no   When did you begin and for how many minutes daily?_____

How many days per week?_____

3. Hours of aerobic exercise weekly _____

4. Contrast showers ❑ yes ❑ no   Skin brushing ❑ yes ❑ no

5. Have you done a cleanse for yeast and parasites? ❑ yes ❑ no

When? _____ What did you use, dosage and for how long _____

6. Have you done a liver cleanse? ❑ yes ❑ no   When? _____

What did you use, dosage and for how long _____

7. Have you done a sauna detoxification program? ❑ yes ❑ no If yes, how many minutes in the sauna each

time and what was the frequency_____ Total hours sauna time to date _____

List supplements used with detox: _____

Attach copy of the Weekly Diet Diary.
Attach copy of the 14-Day Diet Routine Worksheet.
Attach copy of the Daily Therapeutic Amounts of Vitamins and Minerals Chart.

HERBAL FORMULAS

1. Are you taking a lymphatic cleansing formula? Circle which, if any of the following:

Hoxsey Formula   Healthy Breast Formula   Essiac   Floressence

When did you begin? _____ How many drops? _____

How many times daily?_____

2. Are you taking a liver cleansing formula? ❏ yes ❏ no Circle which of the following:

Liver Loving Formula   Milk thistle / Dandelion

Other (list herbs) _____

When did you begin _____ How many drops _____

How many times daily _____

3. Are you taking an immune enhancing formula? ❏ yes ❏ no Circle which of the following:

Immune Power Formula   Astragalus Combo (St. Francis Herbs)

Other (list herbs) _____

When did you begin _____ How many drops _____

How many times daily _____

4. List other therapies you may be doing or taking for breast health. (Attach another sheet if necessary)

_____

_____

_____

_____

_____

_____

5. Please comment on which therapies you feel are most beneficial to you and how you are feeling overall.

_____

_____

_____

_____

6. Is there anything else you think should be included in your healthy breast program?

_____

_____

_____

_____

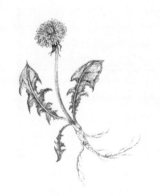

Guidelines for Healthcare Professionals

The following guidelines provide a convenient, practical review of the breast care program described in this book for both practitioners and patients, and suggest how you, the patient, can cooperate with your healthcare professional to make this program work for you. When both you and your healthcare professional understand the approach, prevention and treatment of breast cancer is optimized.

Every woman will differ in the pace at which she can proceed through the following steps. Her degree of willingness to do so will also vary. Healthcare professionals need to use gentle encouragement to keep incorporating positive changes.

Some of these 'visits' will require more than one appointment, depending on the patient and the order can be changed according to need. When the patient has established the components of the program in her everyday life, or at least is familiar with them, consider scheduling visits every three months rather than once monthly.

The visits in these guidelines correspond to the structure of the book.

Assessing Risk Factors

Visit 1 (1½ hours)

❑ Have patient fill out a standard intake form and the Breast Health Data Sheet from this book before the visit. At the end of the visit, ask her to complete the Breast Health Balance Sheet, Diet Diary, and BBT chart at home before the next visit. Make copies of these forms before hand or mark them in the patient's copy of the book.

❑ Take patient history, including family history. Listen to the whole story. Record specifics about any breast tumors and past breast history. Keep homeopathic remedies in mind and repertorize for subsequent visit. Obtain copies of pathology reports and bloodwork.

❑ Ask about emotional links to their breast health: what happened before the appearance of the tumor; was there an unresolved conflict that preceded it?

❑ Ask about environmental history and exposure to specific xenoestrogens; e.g., farm work, lindane in lice shampoo, live near a dump or plastic factory, solvent exposure, hair dyes, etc.

❑ Assess possible dental toxicity, history of root canals, number of mercury fillings, and encourage conscientious removal and replacement with ceramic. Refer to a biological dentist.

❑ Ask about any medications or supplements they have been taking so far; list dosages.

❑ Physical exam; demonstrate, teach, and perform breast exam and breast mapping. Give patient a copy of your breast map for them and ask that patient do breast self-exam each month to update it. Set up clinical breast exam for patient every 6-12 months, recording the next date for both of you.

❑ Review the structure of this breast health program with the patient and ask her to tell you in the next visit how much she can do or if she is uncomfortable or has questions about any piece. Set a tentative schedule for each component, so you both agree upon the road map.

❑ Educate patient about any other breast health resources and support groups available in your area.

Prescribe:

❑ Diet Changes: Give the patient a copy of the Recommended Healthy Breast Diet and ask her to begin to implement dietary changes. Specifically, prescribe kelp or seaweeds, turmeric/curcumin, flaxseed oil and freshly ground flaxseeds (2 tbsp minimum of each). Consider psyllium seed powder or other bowel cleansing formula, Greens + or other green powdered supplement containing spirulina.

Cautions:

❑ Hypothyroidism and the Brassicas: If hypothyroid, monitor the effect of soy and the raw brassicas on TSH and thyroid function (TSH sometimes goes up after consistent intake of soy and raw brassicas). Make sure they are including sea vegetables and/or kelp tablets with these foods to counteract their potential goitrogenic effect.

❑ Soy Allergy: If allergic to soy, increase other phytoestrogens, decrease soy. Miso and tempeh may be easier for some individuals to digest as long as there is not a Candida problem.

❑ Wheat Allergy: If allergic to wheat bran, increase psyllium.

Homework for the Patient:

❑ Fill out Breast Health Data Sheet and Breast Health Balance Sheet found in this book.

❑ Complete a BBT chart for at least two weeks to screen thyroid function; if low, continue to monitor progress.

❑ Complete a Diet Diary for at least one week.

❑ Review the Healthy Breast Diet.

Homework for the Practitioner:

❑ Review the patient's present supplement protocol and ensure that the following nutrients are provided: CoQ10 (100-400 mg), antioxidant formula (containing vitamin C plus bioflavonoids, vitamin E, zinc, selenium, grapeseed), alpha lipoic acid, chromium, niacin, folic acid, B complex, curcumin, DIM, NAC or reduced glutathione, clean fish oil, bromelain, or protease between meals. Consider what is known about pros and cons of antioxidants during chemo and radiation and evaluate dosages.

❑ Fill out the Daily Therapeutic Amounts of Vitamins and Minerals chart found in this book for the patient with what you are recommending at this time, listing dosages and brand names if known. Be prepared to explain to her what each supplement is used for.

❑ Herbal Medicine: Lymphatic formula (Floressence, Hoxsey or Healthy Breast Formula), liver formula (Milk Thistle Combo or Liver Loving Formula), immune tonic (Astragalus Combo or Immune Power Formula). If breast cancer is present, all three should be done simultaneously. If needing prevention, do a lymphatic formula with a liver formula consistently and use an immune formula only if there seems to be an immune weakness from the history. If there is active breast cancer, consider adding goldenseal, echinacea, bloodroot, juniper, and Chinese herbal formulas as well as a medicinal mushroom product.

❑ Consider: potassium, inositol and IP6, melatonin (if estrogen receptor positive tumor or if on Tamoxifen), thymus extract or thymuline 9CH, modified citrus pectin, digestive enzymes, bromelain, Maitake D-fraction, MGN-3, quercetin, ellagic acid, extra niacin, garlic, beta-sitosterol.

❑ Homeopathic Differential Diagnosis: Come up with one.

Hormones

Visit 2

❑ Review Breast Health Balance Sheet and counsel as to ways to decrease breast cancer risk. Start with a few changes and set target dates for the implementation of those changes (for example, sleep in a dark room, decrease exposure to electromagnetic fields in specific ways, begin exercising more, wear a less restrictive bra, assess dental fillings, eliminate use of plastic packaging on foods, use water filter, etc.) Keep coming back to this chart in repeat visits until all the possible changes have been made.

❑ Review Diet Diary and suggest a few simple changes. Be sensitive to the patient's capacity for change. Instruct that you will do a more thorough diet review in the next visit.

❑ Review BBT and thyroid function. Check if BBT is consistently below 97.8° F. Ask about previous thyroid tests and physical symptoms associated with low thyroid (easy weight gain, hair loss, cold, constipated, depression, heavy prolonged menses, insomnia or needing to sleep a lot, infertility, dry skin, eczema, headaches, high cholesterol). If temperature is low or high, complete thyroid tests which include TSH, free T3, free T4, reverse T3, antithyroglobulin antibodies and antimicrosomal antibodies. All of these need to be done to see where the problem lies in the thyroid system. Also check adrenal function through the Koenigsburg test or salivary cortisol. Check salivary progesterone and possible anemia. A low temperature could be related to one or all of these (thyroid, adrenals, progesterone, anemia).

❑ Talk about the importance of long, deep breathing in correcting and maintaining balanced rhythms in the mind-body. Teach patient how to breathe and encourage meditation before bed or refer to a meditation class.

❑ Assess potential risk and necessity for sauna detoxification in future if chronically exposed to environmental estrogens or carcinogens.

❑ Ask any questions for the homeopathic differential diagnosis.

Prescribe:
- ❑ Lifestyle changes to improve the score on the Breast Health Balance Sheet.
- ❑ Daily breathing exercises.
- ❑ Complete Daily Therapeutic Amounts of Vitamins and Minerals form.
- ❑ Continue with BBT and Diet Diary.
- ❑ If low thyroid function is apparent, then assist thyroid, progesterone and adrenals; reduce estrogen dominance following guidelines in Chapters 3 and 5.
- ❑ If a fibrocystic breast condition or breast swelling is present, recommend supplements as described in Chapter 10.
- ❑ Assess necessity to do saliva tests for hormone levels and recommend the following if affordable: estradiol, estrone and estriol and estrogen quotient; C2 and C16 estrogen ratio; progesterone; testosterone; melatonin; IGF-1, cortisol; and blood tests for insulin, prolactin, TSH, free T3, free T4, reverse T3, antithyroglobulin antibodies and antimicrosomal antibodies.
- ❑ If breast cancer is present, also have blood tests for plasma viscosity, plasma fibrinogen, plasma fibrin-D-dimers; assess immune function with natural killer cell activity test and T/B/natural killer cell immune panel.

Visit 3 (1 hour, 1-3 weeks later)

Diet and Digestion

- ❑ Review how the patient is doing physically and emotionally and if she is having any difficulties with the program so far.
- ❑ Ask about meditation/breathing exercises before bed and reinforce their importance.
- ❑ Go over the details of the Healthy Breast Diet and assess what is possible and helpful to this particular patient. Come up with compromises if they are unable to do pieces of it. Avoid being rigid but be firm.
- ❑ Assess whether there may be a deficiency of HCl (trouble digesting beans, bloating, undigested food in stool, low mineral absorption, constipation, weak nails, pH of urine >7.2). Test HCl using the gastro-test, available from HDC Corporation (tel. 408-954-1909 or fax. 408-954-0340) or HCl challenge as needed. Do oral zinc test.
- ❑ Explain how estrogen metabolism can be manipulated in a positive way through diet, exercise, and supplements, using guidelines in Chapters 3 and 5.
- ❑ Provide recipes or cookbook suggestions to patient.
- ❑ Assess bowel function. Keep track of number of bowel movements daily or weekly and adjust diet, supplements, or exercise to ensure at least two per day. Three is ideal.
- ❑ Assess pH balance through daily testing of a.m. urine and saliva or 24 hour urine for several weeks. Correct through acid/alkaline food chart, alkaline powder or potassium/magnesium supplementation.
- ❑ Assess fiber intake and figure out what she needs to do to get 30 g per day.
- ❑ Assess fat intake and counsel regarding the protective fats

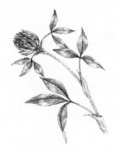

(olive, flaxseed and pure fish oils) and how cooking practices and diet can be changed to utilize these. Restrict saturated and other unhealthy fats to less than 15% of calories or eliminate them altogether. Achieve a ratio of 2:1 Omega 3: Omega 6 oils. Include minimum of 2 tbsp of unheated flaxseed oil in diet daily. Assess the amount of Omega 6 oils she consumes through nuts, and seeds, vegetable oils or evening primrose oil and reduce these if necessary.

❏ Talk about water intake and water filters and recommend an affordable filter; for example, reverse osmosis or carbon block filter. Ensure that she drinks at least 2 liters or quarts of water daily, up to 3 liters or quarts during chemotherapy and radiation.

❏ Assess mineral content of foods and suggest a hair analysis to reflect mineral status. Pay attention to toxic minerals and deficiencies of zinc, selenium, iodine, boron, magnesium, chromium, molybdenum, manganese. When hair analysis comes back, recommend ways to balance mineral status or remove toxic minerals.

Prescribe:

❏ Suggest homeopathic remedy based on constitution and location and quality of the tumor.

❏ Refer to a breast cancer support group or individual therapist. This will increase life expectancy and quality of life according to studies.

❏ If low HCl, supplement with a few drops of wormwood or gentian tincture or bitter foods before meals or mindfulness to increase HCl. Relax before eating and chew well. Consider enzymes.

Homework for the Patient:

❏ Continue making changes to incorporate the Healthy Breast Diet. Keep a Diet Diary for one week each month and bring this to your naturopathic doctor or health practitioner.

❏ Fill out the Dietary Tips for Breast Health Chart for two weeks and bring it to the next visit. Attempt to do more of it over time; don't expect to do it all at once.

❏ Keep monitoring thyroid function through the BBT Chart.

Detoxification

Visit 4 (1 hour; 1-4 weeks later)

❏ Review how patient is doing physically and emotionally, and question if she is having any difficulties with the program. Praise her for everything she has done so far; acknowledge how difficult it is.

❏ Educate the patient in the body's methods of detoxification. Show pictures of liver, bowel, and kidneys. Assess whether there may be a problem in Phase 1 or Phase 2 detoxification and recommend appropriate strategies using guidelines in Chapter 5.

❏ Review what she has been doing so far to detoxify: liver formula, increased fiber, blood cleansing herbs, water.

❏ Review the protocol for sauna detoxification and talk about what would be realistic for the patient. Create a plan for sauna detoxification aiming for 100 hours of sauna time. Consider measuring DDE and PCB levels in blood or fat before and after sauna detoxification.

❑ Recommend any other supplements needed for detoxification of the liver, kidneys, or lymph.

❑ Review the need for and use of enemas and judge whether in your opinion this patient would benefit from coffee enemas or other enemas and decide upon a frequency schedule; if not using enemas, ensure that she is having at least three bowel movements daily and is taking a herbal fiber supplement which may include bentonite.

❑ Assess whether yeast and parasites may be a problem for this patient, and if so, suggest a cleanse for a limited amount of time, following strategies in the book to do so if necessary. Consider recommending a yeast and parasite cleanse once or twice a year for three months as a matter of course, using your clinical judgement. Consider a comprehensive digestive stool analysis and parasitology with Great Smokies Diagnostic Laboratory if digestive symptoms are present.

❑ Review the patient's supplements; any questions or concerns.

Prescribe:

❑ Possible supplementation with probiotics and FOS, the use of the gemmotherapies Juniperus and Rosmarinus for improved liver drainage and repair, antiparasitic and antifungal formulas.

❑ Implement a sauna detoxification program and/or enemas if they were recommended.

❑ Implement a detoxification program

❑ Implement a yeast/parasite cleanse if it was recommended.

❑ Ask her to keep a diet diary for one week and bring it to the next visit.

Visit 5 (1 hour, 2-4 weeks later)   Lymphatics

❑ Review Diet Diary and suggest changes.

❑ Review patient's ability to practice the breathing exercises or meditation. Suggest a class if she is having difficulty. Recommend her to a relaxation/visualization/meditation program.

❑ Ask about how the patient is feeling physically and emotionally.

❑ Monitor progress during the sauna detox, liver detox, and the intestinal cleansing.

❑ Educate patient about the function of the lymphatic system and the importance of regular exercise and deep breathing.

❑ Assess how much aerobic exercise the patient does weekly, outside of normal activity. Impress upon her that what is needed is 4 hours of exercise weekly or 35 minutes a day. This will decrease breast cancer risk 30-60% and improve estrogen metabolism. Help the patient set up an aerobic exercise program that will be enjoyable and which she can maintain for life. It may be walking, rebounding, cycling, a fitness class, dancing, jogging, etc. Consider asking patient to fill out a 2-week Exercise Log.

❑ Talk about the value of rebounding for improved lymphatic circulation and breast health. If possible, demonstrate rebounding exercises and suggest she practice. Recommend a rebounding and yoga program.
❑ Discuss the importance of wearing a bra that it is not too restrictive. After removing one's bra, there should be no red marks from increased pressure. This will impede lymphatic circulation.
❑ Review with the patient the methodology of skin brushing and contrast showers and encourage her to practice them daily. Demonstrate how to use a skin brush.
❑ Recommend use of Healthy Breast Oil, and breast self-massage 3 or more times weekly.

Homework for the Patient:
❑ Begin a daily exercise program that can be maintained for life, exercising at least 4 hours weekly. Keep a 2-week Exercise Log and bring it to the next visit.
❑ Begin rebounding daily for whatever length of time you can sustain, increasing it to at least 15 minutes daily over time.
❑ Purchase a bra that is not restrictive.
❑ Integrate skin brushing and contrast showers into your daily routine.
❑ Keep a diet diary for one week.
❑ Begin using Healthy Breast Oil for your breast self-massage or use essential oils of palmarosa, lavender, juniper, rosemary, frankincense, lemon.

Immune System and Traditional Chinese Medicine

Visit 6 (1 hour, 2-4 weeks later)

❑ Assess diet, breathing practice, exercise, sauna detoxification, review supplements.
❑ Ask patient to draw a large outline of her body. Review the components of the immune system one at a time and ask her to draw them on the picture (thymus gland, spleen, bone marrow, hypothalamus, pituitary, macrophages, T-helper cells, T-killer cells, T-suppressor cells, Kupffer cells, etc.) Read the statements in the book about each of these and do the arm movements or make up arm movements for them while repeating the phrase. Then draw each one in the picture. The various types of white blood cells can be drawn along the side. Explore with the patient how she can use imagery to make these immune system components work better. The imagery should involve as many senses as possible and use cues from her everyday environment. Help the patient find a metaphor for her T-helper cells and her T-killer cells that is personal yet powerful. Include in the drawing symbols for the supplements she is taking that energize her immune system. Work out guidelines for a script for the patient to use in a regular visualization. Include references to the supplements she is using in the script. For homework, ask the patient to write out her script and make her own visualization tape, using the one in the book as a reference. Listen to the tape daily.

- Assess pulse, tongue and history and evaluate patterns of disharmony according to TCM. Recommend any additional herbal formulas or acupuncture to correct patterns of disharmony. If on chemo or radiation, recommend tonics — e.g., royal jelly and ganoderma, caulis millettia tablets, astragalus/oldenlandria tea. Create a plan for acupuncture treatments or refer to a TCM practitioner for a series of treatments. You may also recommend regular classes in Qiqong or yoga.
- Recommend Darkfield Microscopy and/or BTA to assess the condition of the blood and body fluids and use appropriate therapies to adjust, such as the Sanum remedies. Repeat this testing every 3 months.

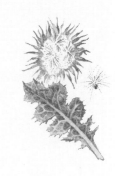

Homework for the Patient:
- Write out a visualization script and make a visualization tape and bring them to the next visit.
- Begin treatments in acupuncture, Qiqong and/or yoga, if recommended.

Visit 7 (1 hour, 2-4 weeks later; may take several visits)

Emotional Issues

- Review the Visualization Script and suggest any changes that might improve it. Ask what her response has been to listening to the tape. Ask her what cues she can place in her environment to remind her of her own innate capacity to heal and of the strength of her immune system. This may include pictures on the wall, affirmations, plants, photographs, places she visits, healing foods, token objects to touch, massage oil, music or specific sounds, smells, essential oils.
- Explore issues around family, nurturing, abandonment, guilt, loss, sexuality, separation, intimacy to uncover any buried emotions that may be connected to the appearance of the tumor or to her breasts in general. Explore ways to heal any of these, perhaps referring to a therapist or body-worker.
- Assess whether the patient feels trapped in an unhappy situation with no way out. Suggest counseling sessions so that she can seek resolution, discover unrecognized options, and be supported through psychological change. Women in either group or individual therapy have a longer life expectancy and better quality of life than control groups.
- Review the chart Limiting Beliefs / Healthy Beliefs Chart and examine which of the limiting beliefs feel true to the patient. Have her read the healthy belief to replace it. Read the healthy belief back to the patient, using the word 'you' and ask her how it feels to receive that statement. Ask her for examples of how in her life she displays the limiting belief and how her thoughts and actions would be different if she lived the healthy beliefs. Have her write out the healthy beliefs she needs as affirmations and repeat them 3 x daily, out loud, in front of a mirror for 40 days. Suggest that she take risks to act out the healthy beliefs.
- Examine issues of buried anger with the patient and help her to bring these out and allow safe expression of them. Encourage a

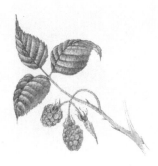

process (it may take several months) of moving from anger to forgiveness. This may require referral to a therapist.

❑ Assess whether this patient is able to act assertively or not. If not, review the assertive model and encourage her to use this model at least three times before the next visit.

❑ Consider homeopathic remedies or flower essences to help the patient on the emotional level.

Homework for the Patient:

❑ Re-do visualization tape if necessary, listen to it one or more times daily. Place cues in your environment to remind you of your innate capacity to heal.

❑ Create a plan to improve your emotional well-being, working with the above issues with your naturopathic doctor, therapist or body-worker.

❑ Read your healthy beliefs out loud while looking in the mirror, at least three times daily for forty days. Begin to take risks to act on the healthy beliefs.

❑ Acknowledge anger, express it, identify steps to resolve it and move to forgiveness with assistance from someone skilled in helping with this process.

❑ Act assertively at least three times before your next visit.

Meaning Mandala

Visit 8 (1 hour, 2-4 weeks later; may take several visits)

❑ Review with patient how she is changing emotionally. Discuss her attempts to act assertively and the outcome of these attempts. Role-play with her, allowing her to act assertively with you in a particular situation that is difficult for her.

❑ Review the healthy beliefs, and how much closer she feels she has moved to accepting them.

❑ Ask her to write out a list of the things that bring her the most joy, through both 'being' and 'doing' states.

❑ Ask her to write out another list of her gifts, talents, and capabilities.

❑ Ask her to write out a third list of the things about which she feels the most passionate, that contribute to the meaning in her life and give her a sense of purpose and fulfillment. This will include both 'things to do' and 'ways of being'. (These may be given as homework the previous visit)

❑ Ask the patient to make yet another list of the things that need 'letting go' in her life. Included in this list are specific limiting beliefs, relationships, addictions, guilt, social obligations, expectations, negative emotions and anything else she can think of. Over time, check in to see what progress is being made with this list. Ask her to focus on one at a time for several weeks.

❑ Give the patient a large piece of paper with markers and other colored materials and have magazines and scissors and glue available to cut out and paste pictures. Show her the diagram for the Meaning Mandala and have her begin to make her own, first with words, then with drawings or cut out pictures. Have

her finish it at home or in the next visit. Suggest that she put the Meaning Mandala up on a wall where she can see it while she does her rebounding. Ask her to bring the mandala back in the future (at least every 3 months) and keep encouraging her to act in the areas her energy wants to move.
❑ Review the types of prayer and explore whether this patient might find a practice of prayer acceptable or beneficial. If so, encourage her to find or to create prayers that resonate with her belief system.

Homework for the Patient:
❑ Complete a Meaning Mandala and hang it where you can see it regularly. Seek to actualize more of the meaning mandala each month, with organized action steps.
❑ Find a form of prayer that works for you and integrate it into your life.

Guidelines for Follow-Up Visits:
❑ Ask that your patient complete a Diet Diary for one week each month and review it at least once every three months.
❑ Perform a clinical breast exam on your patient twice yearly and request that she bring in her Breast Map to these visits.
❑ Perform a hair analysis annually.
❑ Check saliva and thyroid hormone levels annually for a few years, then less often if they are stable.
❑ Keep coming back to the Meaning Mandala in follow-up visits.
❑ Check the condition of the blood and body fluids with Darkfield Microscopy and the BTA every 3-6 months.
❑ After the first year, if the patient is stable in the program, schedule visits every 3 months or so.
❑ Assess whether a yeast and parasite cleanse may be beneficial for three months once or twice yearly.
❑ After the initial sauna detoxification is complete, recommend a weekly sauna as an ongoing practice.
❑ Let your patient know about Rachel Carson Day and about ways in which she can contribute to environmental reform.
❑ Link up to other women following this healthy breast program through the support group directory listed on the web site: www.healthybreastprogram.on.ca and help set up new support groups.
❑ Continue following the program, adjusting the supplements annually.

Summary

While we can achieve a great deal working by ourselves or in groups to prevent breast cancer, working with the support of an informed healthcare professional will ease the load and remind us to keep on track. Preventing breast cancer is a life-long task. We can utilize many resources and people to help us along.

Resources Directory

Clinical Laboratories

Saliva Testing Laboratories
Rocky Mountain Analytic, Unit A 253147
Bearspaw Rd. NW, Calgary, Alberta, T3L 2P5,
Tel: (403) 241-4513, Fax: (403) 241-4516
www.rmalab.com, info@rmalab.com.

Aeron Life Cycles Clinical Laboratory
1933 Davis St., Ste. 310, San Leandro,
California, 94577
Tel: (510) 729-0375, Fax: (510) 729-0383
www.aeron@aeron.com.

Pharmasan
373 280th St., Osceola, Wisconsin, 54020
Tel: (715) 755-3995, or 1-888-342-7272
FAX: (715) 294-3921, www.pharmasan.com.

ZRT Laboratory
12505 NW Cornell Rd., Portland, Oregon, 97229
Tel: (503) 469-0741, Fax: (503) 469-1305
www.salivatest.com.

Toxic Chemicals Testing
Accu-Chem Laboratories, 990 N. Bowser Rd.,
Suite 800, Richardson, Texas, 75081
Tel: 1-800-451-0116, www.accuchem.com.

National Medical Services
3701 Welsh Rd., Willow Grove,
Pennsylvania, 19090
Tel: 1-800-522-6671.

Pacific Toxicology Laboratories
6160 Variel Ave., Woodland Hills,
California, 91367
Tel: 1-800-328-6942.

AMAS Test

Oncolab
36 the Fenway, Boston, Massachusetts, 02215
Tel: (617) 536-0805 or 1-800 9 CATEST,
Fax: (617) 536-0657. Call to order the anti-
malignin antibody test.

Food Sensitivity Testing

Immuno Laboratories
1620 West Oakland Park Blvd.,
Fort Lauderdale, Florida, 33311
Tel: 1-800-231-9197 or (954) 486-4500,
Fax: (954) 739-6563.

Testing Supplies

Gastro Test
From HDC Corporation, 688 Gibraltar Court,
Milpitas, California, 95035
Tel: (408) 942-7340 or 1-800-227-8162,
www.hdccorp.com. Measures pH of the
stomach with a string test.

pH Paper
Micro Essential Laboratory Inc., 4224 Avenue H,
Brooklyn, New York, 11210
Tel: 1-800-227-8162.

Herbal Suppliers

Healthy Breast Products
235 9th St. E. Owen Sound, Ontario. N4K 1N8
Tel: (519) 372-9212, Fax: (519) 372-2755.
www.healthybreastprogram.on.ca. Call to order
the Healthy Breast Formula, Liver Loving
Formula, Immune Power Formula, Healthy
Breast Oil.

St. Francis Herb Farm
104 Maika Road, P. O. Box 29, Combermere,
Ontario, K0J 1L0
Tel: (613) 756-6279, Fax: (613) 756-0002.
www.stfrancisherbfarm.com. For excellent
quality single tinctures or herbal formulas.

Poya Naturals
21-B Regan Road, Brampton, Ontario, L7A 1C5
Tel: (905) 840-5459 or 1-877-255-7692,
Fax: (905) 846-1784, www.poyanaturals.com.
To order excellent quality essential oils.

Herb Pharm
P. O. Box 116, Williams, Oregon 97544
Tel: 1-800-348-4372, www.herb-pharm.com.
For the Hoxsey formula and other single herbs
or blends in tincture form.

Carnivora Research Inc.
Santa Rosa, California, Fax: (707) 568-7468, www.carnivora.com. Call to order the herb, Carnivora.

Avena Botanicals
Tel:(207) 594-0694. www.avenaherbs.com. Sells phytolacca and calendula herbal oils.

Chinese Herbal Suppliers

Eastern Currents
#200A-3540 West 41st Avenue, Vancouver, British Columbia, V6N 3E6
Tel: (604) 263-5042, Fax: (604) 263-8781.

Institute for Traditional Medicine
ITM, 2017 SE Hawthorne Blvd., Portland, Oregon, 97214
Tel: (503) 233-4907, Fax: (503) 233-1017, E-mail: itm@itmonline.org, www.itmonline.org. Chinese herbal formulas can be ordered from ITM.

Crane Herb
E-mail: info@craneherb.com, www.craneherb.com

Medicinal Mushroom Suppliers

Wylie Mycologicals
R.R.#1, Wiarton, Ontario, N0H 2T0
Tel: (519) 534-1570, Fax: (519) 534-9045, E-mail: wylie@interlog.com, www.wyliemycologicals.ca. Call to order Shitake, Maitake and other medicinal mushroom growing kits.

Fungi Perfecti
P.O. Box 7634, Olympia, Washington, 98507
Tel: 1-800-780-9126 or (360) 426-9292, Fax: (360) 426-9377, E-mail: mycomedia@aol.com, www.fungi.com. Shitake and Maitake growing kits, tinctures, capsules and teas.

Sauna Manufacturers

Saunacore
71 Strada Drive, Suite 8, Woodbridge, Ontario, L4L 5V8
Tel: (800) 361-9485, www.saunacore.com.

Heavenly Heat
Tel: 1-800-653-8881 or (845) 679-2490.

Composting Toilets

Sun-Mar Composting Toilets
Burlington, Ontario, Tel: (905) 332-1314.

Storburn Pollution Free Toilet
Brantford, Ontario, Tel: 1-800-876-2286.

BioLet
TEL: 1800-6BIOLET.

Envirolet Composting Toilet Systems
Scarborough, Ontario, Tel: 1-800-387-5245.

Clivus Multrum
Tel: 1-800-4CLIVUS.

Environmental Films

Exposure: Environmental Links to Breast Cancer can be ordered from the
Women's Healthy Environments Network
24 Mercer St., Suite 102, Toronto, Ontario, M5V 1H3, Tel: (416) 928-0880, Fax: (416) 928-9640, E-mail when@web.ca, www.whenvironments.ca.

Hormone Copy-Cats can be ordered from the
World Wildlife Fund Canada
90 Eglinton Ave E, Ste 504, Toronto, Ontario, M4P 2Z7, Tel: (416) 489-8800 or 1-800-26-PANDA, Fax: (416) 489-3611.

Everyday Carcinogens: Acting in the Face of Scientific Uncertainty, with biologist and author Sandra Steingraber, can be ordered from the
Breast Cancer Prevention Coalition
23 Lynden Hill Cres., Brantford, Ontario, N3P 1R1, Tel: (519) 751-2560, www.stopcancer.org.

Rachel's Daughters is available from
Light-Saraf Films
264 Arbor St, San Francisco, California, 94131, Tel: (415) 469-0139.

Blue Vinyl can be ordered from
Transit Media
Attn: Bernie:Blue Vinyl, 22-D Hollywood Ave., Hohokus, New Jersey, 07423, Tel: 800-343-5540, Fax: 201-652-1973, www.bluevinyl.org .

The Next Industrial Revolution and many more very fine inspiring and educational films are available from
Bullfrog Films
P.O. Box 149, Oley, Pennsyvania, 19547
Tel: (610) 779-8226, Fax: (610) 370-1978, www.bullfrogfilms.com.

Naturopathic Associations

Canadian Naturopathic Association
Tel: (416) 496-8633 or 1-800-551-4381,
Fax: (416) 496-8634, www.naturopathicassoc.ca.

American Association of Naturopathic Physicians
Tel: (206) 298-0125, www.naturopathic.org.

American Naturopathic Medical Association
Tel: (702) 897-7053, www.anma.com.

For Naturopathic Doctors Trained in the Healthy Breast Program, www.healthybreast-program.on.ca.

Breast Cancer Organizations

Canadian Breast Cancer Network
207 Bank St., Suite 102, Ottawa, Ontario, K2P 2N2, Tel: (613) 788-3311, Fax: (613) 233-1056. Can link you to other breast cancer support groups in Canada.

Breast Cancer Research and Education Fund
266 St. Paul St., St. Catharines, Ontario, L2R 5N2, Tel: (905) 687-3333. Great newsletter focusing on natural therapies and environmental links to breast cancer.

Willow: Ontario Breast Cancer Support and Resource Center
785 Queen St. E., Toronto, Ontario, M4M 1H5, Tel: (416) 778-5000, Fax: (416) 778-8070. Provides resources for women with breast cancer.

Cancer Information Service of the Canadian Cancer Society
Tel: 1-888-939-3333, www.cancer.ca. Provides information on all aspects of breast cancer.

AMC Cancer Research Center's Cancer Information and Counseling Line
Tel: 1-800-525-3777. Provides information on cancer.

American Cancer Society
1599 Clifton Rd. N.E., Atlanta, Georgia, 30329, Tel: 1-800-227-2345. Provides information on support groups, educational materials, financial aid, loans and medical equipment.

Cancer Care Inc.
1180 Avenue of the Americas, 2nd Floor, New York, New York, 10036, Tel: 1-800-813-HOPE, www.cancercare.org.

Cancervive
6500 Wilshire Boulevard, Suite 500, Los Angeles, California, 90048, Tel: (310) 203-9232. Support groups, fund-raising, insurance information and advocacy for cancer patients.

Commonweal
P.O. Box 316, Bolinas, California, 94924, Tel: (415) 868-0970. Offers workshops for people with cancer and for health care professionals working with cancer patients.

Healing Journeys
P.O. Box 250, Aptos, California, 95001, Tel: 800-423-9882, www.healingjourneys.com. Sponsors a free two-day conference for women with cancer in Northern California, "Cancer as a Turning Point: From Surviving to Thriving.

National Alliance of Breast Cancer Organizations
9 E. 37th St., New York, New York, 10016, Tel: 800-719-9154. Central resource for a network of 375 organizations providing detection, treatment and care.

National Breast Cancer Coalition
1707 L St. N.W., Suite 1060, Washington, D.C., 20036, Tel: 1-800-622-2838. Advocacy group of over 300 member organizations dedicated to the eradication of breast cancer through action, advocacy and public education.

Alternative Cancer Clinics

Klinik St. Georg
Bad Aibling/Germany, Tel: int. +49 (0) 8061-398-0, Fax: int. +49 (0) 8061-398-454. The Integrative Cancer Therapy Concept practiced at St. George Hospital combines the essential standard methods of treatment (i.e. radiation treatment, chemotherapy) with complementary methods

(immune biological program, nutrition, supplementation of antioxidants, hyperthermia, psychotherapy) to provide a complete cancer therapy.

Biological Medicines Network
Kestrels, Witherenden Hill, Etchingham, East Sussex TN19 7JP, UK, Tel: +44 (0)1435 883225, Fax: +44 (0)1435 883642, E-mail: info@bmnuk.net, www.bmnuk.net. The Paracelsus Clinic specializes in the treatment of chronic, degenerative and tumor diseases. The advanced diagnostic tests include darkfield microscopy, biological terrain assessment, electro-acupuncture (Voll), thermography, dental panoramic x-rays, heavy metal evaluation, heart rate variability testing, hair mineral analysis and many others. Centres located in: Paracelsus Clinica Al Rone, Castaneda, Southern Switzerland; Clinica Paracelsus, Raima de Mallorca, Spain; Paracelsus Foxhollow Clinic, Crestwood, Kentucky, USA.

Hippocrates Health Institute
1443 Palmdale Court, West Palm Beach, Florida, 33411, Tel: (561) 471-8876, Reservations: 1-800-842-2125, Fax: (561) 471-9464. E-mail: info@hippocratesinst.com, www.reservations@hippocratesinst.com. The Hippocrates philosophy is dedicated to the belief that a pure enzyme-rich diet, complemented by positive thinking and non-invasive therapies, are essential elements on the path to optimum health.

The Gerson Institute
1572 Second Avenue, San Diego, California, 92101, Tel: (619) 685-5353, or 1-888-4-GERSON, www.gerson.org. The Gerson Therapy seeks to regenerate the body to health, supporting each important metabolic requirement by flooding the body with nutrients from almost 20 pounds of organically grown fruits and vegetables daily. Most is used to make fresh raw juice, one glass every hour, 13 times per day. Raw and cooked solid foods are generously consumed. Oxygenation is usually more than doubled, as oxygen deficiency in the blood contributes to many degenerative diseases. The metabolism is also stimulated through the addition of thyroid, potassium, and other supplements, and by avoiding heavy animal fats, excess protein, sodium, and other toxins.

Bio-Medical Center
Hoxsey clinic, PO Box 727, 615 General Ferreira, Colonia Juarez, Tijuana, B.C. Mexico, Tel: 52 814 9011.

Aidan Incorporated
850 West Elliot Road, Tempe, Arizona, 85284, Tel: (480) 756-8900, or 1-800-529-0269, Fax: (480) 756-8906, E-mail: aidan@aidan-az.com. Aidan has developed and pioneered a unique treatment approach designed to help stimulate a person's own immune system to recognize and attack tumor cells.

Chronic Disease Control and Treatment Center
Dr. Helmut Keller, Am Reuthlein, D-8675 Bad Steben, den, Germany, Tel: 011-49-9288-5166 or 011-49-9267-1702, Fax: 011-49-9267-1040 or 011-49-9288-7815, www.cancer2000.com. Specific treatment modalities include: Photodynamic Therapy enhanced with a laser light source that includes the frequencies according to Rife; Galvano Therapy; Moderate Whole Body Hyperthermia together with oxygen in order to change the tumor cell proteins form body-own to body-foreign. Carnivora is utilized to block the protein kinases of tumor cells and deplete the ATP content (energy source) of malignant cells. Monoclonal Antibodies, Antitumor Vaccines, Cytokines, and other primary and adjuvant therapies are employed.

Macrobiotics
Kushi Inst, PO Box 7, Beckett, Massachusetts, 01223, Tel: 413 623 5741, www.macrobiotics.org.

American Biologics, Mexico, S.A. Medical Center
International Admissions Office, 1180 Walnut Avenue, Chula Vista, California, 91911. Tel: (800) 227-4458 (619) 429-8200. www.abmex.com (Note: This is the contact office. The clinic is in Mexico.)

Burzynski Research Institute
6221 Corporate Drive, Houston, Texas, 77036, Tel: (713) 777-8233, www.catalog.com/bri/bri.htm.

HEALTHY BREAST PRODUCTS ORDER FORM

Name

Address:

City   Prov/State   Postal Code/Zip:

Tel: Fax: E-mail:

DESCRIPTION	QTY.	UNIT PRICE (Can + U.S.)	SHIPPING	TOTAL
The Complete Natural Medicine Guide to Breast Cancer		$25.00 Cdn $19.00 U.S.	$6.50 Cdn $7.00 U.S.	
Recovering from Breast Cancer: A Guided Visualization Audiotape		$12.00 Cdn $9.00 U.S.	$4.00 Cdn $5.00 U.S.	
The Healthy Breast Kundalini Yoga and Rebounding Video		$25.00 Cdn $19.00 U.S.	$5.00 Cdn $6.00 U.S.	
The Healthy Breast Formula				
250 ml bottle		$55 Cdn/40 U.S.	$6. Cdn/U.S.	
500 ml bottle		$90 Cdn/65 U.S.	$7. Cdn/U.S.	
Liver Loving Formula				
250 ml bottle		$55 Cdn/40 U.S.	$6. Cdn/U.S.	
500 ml bottle		$90 Cdn/65 U.S.	$7. Cdn/U.S.	
Immune Power Formula				
250 ml bottle		$55 Cdn/40 U.S.	$6. Cdn/U.S.	
500 ml bottle		$90 Cdn/65 U.S.	$7. Cdn/U.S.	
Healthy Breast Oil				
250 ml bottle		$55 Cdn/40 U.S.	$6. Cdn/U.S.	
500 ml bottle		$90 Cdn/65 U.S.	$7. Cdn/U.S.	
			SUBTOTAL	
		7% GST (Can. only)		
			TOTAL DUE	

Payment by cheque, money order or Visa to:
Healthy Breast Products
235 9th Street East, Second Floor
Owen Sound, Ontario N4K 1N8
Please allow 3 weeks for delivery

VISA (we do not accept Mastercard or American Express)

Card No._____Exp Date_____

Signature_____

To order by fax please call **(519) 372-2755** or by phone **(519) 372-9212**. For other products from The Healthy Breast Program please visit our web site at **www.healthybreastprogram.on.ca** or request an order form by phone or fax. Email us at **sdk@log.on.ca**. Prices subject to change without notice.

Workshops: Please consult the website for upcoming workshops in The Healthy Breast Program and the Healthy Breast Teacher Training Program. We would also be pleased to teach in your area.

References

Chapter One: What Is Your Risk of Developing Breast Cancer

1. Ferlay, J. et al. GLOBOCAN 2000: *Cancer Incidence, Mortality and Prevalence Worldwide*. Version 1.0. IARC CancerBase No. 5. Lyon:IARC Press (2001). Limited version available online at www-dep.iarc.fr/globocan/globocan.html.

2. Ferlay, J. et al. GLOBOCAN 2000: *Cancer Incidence, Mortality and Prevalence Worldwide*. Version 1.0. IARC CancerBase No. 5. Lyon:IARC Press (2001). Limited version available online at www-dep.iarc.fr/globocan/globocan.html.

3. Thornton, J. *Human Health and the Environment: The Breast Cancer Warning*. Washington, DC: Greenpeace, 1993.

4. Harris, J.M. Lippman, et al. *Breast Cancer. New England Journal of Medicine*, 1992;327:319-28.

5. *Cancer Facts and Figures 2003*. American Cancer Society. www.cancer.org.

6. *Canadian Cancer Statistics 2003*. Toronto, ON: National Cancer Institute of Canada, www.hc-gc.ca.

7. Canadian Cancer Statistics 1998:55. Ferlay, J. et al. GLOBOCAN 2000: *Cancer Incidence, Mortality and Prevalence Worldwide*. Version 1.0. IARC CancerBase No. 5. Lyon:IARC Press (2001). Limited version available online at www-dep.iarc.fr/globocan/globocan.html.

8. Willett, W. The search for the causes of breast and colon cancer. *Nature*, 1989;338:389-93.

9. Breast Cancer Risk Factors: Are They Taken Too Seriously? *Health Facts*, September 1993.

10. Anderson, D. A genetic study of human breast cancer. *J Natl Cancer Inst*, 1972;48:1029.

11. Ottman, R. Practical guide for estimating risk for familial breast cancer. *Lancet*, 1983;2:556.

12. Anonymous. Breast cancer: A reassuring look at your odds. *Health*, January 1993.

13. Barkardottir, R.B. et al. Haplotype analysis in Icelandic and finnish BRCA2 999del5 breast cancer families. *Eur Hum Genet*, 2001.

14. Grzybowska E., et al. High frequency of recurrent mutations in BRCA1 and BRCA2 genes in Polish families with breast and ovarian cancer. *Hum Mutat*, 2000; Dec;16(6):482-90.

15. Fackelmann, K. Breast cancer Risk and DDT: No Verdict Yet. *Science News*, April 23, 1994.

16. Tulinius, H., Egilsson, V., Olafsdottir, Gudrider, Sidvaldason. Risk of prostate, ovarian, and endometrial cancer among relatives with breast cancer. *BMJ*, Oct.10,1995.855-57.

17. Einbeigi, Z. et al. Clustering of individuals with both breast and ovarian cancer – a possible indicator of BRCA founder mutations. *Acta Oncol*, 2002; 41(2):153-57.

18. *Lifetime Health Letter*, University of Texas. October, 1992.

19. Payson, R.A. Regulation of a promoter of the fibroblast growth factor 1 gene in prostate and breast cancer cells. *J Steroid Biochem Mol Biol*. 1998 Aug;66(3):93-103.

20. Li, S.L. et al. Expression of insulin-like growth factor (IGF)-II in human prostate, breast, bladder, and paraganglioma tumors. *Cell Tissue Res*, Mar;291(3):469-79.

21. Ekbom, A. Growing evidence that several human cancers may originate in utero. *Semin Cancer Biol*, 1998. Aug;8(4):237-44.

22. Saltzstein, S.L. The association of ethnicity and the incidence of mammary carcinoma in situ in women: 11,436 cases from the California Cancer Registry. *Cancer Detect Prev*, 1997;21(4):361-9.

23. Paskett, E.D., et al. Cancer screening behaviors of low-income women: the impact of race. *Women's Health*, 1997. Fall-Winter;(3-4): 203-26.

24. Vatten, L.J. et al. Birth weight as a predictor of breast cancer: a case control study in Norway. *Br J Cancer*, 2002; Jan;86(1):89-91.

25. McCormack, V.A. et al. Fetal growth and subsequent risk of breast cancer:results from long term follow up of Swedish cohort. *British Medical Journal*, 2003; Feb 1;326:248.

26. Bauer, M.K. et al. Fetal growth rate and placental function. *Mol Cell Endocrinol*, 1998; May 25;140(1-2):115-20.

27. Clapp, J.F. Maternal carbohydrate intake and pregnancy outcome. *Proc Nutr Soc*, 2002; Feb; 61(1):45-50.

28. Owens, J.A. Endocrine and substrate control of fetal growth:placental and maternal influences and insulin-like growth factors. *Reprod Fertil Dev*, 1991;3(5):501-17.

29. Parks, J.S. The ontogeny of growth hormone sensitivity. *Horm Res*, 2001; 55 Suppl 2:27-31.

30. Reddy, S. et al. The influence of maternal vegetarian diet on essential fatty acid staus of the newborn. *Eur J Clin Nutr*,1994; May;48(5):358-68.

31. Anonymous. Breast cancer and body shape. *Annals of Internal Medicine*, 1990;112:182-86.

32. MacDonald, P. Effect of obesity on conversion of plasma androstenedione to estrone in post-menopausal women with and without endometrial cancer. *Am J Obstet Gyneco*, 1978;130:448.

33. Van den Brandt, P.A., et al. Pooled analysis of prospective cohort studies on height, weight, and breast cancer risk. *Am J Epidemiol*, 2000 Sep15; 152(6):514-27.

34. Petrelli, J.M., et al. Body mass index, height, and postmenopausal breast cancer mortality in a prospective cohort of U.S. women. *Cancer Causes and Control*, 2002; May; 13(4):325-32.

35. Huang, Z. Waist circumference, waist:hip ratio, and risk of breast cancer in the Nurses' Health Study. *Am J Epidemiol*, 1999; Dec15;150(12):1316-24.

36. Kaaks, R. et al. Breast cancer incidence in relation to height, weight and body-fat distribution in the Dutch "DOM" cohort. *Int J Cancer*, 1998; May 29;76(5):647-51.

37. Schmitz, K.H. Effects of a 9-month strength training intervention on insulin, insulin-like growth factor (IGF)-1, IGF-binding protein (IGFBP)-1, and IGFBP-3 in 30-50-year–old women. *Cancer Epidemiol Biomarkers Prev*, 2002, Dec;11(12):1597-1604.

38. Huang, Z. Waist circumference, waist:hip ratio, and risk of breast cancer in the Nurses' Health Study. *Am J Epidemiol*, 1999; Dec15;150(12):1316-24.

39. Hoy, C. The Truth about Breast Cancer. Don Mills, ON: Stoddart, 1995.

40. Love, S. *Dr. Susan Love's Breast Book*. Don Mills, ON: Addison-Wesley Publishing Co.,1995:128.

41. Kelly, P. *Understanding Breast Cancer Risk*. Philadelphia, PA: Temple University, 1991.

42. Ungar, S. What about Estriol? *Menopause News*, March/April 1998 Vol.8 Issue 2, Madison Pharmacy Associates Inc.

43. Anonymous. *New England Journal of Medicine*, 1993;328:176.

44. Chris, J. Women who breastfeed. *American Health*, April, 1994.

45. Galetin-Smith, Pavkov, S. and Roncevic, N. DDT and PCBs in human milk: implication for breast-feeding infants. *Bulletin of Environmental Contaminant Toxicology*. 1989;43:641-646.

46. Allsopp, M., R. Stringer, P. Johnston. *Unseen Poisons: Levels of Organochlorine Pollutants in Human Tissues*. Exeter, UK: Greenpeace Research Laboratories, Dept. of Biological Sciences, University of Exeter, 1998:33.

47. Yurko, J., J. Millington. Increased breast milk toxicity in women of the Arctic: causes and methods for reduction. Toronto, ON: Canadian College of Naturopathic Medicine, April, 1999.

48. Colborn, Theo, D. Dumanoski, J. Peterson Myers. *Our Stolen Future*. New York, NY: Penguin, 1996: 107.

49. Colborn, Theo, D. Dumanoski, J. Peterson Myers. *Our Stolen Future*. New York, NY: Penguin, 1996:107.

50. Steingraber, Sandra. *Living Downstream: An Ecologist Looks at Cancer and the Environment*. Reading, MA: Addison-Wesley Publishing Co. Ltd., 1997:238.

51. Anonymous.Toxins found in breast milk. *Owen Sound Sun Times*, Dec. 26, 1998. From research published in the Dec. 20 edition of *Chemical Research in Toxicology*.

52. Greenpeace. *Death in Small Doses. The Effects of Organochlorines on Aquatic Ecosystems*. 1992.

53. Coleman, C., D. Lerman. Environmental toxins in breast milk. Toronto, ON: Canadian College of Naturopathic Medicine, April, 1999.

54. Moller Jensen, O, B. et al. *Atlas of Cancer Incidence in the Nordic Countries*. Helsinki, Finland: Nordic Cancer Union, 1988.

55. Translation of a German study presented to me by Bernd Rohlf from Bona Dea Ltd., Dec. 8, 1999. The original study was done by Dr. Maiwald of Wurzburg, Germany.

56. Kelsey, J. and M. Gammon. The epidemiology of breast cancer. *A Cancer Journal for Clinicians*, 1991;41:146-65.

57. Willet, W. The search for the causes of breast and colon cancer. *Nature*, 1989;338:389-93.

58. LaCecchia, C.L. et al. Reproductive factors and breast cancer: An overview. *Soz Praventivmed*, 1989;34:101-107.

59. National cancer Institute. Surveillance, Epidemiology, and End Results Program, 1973-1996, Division of Cancer Control and Population Sciences, *National Cancer Institute*, DEVCAN Software, Version 4.0, National Cancer Institute.

60. Boyd, N.F. et al. Heritability of mammographic density, a risk factor for breast cancer. *N Engl J Med*, 2002, Sept.,19;347(12):886-94.

61. Boyd, N.F. et al. Heritability of mammographic density, a risk factor for breast cancer. *N Engl J Med*, 2002, Sept.,19;347(12):886-94.

62. Byrne, C. Plasma insulin-like growth factor (IGF) 1, IGF-binding protein 3, and mammographic density. *Cancer Res*, 2000, July;15;60(14):3744-48.

63. Vachon, C.M., et al Association of mammo-graphically defined percent breast density with epidemiological risk factors for breast cancer. *Cancer Causes Control*, 2000, Aug:11(7):653-62.

64. Sala, E. et al. High risk mammographic parenchymal patterns and diet: a case-control study. *Br J Cancer,*2000, July:83(1):121-26.

65. Vachon, C.M., et al Association of mammo-graphically defined percent breast density with epidemiological risk factors for breast cancer. *Cancer Causes Control*, 2000, Aug:11(7):653-62.

66. Knight, J.A. Macronutrient intake and change in mammographic density at menopause:results from a randomized trial. *Cancer Epidemio Biomarkers Prev.* 1999, Feb.;8(2):123-28.

67. Brisson, J. Diet, mammographic features of breast tissue, and breast cancer risk. *Am J Epidemiol*, 1989, July,130(1):12-24.

68. Thune, Inger, T. Brenn, E. Lund, M. Gaard. Physical activity and the risk of breast cancer. *New England Journal of Medicine*, May 1, 1997;336(18):1269-1275, 1311.

69. Jancin, B. Exercise study may point to hor-mones as the breast cancer culprit. *Family Practise News.* 1994;Nov.1;5.

70. Marcus, P.M., et al. Physical activity at age 12 and adult breast cancer risk (United States). *Cancer Causes Control*, 1999;Aug;10(4):293-302.

71. Schmitz, K.H. Effects of a 9-month strength training intervention on insulin, insulin-like growth factor (IGF)-1, IGF-binding protein (IGFBP)-1, and IGFBP-3 in 30-50-year–old women. *Cancer Epidemiol Biomarkers Prev*, 2002, Dec;11(12):1597-1604.

72. Brandes, L.J. Stimulation of malignant growth in rodents by antidepressant drugs at clinically relevant doses. *Cancer Research*, 1992;52:3796-3800.

73. *Physician's Desk Reference.* Montvale, N.J.: Medical Economics Data Production Company, 1996:1577-1579.

74. Anonymous. Depressing News. Toronto *Globe and Mail*, Thursday, Feb 14, 2002.

75. Williams, R.R., et al. Case-control study of anti-hypertensive and diuretic use by women with malignant and benign breast lesions detected in a mammography screening program. *Journal of the National Cancer Institute*, 1978;61:327-335.

76. Fitzpatrick, A.L. Use of calcium channel block-ers and breast carcinoma risk in post-menopausal women.*Cancer*, 1997, Oct. 15;80(8):1435-47.

77. Danielson, D.A., et al. Metronidazole and can-cer. *Journal of the American Medical Association*, 1982;247(18):2498-2499.

78. Erturk, E., et al. Transplantable rat mammary tumors induced by 5-nitro-2-furaldehyde semi-carbazone and by formic acid 2[4-(5-nitro-furyl)-2-thiazolyl]hydrazyde. *Cancer Research*, 1970;30:1409-12.

79. Stoll, B.A. (ed.) *Psychosomatic Factors and Their Growth from Risk Factors in Breast Cancer.* Chicago: Yearbook Medical Publishers, 1976:193.

80. *Breast Cancer: Research and Programs.* National Cancer Institute, June, 1993.

81. Sneden, Suzanne. Bioassays: Examples of chemicals that cause breast cancer tumors in laboratory animals. Program on Breast Cancer and Environmental Risk Factors in New York State. April 26, 2003. http://envirocancer.cor-nell.edu//FactSheet/General/fs45.chemical.cfm.

82. Newman, T.B. and S.B. Hully. Carcinogenicity of lipid-lowering drugs. *Journal of the American Medical Association,* 1996;275(1):55-60.

83. Smedley, H.M. Malignant breast change in man given two drugs associated with breast hyper-plasia. *Lancet,*1981;2:638-639.

84. Fackelmann, K.A. Do antihistamines spur can-cer growth? *Science News*, 1994, May 21:324.

85. Hong, C.H. et al. Evaluation of natural products on inhibition of inducible cyclooxygenase (COX-2) and nitric oxide synthase (iNOS) in cultured mouse macrophage cells. *J Ethnopharmaol* 2002; Nov;83(1-2):153-159.

86. Lin, N. et al. Triptolide, a novel diterpenoid triepoxide from Tripterygium wilfordii Hook, f., suppresses the production and gene expression of pro-matrix metalloproteinases 1 and 3 and augments those of tissue inhibitors of metallopro-teinases 1 and 2 in human synovial fibroblasts. *Arthritis Rheum*, 2001, Sept.;44(9):2193-2200.

87 Danz,H. et al. Quantitative determination of the dual COX-2/5-LOX inhibitor trytanthrin in Isatis tinctoria by ESI-LC-MS. *Planta Med*, 2002, Feb.;68(2):152-157.

88. Chrubasik, S. et al. Treatment of low back pain with a herbal or synthetic anti-rheumatic: a randomized controlled study. Willow bark extract for low back pain. *Rheumatology (Oxford)*, 2001, Dec.;40(12):1388-1393.

89. Picard, A. Ibuprofen can cut breast cancer risk, study says. Toronto *Globe and Mail* , April 9 2003, A1- A2.

90. Petrakis, N.L. & E.B. King. 1981. Cytological abnormalities in nipple aspirates of breast fluid from women with severe constipation. *Lancet*, 1981;ii:1203-05.

91. Ross, W.S. Crusade: The Official History of the American Cancer Society. New York: Arbor House, 1987:96

92. Smigel, K. Perception of risk heightens stress of breast cancer screening. *Journal of the National Cancer Institute*, 1993;85(7):525-26.
93. Gastrin, G., et al. Preliminary results of primary screening for breast cancer with incidence and mortality from breast cancer in the Mama program. *Sozial- und Praventivmedizin*, 1993:38(5):280-87.
94. Egan K.M. et al. Active and passive smoking in breast cancer: prospective results from the Nurses' Health Study. *Epidemiology*, 2002, March;13(2):138-145.
95. Khuder, S.A. Is there an association between passive smoking and breast cancer? *Eur J Epidemiol* 2000;16(12):1117-1121.
96. Sorensen, L.T. et al. Smoking as a risk factor for wound healing and infection in breast cancer surgery. *Eur J Surg Oncol*, 2002, Dec;28(8):815-820.
97. Epstein, S. and D. Steinman. *The Breast Cancer Prevention Program*. New York, NY: Macmillan, 1997:226-31
98. Epstein, S. and D. Steinman. *The Breast Cancer Prevention Program*. New York, NY: Macmillan, 1997:133-41.

Chapter 2: Getting to Know Our Breasts

1. Harvey, B.J., A. Miller, C. Baines, P. Corey. Effects of breast self-examination on the risk of death from breast cancer. *Can Med Assoc J*, Nov.1, 1997:157 (9), 1205-12, 1225-26.
2. Canadian Medical Association. Clinical practice guidelines for the care and treatment of breast cancer. *Can Med Assoc J*, Feb. 10, 1998;158 (3 Suppl)S5.
3. Sem, B.C. Pathologico-anatomical and clinical investigations of fibroadenomatosis cystica ammae, and its relation to other pathological conditions in mammae especially cancer. *Acta Chir Scand.*, 1928;64(suppl 10):1-484.
4. Kramer, W.M., B.F. Rush, Jr. Mammary duct proliferation in the elderly; a histopathologic study. *Cancer*, 1973;31:130-37.
5. Peters, F., W. Schuth, B. Schevrich, M. Breckwoldt. Serum prolactin levels in patients with fibrocystic breast disease. *Obstet. Gynecol*, 1984;64:381-85.
6. Ciatto, S., et al. Risk of breast cancer subsequent to proven gross cystic disease. *Eur Jour Cancer*, 1990;26(5):555-57.
7. Modan, B., et al. Breast cancer following benign breast disease - a nationwide study. *Breast Cancer Research and Treatment*, 1997;46(1):45.
8. Guiltinan, J. Naturopathic management of fibrocystic breast disease. *The Journal of Naturopathic Medicine*, 1997;7(1):95-98.
9. Vishnyakova, V.V., N. Murav-yeva. On the treatment of dyshormonal hyperplasia of mammary glands. *Vestn USSR Akad Med Sci*, 19666;21:26-31.
10. Furlanetto, T.W. Estradiol increases proliferation and down-regulates the sodium/iodide symporter gene in FRTL-5 cells. *Endocrinology.* 1999 Dec.;140(12):5705-5711.
11. Eskin, B.A. et al. Different tissue responses for iodine and iodide in rat thyroid and mammary glands. *Biological Trace Element Research.* 1995; 49:9-19.
12. Krouse, B. et al Age –related changes in resembling fibrocystic disease in iodine-blocked rat breasts. *Arch Pathol Lab Med.* 1979, Nov.;103:631-634.
13. Minton, J. Caffeine, cyclic nucleotides and breast disease. *Surgery*, 86,1979:105.
14. Brooks, P. Measuring the effect of caffeine restriction on fibrocystic breast disease. *J Reprod Med*, 1981; 26:279.
15. Goldin, B., H. Adlerkreutz, J. Dwyer, et al. Effect of diet on excretion of estrogens in pre and post-menopausal women. *Cancer Res*, 1981;41:3771-73.
16. Love, S. *Dr. Susan Love's Breast Book*. New York, NY: Addison-Wesley Publishing Co. 1995:130-17. Page, D.L., Dupont, W.D. Intraductal carcinoma of the breast. *Cancer*, 1982; 49:751.
18. Wheeler, J.E.W., et al. Lobular carcinoma in situ of the breast: Long term follow-up. *Cancer*, 1974;34:554.
19. Rosen, P.P., Lieberman, P.H., Braun, D.W. Lobular carcinoma of the breast. *American Journal of Surgical Pathology.* 1987; 2:225.
20. Breast Cancer: grading and staging. http://medlib.med.utah.edu/WebPath/TUTORI-AL/BREAST/BREAST.html. May 13,2003.
21. Breast Cancer: grading and staging. http://medlib.med.utah.edu/WebPath/TUTORI-AL/BREAST/BREAST.html. May 13,2003.
22. Love, Susan. *Dr. Susan Love's Breast Book*. New York, N.Y. Perseus Publishing, 2000: 343.
23. Von Tempelhoff, G.F., F. Nieman, L. Heilmann, G. Hommel. Association between blood rheopogy, thrombosis and cancer survival in patients with gynecologic malignancy. *Clin Hemorheol Microcirc*, 2000; 22(2):107-130.
24. Dirix, L.Y. et al. Plasma fibrin D-dimer levels correlate with tumor volume, progression rate and survival in patients with metastatic breast cancer. *Br J Cancer*, 2002, Feb. 1;86(3):389-395.

25. Simpson-Haidaris, P.J., B. Rybarczyk. Tumors and fibrinogen. The role of fibrinogen as an extracellular matrix protein. *Ann N Y Acad Sci*, 2001; 936:406-425.

26. Breast Cancer: grading and staging. http://medlib.med.utah.edu/WebPath/TUTORIAL/BREAST/BREAST.html. May 13,2003.

27. Health Canada. Clinical practise guidelines for the care and treatment of breast cancer: a Canadian consensus document. *Can Med Assoc J.*, Feb. 10, 1998;1158 (3 Supp)S5.

28. Love, S. What we really know about breast cancer and HRT. *Alternative Therapies*, Sept, 1997:3(5)82-90.

29. Health Canada. Clinical practise guidelines for the care and treatment of breast cancer: a Canadian consensus document. *Can Med Assoc J.*, Feb. 10, 1998;1158 (3 Suppl)S5.

30. Love, S. What we really know about breast cancer and HRT. *Alternative Therapies*, Sept 1997:3(5)82-90.

31. Whitaker, Julian. Preventing breast cancer: Let's clear up the confusion on mammograms. *Alive*, April, 1999:16-17.

32. Love, S. *Dr. Susan Love's Breast Book*. Don Mills, ON: Addison-Wesley Publishing Co.,1995:128.

33. Baines, C. et al. Impact of menstrual phase on false-negative mammograms in the Canadian National Breast Screening Study. *Cancer,* 1997 August 15;80(4):720-24.

34. Health Canada. Clinical practise guidelines for the care and treatment of breast cancer: a Canadian consensus document. *Can Med Assoc J.*, Feb. 10, 1998;1158 (3 Supp)S3.

35. Clorfene-Casten, Liane. *Breast Cancer: Poisons, Profits and Prevention*. Monroe, ME: Common Courage Press, 1996:107.

36. Thornwaite, J.T. Anti-malignin antibody in serum and other tumor marker determination in breast cancer. *Cancer Letters,* 2000, Jan.1, 148(1):39-48.

37. Abstract #3318. Scientific Proceedings. 87th Annual Meeting of the American Association for Cancer Research. Washington, DC., 1996, April 20-24.

38. Botti, C., A. Martivetti, S. Nerini-Molteni, L. Ferrari. Anti-malignin antibody evaluation: a possible challenge for cancer management. *Int J Biol Markers*, 1997, Oct.-Dec;12(4):141-47.

39. Requisition for AMAS Determination and information sheet from Oncolab, Boston; 1-800-9-CATest.

40. Ultra-sensitive breast cancer blood test developed. PRNewswire. Huntington Valley, PA., Feb. 20, 1999.

41. Infrared imaging as a useful adjunct to mammography. *Oncology News International*, Sept, 1997:6(9).

42. Leandro, P. Position paper on digital infrared imaging of the breast. http://www.meditherm.com/breasthealth/research.htm. 1999:1-7.

43. Head, J.F., F. Wang, R.L. Elliott. Breast thermography is a noninvasive prognostic procedure that predicts tumor growth rate in breast cancer patients. *Ann N Y Acad Sc*, 1993:Nov.30;698:153-58.

44. Sterns, E.E., B. Zee, S. SenGupta, F.W. Saunders. Thermography. Its relation to pathologic characteristics, vascularity, proliferation rate, and survival of patients with invasive ductal carcinoma of the breast. *Cancer*, 1996:Apr 1;77(7):1324-28.

45. Turnbull, Barbara. Laser detects breast cancer. *Toronto Star*, Jan. 27, 2000:A2.

46. Grable, R. Medical optical imaging: A status review. http://www.imds.com/moi.htm. July 1997:3.

47. Hindle, William. Fine needle aspiration of a palpable breast mass: current technology and techniques. Ottawa, ON: World Conference on Breast Cancer, oral presentation, July, 1999.

48. Molina, R., et al. C-erbB-2, CEA and CA 15.3 serum levels in the early diagnosis of recurrence of breast cancer patients. *Anticancer Res*, 1999:Jul-Aug;19(4A):2551-55.

49. Ebeling, F.C., et al. Tumor markers CEA and CA 15-3 as prognostic factors in breast cancer - univariate and multivariate analysis. *Anticancer Res*, 1999:Jul-Aug;19(4A):2545-50.

50. Fogel, M. et al. CD24 is a marker for human breast carcinoma. *Cancer Letters*, 1999:Aug 23;143(1).

Chapter 3: Understanding the Hormone Puzzle

1. Meyer, F., et al. Endogenous sex hormones, prolactin, and breast cancer in premenopausal women. *J Natl Cancer Inst*, 1986 Sep;77(3):613-16.

2. Katzenellenbogen, B.S. Biology and receptor interactions of estriol and estriol derivatives in vitro and in vivo. *J Steroid Biochem*, 1984, Apr;20(4B):1033-37.

3. Gillson, G., Marsden, T. *You've Hit Menopause: Now What?* Calgary, Alberta. Blitzprint, 2003. p. 39.

4. Shiuan, C. Aromatase and breast cancer. *Frontiers in Bioscience,* 1998 Aug 6; 3:d922-933.

5. Kellis, J.T., L.E. Vickery. Inhibition of human estrogen synthetase (aromatase) by flavones. *Science,* 1984 Sep; 225(4666):1032-1034.

6. Saarinen, N.M. et al. Enterolactone inhibits the growth of 7,12-dimethylbenz(a) anthracene-induced mammary carcinomas in the rat. *Mol Cancer Ther,* 2000 Aug; 1(10):869-876.

7. Om, A.S., K.W. Chung. Dietary zinc deficiency alters 5 alpha-reduction and aromatization of testosterone and androgen and estrogen receptor in rat liver. *J Nutr,* 1996 Apr; 126(4):842-848.

8. Follingstead, A.H., Estriol: The forgotten estrogen? *JAMA,* Jan. 2, 1978; 239,1:29-30.

9. Zumoff, B. Hormone profiles in hormone-dependent cancers. *Cancer Res,* 1975;35:3365.

10. Fractionated Estrogen, 1998. Handout from Meridian Valley Clinical Laboratory.

11. Bradlow, H.L. et al. Long-term responses of women to indole-3-carbinol or a high fiber diet. *Cancer Epidemiol Biomarkers Prev,* 1994 Oct-Nov; 3(7):591-595.

12. Lemon, H.M. Pathophysiologic considerations in the treatment of menopausal patients with oestrogens: the role of oestriol in the prevention of mammary carcinoma. *Acta Endocrinol (Copenh),* 1980;233:S17-S27.

13. Longcope, C. Estriol production and metabolism in normal women. *J Steroid Biochemistry,* 1984;20:959-62.

14. Cos S., E.J. Sanchez-Barcelo. Melatonin inhibition of MCF-7 human breast-cancer cells growth: influence of cell proliferation rate. *Cancer Lett,* 1995;Jul 13(2):207-12.

15. Barnard, N.D., A.R. Scialli, D. Hurlock, P. Bertron. Diet and sex-hormone binding globulin, dysmenorrheal, and premenstrual symptoms. *Obstet Gynecol,* 2000 Feb; 95(2):245-250.

16. Cassidy, A. Potential tissue selectivity of dietary phytoestrogens and estrogens. *Curr Opin Lipidol,* 1999; 10:47-52.

17. Longcope, C. Estriol production and metabolism in normal women. *J Steroid Biochemistry,* 1984;20:959-62.

18. Arnold, S. et al. Synergistic activation of estrogen receptor with combination of environmental chemicals *Science,* vol 272, June 7, 1966:1489-91.

19. Body burden: The pollution in people. Executive summary: What we found. Environmental Working Group, 2003. Washington, D.C. http://www.ewg.org/reports/bodyburden/es.php.

20. Dewaillly, E, et al. Could the rising levels of estrogen receptors in breast cancer be due to estrogenic pollutants? *Journal of the National Cancer Institute,* 1997;89(12):888.

21. Ho, GH, XW Luo, CY Ji, EH Ng. Urinary 2/16 alpha-hydroxyestrone ratio: correlation with a serum insulin-like growth factor binding protein-3 and a potential marker of breast cancer risk. *Annual Acad Med Singapore,* 1998. Mar;27(2):294-99.

22. Schneider, J., D. Kinne, A. Fracchia, et al. *Proceedings of the National Academy of Sciences,* 1982;79:3047-51.

23. Michnovicz, J. *How to Reduce Your Risk of Breast Cancer.* New York, NY: Warner Books, 1994:82.

24. Davis, D. L. & H. Bradlow. Can environmental estrogens cause breast cancer? *Scientific American,* Oct. 1995:168.

25. Pizzorno, J., and M. Murray. *A Textbook of Natural Medicine.* Seattle, WA: John Bastyr College Publications,1987: IV-2 Immune Support.

26. Davis, D.L., & H. Bradlow. Can environmental estrogens cause breast cancer? *Scientific American,* Oct. 1995:168.

27. Gorbach, S. Estrogens, breast cancer and intestinal flora. *Rev Infect Dis 6 (Suppl I),* 1984:S85.

28. Goldin, B. Estrogen excretion patterns and plasma levels in vegetarian and omnivorous women. *N Engl J Med,* 1982;307:1542.

29. Goldin, B. Estrogen excretion patterns and plasma levels in vegetarian and omnivorous women. *N Engl J Med,* 1982;307:1542.

30. Goldin, B. Estrogen excretion patterns and plasma levels in vegetarian and omnivorous women. *N Engl J Med,* 1982;307:1542.

31. Cohen, L.A., et al. Wheat bran and psyllium diets: Effects on N-methylnitrosoura-induced mammary tumorigenesis in F344 rats. *J Natl Cancer Inst,* 1996 Jul;88(13):899-907.

32. Waalaszek, Z., et al. Dietary glucarate as anti-promoter of 7,12-dimethylben(a)anthracene-induced mammary tumorigenesis. *Carcinogenesis,* 1986 Sep;7(9):1463-66.

33. Lemon, H.M. Pathophysiologic consideration in the treatment of menopausal patients with oestrogens; the role of oestriol in the prevention of mammary carcinoma. *Acta Endocrinol(Copenh),* 1980;233:S17-S27.

34. Head, K. Estriol: Safety and efficacy. *Alternative Medicine Review,* 1998;3(2):101-13.

35. Pratt, J.H., C. Longcope. Estriol production rates and breast cancer. *J Clin Endocrinol Metab,* 1978;46:44-47.

36. Lemon, H.M. et al. Reduced estriol excretion in patients with breast cancer prior to endocrine therapy. *JAMA,* April 21,1978;249(16):1638-41.

37. More about that 1 in 8 breast cancer statistic, *Health Facts*, May, 1993.
38. Clavel-Chapelon, F., G. Launoy, A. Auquier et al. Reproductive factors and breast cancer risk. Effect of age at diagnosis. *Ann Epidemiol*, 1995;5:315-20.
39. Kagawa, Y. Impact of westernization on the nutrition of the Japanese: Changes in physique, cancer, longevity and centenarians. *Prev Med J*, 1978;7:205.
40. Frommer, D. Changing age of menopause. *Br Med J*, 1964;2:349.
41. Armstrong, B. Diet and reproductive hormones: a study of vegetarian and non-vegetarian post-menopausal women. *JNCI*, 1981;67:761.
42. Staszewski, J. Age at menarche and breast cancer. *J Natl Cancer Inst*, 1971;47:935.
43. Trichopoulos, D. Menopause and breast cancer risk. *J Natl Cancer Inst*, 1972;48:605.
44. National Research Council. *Biomarkers in Reproductive Toxicology*. Washington, DC: National Academy of Sciences, 1991.
45. *Rachel's Environment and Health Weekly*. Environment Research Foundation, Oct. 2, 1997, #566.
46. Herman-Giddens, M., et al. Secondary sexual characteristics and menses in young girls seen in office practice: A study from the pediatric research in office settings network. *Pediatrics*, 1997;99(4):505-12.
47. MacMahon, B, D. Trichopoulos, D. Brown et al. Age at menarche, urine estrogens and breast cancer risk. *Int J Cancer*, 1982;30:427-31.
48. Stoll, B.A. Western diet, early puberty, and breast cancer risk. *Breast Cancer Research and Treatment*, 1998;49:187-93.
49. Apter, F., M. Reinila, R. Vikho. Some endocrine characteristics of early menarche, a risk factor for breast cancer, are preserved into adulthood. *Int J Cancer*, 1989;44:783-87.
50. Boyce, Nell. Growing up too soon. *New Scientist*, Aug. 2, 1997:5.
51. Colon, I., et al Identification of phthalate esters in the serum of young Puerto Rican girls with premature breast development. *Environ Health Perspect*, 2000 Sep; 108(9):895-900.
52. Apter, D, I. Sipila. Development of children and adolescents; physiological, pathophysiological and therapeutic aspects. *Curr Opin Obstet Gynec*, 1993;51:764-73.
53. Stoll, B.A. et al. Does early physical maturity increase breast cancer risk? *Acta Oncologica*, 1994;33(2); 171-76.
54. Apter, D. Hormonal events during female puberty in relation to breast cancer risk. *European Journal of Cancer*, 1996;5(6):476-82.

55. Brown, H. The other reward of exercise. *Health*, July, 1994.
56. Whelan, E. Menstruation and reproductive history study. *American Journal of Epidemiology*, December 15, 1994.
57. Pill ups cancer risk in young women. *Science News*, June 10, 1995.
58. Oral contraceptive use and breast cancer risk in young women. *Lancet*, 1989:973-82.
59. Rinzler, C. *Estrogen and Breast Cancer: A Warning to Women*. London, UK: Macmillan,1993.
60. Stanford, J. & D. Thomas. Exogenous estrogens and breast cancer. *Epidemiological Reviews*, 1993;15(1):98-105.
61. Beral, V., D. Bull, R. Doll, T. Key, G. Reeves. Breast cancer and hormone replacement therapy: collaborative reanalysis of data from 51 epidemiological studies of 52,705 women with breast cancer and 108,411 women without breast cancer. *Lancet*, 1997;350:1047-58, 1042-43.
62. Lee, John R. *What Your Doctor May Not Tell You About Menopause*. New York, NY: Time Warner, Inc., 1996:323.
63. Venn, A., et al. Risk of cancer after use of fertility drugs with in-vitro fertilization. *Lancet*, 1999 Nov 6; 354(9190):1586-90.
64. *National Women's Health Network News*, May/June 1990.
65. Colborn, Theo, D. Dumanoski, J. Peterson Myers. *Our Stolen Future*. New York, NY: Penguin, 1996:65.
66. Ekbom, A., D. Trichopoulous, et al. Evidence of prenatal influences on breast cancer risk. *Lancet*, 1992;340:1015-18.
67. Hsieh, C., S. Lan, A. Ekbom, E. Petridou, and H. Adami. (1992) Twin membership and breast cancer risk. *American Journal of Epidemiology*, 136:1321-26.
68. Setchell, K., L. Zimmer-Nchemias, J. Cai, J. Heubi. Exposure of infants to phyto-oestrogens from soy-based infant formula. *Lancet*, July 5, 1997;350:23-27.
69. Lee, John R. *What Your Doctor May Not Tell You About Menopause*. New York, NY: Time Warner, Inc., 1996:323.
70. Cowan, L.D., L. Gordis, J. A. Tonasia, and G,S, Jones. Breast cancer incidence in women with a history of progesterone deficiency. *American Journal of Epidemiology*, 1981;114:209-17.
71. Boulakoud, M.S. et al The toxicological effects of the herbicide 2,4-DCPA on progesterone levels and mortality in Wistar female rats. *Meded Rijksuniv Gent Fak Landbouwkd Toegep Biol Wet*, 2001; 66(2b):891-95.

72. Foster, W.G., et al. Hexachlorobenzene (HCB) suppresses circulating progesterone concentrations during the luteal phase in the cynomolgus monkey. *J Appl Toxicol*, 1992;12:13-17.

73. Bergkvist, L., H.-O. Adami, I. Persson, R. Hoover, and C. Schairer. The risk of breast cancer after estrogen and estrogen-progestin replacement. *New England Journal of Medicine*, 1989;321:293-97.

74. Lee, John R. *What Your Doctor May Not Tell You About Menopause*. New York, NY: Time Warner, Inc., 1996:323.

75. Zava, D., C. Dullbaum, M. Blen. Estrogen and progestin bioactivity of foods, herbs and spices. *Biol Med*, 1998;217(3):369-78.

76. Brun, J., B. Claustrat, M. David. Urinary melatonin, LH, oestradiol, progesterone excretion during the menstrual cycle or in women taking oral contraceptives. *Acta Endocrinol (Copenh)*, 1987, Sept;116(1):145-49.

77. McMichael-Phillips, D.F., et al. Effects of soy supplementation on epithelial proliferation in the histologically normal human breast. *American Journal of Clinical Nutrition*. 1998;68(6 Suppl):1431S-1435S.

78. Phipps, W.R. et al. Effect of flaxseed ingestion on the menstrual cycle. *J Clin Endocrinol Metab*, 1993; 77(5):1215-19.

79. Holmes, P. *The Energetics of Western Herbs*. Vol. II. 2nd. ed. Berkeley, CA: NatTrop Publishing, 1993:753.

80. Erichsen-Brown, C. *Medicinal and Other Uses of North American Plants: A Historical Survey with Special References to the Eastern Indian Tribes*. New York, NY: Dover Publications, Inc., 1995.

81. Reichert, R., Comparing Vitex and vitamin B6 for PMS. *Quarterly Review of Natural Medicine*, 1998;19-20

82. Weed, Susun. *Menopausal Years - The Wise Woman Way*. Woodstock, NY: Ash Tree Publishing, 1992:107-08.

83. Reichert, R. Comparing Vitex and vitamin B6 for PMS. *Quarterly Review of Natural Medicine*. 1998;19-20.

84. Reichert, R., Comparing Vitex and vitamin B6 for PMS. *Quarterly Review of Natural Medicine*, 1998;19-20.

85. Carr, C. Keep your (hormonal) balance. *Conscious Choice: The Journal of Ecology and Natural Living*, 1998;11(2):55.

86. Kamada et al. Effect of dietary selenium supplementaion on the plasma progesterone concentration in cows. *Journal of Veterinary Medicine and Science*, 1998;60(1):133-35.

87. Jato, I. Neoadjuvant progesterone therapy for primary breast cancer: rationale for clinical trial. *Clinical Therapies*, 1997;19(1):56-61, discussion 2-3.

88. Formby, B., T.S. Wiley. Bcl-2, survivin, and variant CD44 v7-v10 are downregulated and p53 is upregulated in breast cancer cells by progesterone: inhibition of cell growth and induction of apoptosis. *Mol Cell Biochem*, 1999 Dec;202(1-2):53-61.

89. Hyder, S.M., C. Chiappetta, G.M. Stancel. Pharmacological and endogenous progestins induce vascular endothelial growth factor expression in human breast cancer cells. *Int J Cancer*, 2001 May 15; vol. 92(4):469-73.

90. Wiebe, J.P. et al. The 4-pregnene and 5alpha-pregnane progesterone metabolites formed in nontumorous and tumorous breast tissue have opposite effects on breast proliferation and adhesion. *Cancer Research*, 2000 Feb 15;60(4):936-43.

91. Meyer, F., et al. Endogenous sex hormones, prolactin, and breast cancer in premenopausal women. *J Natl Cancer Inst*, 1986 Sep;77(3):613-16.

92. Meyer, F., et al. Endogenous sex hormones, prolactin, and mammographic features of breast tissue in premenopausal women. *J Natl Cancer Inst*, 1986 Sep;77(3):617-20.

93. Zumoff, B. Hormonal profiles in women with breast cancer. *Obstet Gynecol Clin North Am*, 1994 Dec;21(4):751-72.

94. Zumoff, B. Hormonal profiles in women with breast cancer.. *Obstet Gynecol Clin North Am*, 1994; 21:751-72.

95. Kleinberg, D.L., W. Ruan, V. Catanese et al. Non-lactogenic effects of growth hormone on growth and IGF-1 messenger mRNA of rat mammary gland. *Endocrinology*, 1990;126:3274-76.

96. Darendeliler, F., P.C. Hindmarsh, M.A. Preece. Growth hormone increases rate of pubertal maturation. *Acta Endocrinol*, 1990;122:414-16.

97. Sharara, F.J., L.C. Giudice. Role of growth hormone in ovarian physiology and onset of puberty. *J Soc Gyne Invest*, 1997;4:2-7.

98. Cauley, J.A., et al. Elevated serum estradiol and testosterone concentrations are associated with a higher risk of breast cancer: Study of osteoporotic fractures research group. *Ann Intern Med*, 1999; 130:270-77.

99. Secreto, G., B. Sumoff. Abnormal production of androgens in women with breast cancer. *Anticancer Res*, 1994; 14:2113-17.

100. Secreto, G., B. Zumoff. Abnormal production of androgens in women with breast cancer. *Anticancer Res,* 1994 Sep-Oct; 14(5B):2113-17.

101. The Doctor's Medical Library. Wilson's Reverse T3 Dominance Syndrome. http://www.medicallibrary.net/sites/-wilson's-syndrome.html. Jan. 15, 1999.

102. Diogo, A., C. Merluza, B. Janczak. Thyroid function and breast cancer. Toronto, ON: Canadian College of Naturopathic Medicine, April, 1999.

103. Kelly, G. Peripheral metabolism of thyroid hormones: a review. *Alt Med Review,* 2000; 5(4):306-33.

104. Brent, G.A. The molecular basis of thyroid hormone action. *New Engl J Med.* 1994; 331:847-53.

105. Pennington, Jean. *Food Values of Portions Commonly Used.* 15th edition. New York, NY: HarperPerennial, 1989: 219-57.

106. Lee, John, David Zava , Virginia Hopkins. *What Your Doctor May Not Tell You About Breast Cancer.* New York, NY: Warner Books Inc., 2002:72.

107. Berkow, R., ed. *The Merck Manual of Medical Information: Home Edition.* New York, NY: Merck and Company Inc., 1997:705.

108. Rose, D.P. Plasma triiodothyronine concentrations and breast cancer. *Cancer,* 1979;43(4):1434-38.

109. Rasmussen, B., et al. Thyroid function in patients with breast cancer. *Eur J Cancer Clin Oncol,* 1986; 22(3):301-07.

110. Gogas, J. et al. *Autoimmune thyroid disease in women with breast carcinoma.* Eur J Surg Oncol, 2001, Nov; 27(7):626-30.

111. Lemaire, M., L. Baugnet-Mahieu. Thyroid function in women with breast cancer. *Eur J Cancer Clin Oncol,* 1986;22(3):301-07.

112. Shering, S.G., et al Thyroid disorders and breast cancer. *Eur J Cancer Prev,* 1996 Dec: 5(6):504-06.

113. Smyth, P.P., et al. A direct relationship between thyroid gland enlargement and breast cancer. *J Clin Endocrinol Metab,* 1996 Mar; 81(3):937-41.

114. Gerson, Max. *A Cancer Therapy: Results of Fifty Cases.* 3rd ed. Del Mar, CA: Totality Books, 1977:100.

115. Kohrle, J. The trace element selenium and the thyroid gland. *Biochimie,* 1999, May;81(5):527-33.

116. Stadel, B.V. Dietary iodine and risk of breast, endometrial and ovarian cancer. *Lancet,* 1976, April 24.

117. Ghent, W.R., et al. Iodine replacement in fibrocystic disease of the breast. *Canc J Surg,* 1993; 36:453-60.

118. Eskin, B.A., Iodine metabolism and breast cancer. *Trans NY Acad Sci,* 1970; 11:911-947.

119. Colborn, Theo, D. Dumanoski, J. Peterson Myers. *Our Stolen Future.* New York, NY: Penguin, 1996:75-80, 188.

120. Colborn, Theo, D. Dumanoski, J. Peterson Myers. *Our Stolen Future.* New York, NY: Penguin, 1996:75-80, 188.

121. Capen, C.C. Mechanisms of chemical injury to the thyroid gland. *Prog Clin Biol Res,* 1994;387:173-91.

122. The Doctor's Medical Library. Wilson's Reverse T3 Dominance Syndrome. http://www.medicallibrary.net/sites/-wilson's-syndrome.html. Jan. 15, 1999.

123. Pizzulli, A, A. Ranjbar. Selenium deficiency and hypothyroidism: a new etiology in the differential diagnosis of hypothyroidism in children. *Biol Trace Elem Res,* 2000 Dec; 77(3):199-208.

124. Colborn, Theo, D. Dumanoski, J. Peterson Myers. *Our Stolen Future.* New York, NY: Penguin, 1996:75-80, 188.

125. Beyssen, M. Antithyroid action of Tamoxifen in the rat: in vivo and in vitro studies. *Pharmacology.* 2000 Jul; 61(1):22-30.

126. Holmes, P. *The Energetics of Western Herbs.* Vol. I. 2nd ed. Berkeley, CA: NatTrop Publishing, 1993: 389-414.

127. DelGiudice, M.E. et al Insulin and related factors in premenopausal breast cancer risk. *Breast Cancer Research Treat,* 1998; 47:111-20.

128. Papa V. et al. Elevated insulin receptor content in human breast cancer. *J Clin Invest,* 1990; 86:1503-10.

129. Nemiroff, H. High insulin associated with breast cancer. *Breast Cancer News,* Dec 7, 2001 e-letter.

130. Kaaks, R. Nutrition, hormones and breast cancer: Is insulin the missing link? *Cancer Causes Control,* 1996; 7:605-25.

131. Kaaka, R. Plasma insulin, IGF-1 and breast cancer. *Gynecol Obstet Fert,* 2001 March; 29(3):185-191.

132. Berrino, F. et al. Reducing bioavailable sex hormones through a comprehensive change in diet: the diet and androgens (DIANA) randomized trial. *Cancer Epidemiol Biomarkers Prev,* 2001 Jan; 10(1):25-33.

133. Kaaka, R. Plasma insulin, IGF-1 and breast cancer. *Gynecol Obstet Fert,* 2001 March; 29(3):185-91.

134. Kaaks, R., A. Lukanova. Energy balance and cancer: the role of insulin and insulin-like growth factor-1. *Proc Nutr Soc,* 2001 Feb; 60(1):91-106.

135. Stoll, B.A. Western nutrition and the insulin resistance syndrome. *Eur J Clin Nutr,* *1999*;Feb;53(2):83-87.

136. Berrino, F. et al. Reducing bioavailable sex hormones through a comprehensive change in diet: the diet and androgens (DIANA) randomized trial. *Cancer Epidemiol Biomarkers Prev,* 2001 Jan; 10(1):25-33.

137. Bereket, A., C.H. Lang, T.A. Wilson. Alterations in the growth hormone-insulin-like growth factor axis in insulin dependent diabetes mellitus. *Hormon Metab Res,* 1999;Feb-Mar;31(2-3):172-81.

138. Shim M., P. Cohen. IGFs and human cancer: Implications regarding the risk of growth hormone therapy. *Hormone Research,* 1999, Nov;51 Suppl S3:42-51.

139. Macaulay, V.M. Insulin like growth factor and cancer. *Br J Cancer,* 1992;65:311-20.

140. Clarke, R.B. et al. Type 1 IGF receptor gene expression in normal breast tissue treated with oestrogen and progesterone. *Br J Cancer,* 1997;75:251-57.

141. Westley, B.R., F.E. May. Role of IGF in steroid-modulated proliferation. *J Ster Biochem Mol Biol.* 1994; 51:1-9.

142. Sachdev, D. and D. Yee. The IGF system and breast cancer. *Endocr Relat Cancer,* 2001 Sept; 8(3):197

143. Hankinson, S. et al. Circulating concentrations of insulin-like growth factor-1 and risk of breast cancer. *Lancet,* 1998;351:1393-96.

144. Yu, H., J. Berkel. Do insulin-like growth factors mediate the effect of alcohol on breast cancer risk? *Med Hypotheses,* 1999;Jun;52(6):491-96.

145. Vadgama, J.V., Y. Yu, G. Datta, H. Khan, R. Chillar. Plasma insulin-like growth factor-1 and serum IGF-binding protein 3 can be associated with the progression of breast cancer, and predict the risk of recurrence and the probability of survival in African-American and Hispanic women. *Oncology,* 1999, Nov;57(4):330-40.

146. Stoll, B.A. Western diet, early puberty, and breast cancer risk. *Breast Cancer Research and Treatment,* 1998;49:187-93.

147. Oh, Y. IGFBPs and neoplastic models. New concepts for roles of IGFBPs in regulation of cancer cell growth. *Endocrine,* 1997, Aug;7(1):111-13.

148. Enriori, P.J. et al. Augmented serum levels of the IGF-1/IGF-binding protein-3 ratio in premenopausal patients with type 1breast cysts. *Eur J Endocrinol,* 2003 Feb; 148(2):177-184.

149. Byrne, C et al. Plasma insulin-like growth factor (IGF) 1, IGF-binding protein 3, and mammographic density. *Cancer Res,* 2000 Jul 15; 60(14):3744-3748.

150. Demori, I., C. Bottazzi, E. Fugassa. Tri-iodothyronine increases insulin-like growth factor binding protein-2 expression in cultured hepatocytes from hypothyroid rats. *J Endocrinol,* 1999;161(3):465-74.

151. Allen, N.E. et al. The associations of diet with serum insulin-like growth factor 1 and its main binding proteins in 292 women meat-eaters, vegetarians and vegans. *Cancer Epidemiol Biomarkers Prev,* 2002 Nov; 11(11):1441-1448.

152. Zava, D. The hormonal link to breast cancer: The estrogen matrix. *Int J Pharmaceut Comp,* 2002 July/Aug; 6(4).

153. Zava, D. The hormonal link to breast cancer: The estrogen matrix. *Int J Pharmaceut Comp,* 2002 July/Aug; 6(4).

154. Turner-Cobb, J.M., et al. Social support and salivary cortisol in women with metastatic breast cancer. *Psychosom Med,* 2000 May-Jun; 62(3):337-345.

155. Sephton, S.E., et al Diurnal cortisol rhythm as a predictor of breast cancer survival. *J Natl Cancer Inst,* 2000 Jun 21; 92(12): 994-1000.

156. Gupta, D., R. Attanasio & R. Reiter. (Eds.) *The Pineal Gland and Cancer.* Tubingen, Germany: Muller and Bass, 1988.

157. Hajdu, S., R. Porro, P. Lieberman & F. Foote. Degeneration of the pineal gland of patients with cancer. *Cancer,* 1972;29:706-09.

158. Lissoni, P., S. Crispino, S. Barni et al. Pineal gland and tumour cell kinetics: serum labelling rate in breast cancer. *Oncology,* 1990;47:3:275-77.

159. Glickman, G, R. Levin, G.C. Brainard. *Ocular input for human melatonin regulation: relevance to breast cancer,* Neuroendocrinology Letter, 2002 Jul., 23 Suppl., 2:17-22.

160. Napoli, M. *Exposure to light at night increases the risk of breast cancer.* Health Facts, Nov. 2001,26(11):3-4.

161. Matsen, Jonn. *The Secrets to Great Health from Your Nine Liver Dwarves.* North Vancouver, B.C.,Goodwin Books, Ltd., 1998:190.

162. Glickman, G, R. Levin, G.C. Brainard. Ocular input for human melatonin regulation: relevance to breast cancer, *Neuroendocrinology Letter,* 2002 Jul., 23 Suppl., 2:17-22.

163. Lissoni, P. et al. Melatonin as a modulator of cancer endocrine therapy. *Front Horm Res.* 1997;23:132-36.

164. Coss, G. Influence of melatonin on invasive and metastatic properties of MCF-7 human breast cancer cells. *Cancer Research,* 1998;58(19):4383-90.

165. Bartsch, C., H. Bartsch, U. Fuchs, et al. Stage-dependent depression of melatonin in patients with primary breast cancer. *Cancer,* 1989;64:426-33.

166. Bartsch, H., C. Bartsch. Effect of melatonin on experimental tumours under different photoperiods and times of administration. *J. Neural. Transm*, 1981;52:269-79.

167. Lissoni, P. et al. Clinical study of melatonin in untreatable advanced cancer patients. *Tumouri*, 1987;73: 475.

168. Lissoni, P., S. Barni, S. Meregalli et al. Modulation of cancer endocrine therapy by melatonin: A phase II study of tamoxifen plus melatonin in metastatic breast cancer patients progression under tamoxifen alone. *Br. J. Cancer*, 1995;71:854-56.

169. MacPhee, A., F. Cole, F. Rice. The effect of melatonin on steroidogenesis by the human ovary in vitro. *J Clin Endocrin Metab*, 1975;40:688-96.

170. Wetterberg, L., J. Arendt, L. Paunier et al. Human serum melatonin changes during the menstrual cycle. *J Clin Endocrin Metab*, 1976;42:185-88.

171. Blask, D., S. Wilson, F. Zalatan. Physiological melatonin inhibition of human breast cancer cell growth in vitro: Evidence for a glutathione-mediated pathway. *Cancer Res*, 1997;57:1909-14.

172. Tamarkin, L., C.J. Baird, O. Almeida. Melatonin: A coordinating signal for mammalian reproduction? *Science*, 1985;227:714-20.

173. Singh, R. *Self-Healing: Powerful Techniques*. London, ON: Health Psychology Associates, 1997:29-30.

174. Singh, R., *Self-Healing: Powerful Techniques*. London, ON: Health Psychology Associates, 1997: 27.

175. Bartsch, C., H. Bartsch. The link between the pineal gland and cancer: an interaction involving chronobiological mechanisms. In Halberg, F. et al. *Chronobiological Approach to Social Medicine*. Rome,Italy: Istitiuto Italiano di Medicina Sociale, 1984:105-26.

176. Carr, D.B., Reppert, S.M. et al. Plasma melatonin increases during exercise in women. *J Clin Endocrinol Metab*, 1981 Jul;53(1):224-25.

177. Rossi, E. *The Psychobiology of Mind-Body Healing*. New York, NY: W.W. Norton, 1986.

178. Shannahoff-Khalsa, D.S., M.R. Boyle, M.E. Buebel. The effects of unilateral forced nostril breathing on cognition. *Int J Neurosci*, 1991;Apr;57(3-4):239-49.

179. Werntz, D.A., R.G, Bickford, D. Shannahoff-Khalsa. Selective hemispheric stimulation by unilateral forced nostril breathing. *Hum Neurobiol*, 1987;6(3):165-71.

180. Massion, A.O., et al. Meditation, melatonin and breast/prostate cancer: hypothesis and preliminary data. *Med Hypothesis*, 1995 Jan;44 (1):39-46.

181. Singh, R. *Self-Healing: Powerful Techniques*. London, ON: Health Psychology Associates, 1997:5.

Chapter 4: Environmental Impact on Breast Health

1. Gregg, E. Radiation risks with diagnostic x-rays. *Radiology*, 1977; 123:447.

2. Gofman, John. *Preventing Breast Cancer: The Story of a Major, Proven, Preventable Cause of This Disease*. 2nd. ed. San Francisco, CA: Committee for Nuclear Responsibility, 1996.

3. Pacini, F., et al. Thyroid consequences of the Chernobyl nuclear accident. *Acta Paediatr Suppl*, 1999 Dec; 88(433):23-27.

4. Bertell, Rosalie. Gulf war syndrome, depleted uranium and the dangers of low-level radiation. www.ccnr.org/bertell_book.html.

5. Stevenson, A.F. Low level radiation exposure the radiobiologists's challenge in the next millennium. *Indian J Exp Biol*, 2002 Jan;40(1):12-24.

6. John, E. and J. Kelsey. Radiation and other environmental exposures and breast cancer. *Epidemiologic Reviews*, 1993;15(1):157-61.

7. Harris, J., M. Lippman, et al. Breast cancer. *New England Journal of Medicine*, 1992;327:319-28.

8. Kelsey, J. and M. Gammon. The epidemiology of breast cancer. *CA: A Cancer Journal for Clinicians*, 1991;41:146-65.

9. Epstein, S. Europe's worries about U.S. meat should be our worry, too. *Los Angeles Times*, January 30,1989:A11.

10. Clorfene-Casten, Liane. *Breast Cancer: Poisons, Profits and Prevention*. Monroe, ME: Common Courage Press, 1996:62.

11. Clorfene-Casten, Liane. *Breast Cancer: Poisons, Profits and Prevention*. Monroe, ME: Common Courage Press, 1996:62.

12. Reported in *JAMA*, 1984.

13. Living at Ground Zero. *Toronto Star*, Sunday, Jan. 10, 1999:B1-2.

14. Clorfene-Casten, Liane. *Breast Cancer: Poisons, Profits and Prevention*. Monroe, ME: Common Courage Press, 1996:70.

15. Clorfene-Casten, Liane. *Breast Cancer: Poisons, Profits and Prevention*. Monroe, ME: Common Courage Press, 1996:72.

16. Greenpeace. Nuclear power, human health and the environment: Breast cancer warning in the Great Lakes region. Toronto, ON: Greenpeace International, 1995.

17. Lansberg, Michele. U.S. war toxins blamed for rise in Iraqi cancers. *Toronto Star*, Nov. 21, 1998:L1.

18. Spears, Tom. Radioactive baby teeth flag cancer rate. *Ottawa Citizen*, July 25, 1999:A1.

19. Brown, J. Childhood cancer in south Florida: Study finds cause in nuclear plant radiation emissions – drinking water most likely source., April 9, 2003. http://www.radiation.org/florida.html.

20. Stewart, T., and N. Stewart. Breast cancer in female flight attendants. *Lancet*, 1995:Nov.25;346:1379.

21. Nystrom, Lennarth, et al. Breast cancer screening with mammography: overview of Swedish randomized trials. *Lancet*, 1993:Apr 17;341(8851):973-978.

22. Tanaka, Y. et al. Application of algal polysaccharides as in vivo binders of metal pollutants. Proc Seventh Int Seaweed Symp, 602-607, Wiley and Sons, 1972.

23. Tanaka, Y. et al. Studies on inhibition of intestinal absorption of radioactive strontium. *Can Med Assoc J*, 1968, 99:169-75.

24. Sukhanov, B.P., et al. Medical and biological evaluation of new food products for children exposed to excessive radiation. *Gig Sanit*, 1994 Sept-Oct; (8):24-26.

25. Dharmananda, S. The nutritional and medicinal value of seaweeds used in Chinese medicine.

26. Walkiw, O., Douglas, D.E. Health food supplements prepared from kelp – a source of elevated urinary arsenic. *Can Med Assoc J*, 1974;111:1301-2 (letter).

27. US Dept Health and Human Services. Dietary aspects of carcinogenesis, Nov. 1981.

28. Gong, Y.F. et al. Suppression of radioactive strontium absorption by sodium alginate in animals and human subjects. *Biomed Environ Sci.*, 1991 Sep; 4(3):273-282.

29. Inano, H., M. Onoda. Radioprotective action of curcumin estracted from Curcuma longa LINN:inhibitory effect on formation of urinary 8-hydroxy-2-deoxyguanosine, tumorigenesis, but not mortality, induced by gamma-ray irradiation. *Int J Radiat Oncol Biol Phys*, 2002 Jul 1; 53(3):735-743.,

30. Kapitanov, A.B., et al. Radiation-protective effectiveness of lycopene. *Radiats Biol Radioecol*

31. Tarbell, N.J., M. Rosenblatt, et al. The effect of N-acetylcysteine inhalation on the tolerance to thoracic irradiation in mice. *Radiother Oncol*, 1986 Sept; 7(1): 77-80.

32. Gorshkov, A.I., Comparative evaluation of radiation protective efficiency of regimens with various contents of calcium, potassium and iron. *Gig Sanit*, 1994 Jun; (6):18-20.

33. Perepelkin, S.R., N.D. Egorova. Prophylactic and therapeutic role of the B group vitamin, mesoinositol, in radiation sckness against a background of the use of a milk and egg diet. *Radiobiologiia*, 1980 Jan-Feb; 20(1):137-139

34. Weed, S. *Breast Cancer? Breast Health!* Woodstock, NY: Ash Tree Publishing, 1996:211-12.

35. Anonymous. Electromagnetic fields and male breast cancer. *Lancet*, December, 1990:336.

36. Anonymous. Health Report, *Time*, June 27, 1994.

37. Fackelmann, K. Do EMFs Pose Breast Cancer Risk? *Science News*, June 18, 1994:388.

38. Caplan, L.S., et al. Breast cancer and electromagnetic fields – a review. *Ann Epidemiol*, 2000 Jan; 10(1):31-44.

39. Weed, S. *Breast Cancer? Breast Health!* Woodstock, NY: Ash Tree Publishing, 1996:19.

40. Greenpeace, Death in Small Doses: The Effects of Organochlorines on Aquatic Ecosystems. 1992.

41. Arnold, S., D. Klotz, B. Collins, P. Vonier, L. Guillette Jr., J. Mclachlan. Synergistic activation of estrogen receptor with combinations of environmental chemicals. *Science*, Vol. 272, June 7, 1996:1489-91.

42. Colborn, Theo, D. Dumanoski, J. Peterson Myers. *Our Stolen Future*. New York, NY: Penguin, 1996:152.

43. Davis, Devra Lee, H.L. Bradlow. Can environmental estrogens cause breast cancer? *Scientific American*, Oct. 1995:172.

44. Davis, Devra Lee, H.L. Bradlow. Can environmental estrogens cause breast cancer? *Scientific American*, Oct. 1995:172.

45. Davis, Devra Lee, H.L. Bradlow. Can environmental estrogens cause breast cancer? *Scientific American*, Oct. 1995:172.

46. Davis, Devra Lee, H.L. Bradlow. Can environmental estrogens cause breast cancer? *Scientific American*, Oct. 1995:172.

47. Steingraber, Sandra. *Living Downstream: An Ecologist Looks at Cancer and the Environment*. Reading, MA: Addison-Wesley Publishing Co. Inc., 1997:133.

48. Sharpe, R., N. Skakkeback. 1993. Are oestrogens involved in falling male sperm counts and disorders of the male reproductive tract? *Lancet*, 341:1392-95.

49. Abell, A., et al. High sperm density among members of organic farmer's association. *Lancet*, 1994 June11; 343:1498.

50. Lee, John. *What Your Doctor May Not Tell You About Menopause*. New York, NY: Warner Books, 1996:55-56.

51. Chilvers, C. et al. Apparent doubling of frequency of undescended testes in England and Wales in 1962-81. *Lancet*, 1984:330-32.

52. Hutson, J. et al. Hormonal control of testicular

descent and the cause of cryptorchidism. *Reproduction, Fertility and Development*, 1994;6:151-56.

53. Davis, Devra Lee, H.L. Bradlow. Can environmental estrogens cause breast cancer? *Scientific American*, Oct. 1995;273(4):166-72.

54. Wasserman, M. et al. Organochlorine compounds in neoplastic and adjacent apparently normal tissue. *Bulletin of Environmental Contamination and Toxicology*, 1976:15:478-84.

55. Mussalo-Rauhamaa, H.E. et al. Occurrence of b-hexachlorocyclohexane in breast cancer patients. *Cancer*, 1990:66:2124-28.

56. Bishop, J., S. Ho, H. Hutchinson, L. Young. Organochlorines and their link to breast cancer. Toronto, ON: Canadian College of Naturopathic Medicine, April, 1999.

57. Environmental Health Committee Newsletter for Family Physicians. Pesticides and Human Health. Toronto, ON: Environmental Health Committee of the Ontario College of Family Physicians, ND.

58. Nikiforuk, Andrew. Rocky Mountain Blight. *The Globe and Mail*, Oct. 17, 1998:D5.

59. Neidert, E., P. Saschenbrecker. Occurrence of pesticide residues in selected agricultural food commodities available in Canada. *Journal of AOAC International*, 1996;79(2):549-66.

60. Steingraber, Sandra. *Living Downstream: An Ecologist Looks at Cancer and the Environment*. Reading, MA: Addison-Wesley Publishing Co. Inc.,1997:161-62.

61. Mussalo-Rauhamaa et al., Occurrence of beta-Hexachlorocyclohexane in breast cancer patients. *Cancer*, 1990;66:2124-28.

62. This list of pesticides is adapted from 'Currently used pesticides linked with breast cancer' by Carolyn Cox, *Journal of Pesticide Reform*, Spring, 1996;16, 1.

63. A handout from WEDO, 'Currently used pesticides linked with breast cancer'.

64. List of known and suspected hormone disruptors. World Wildlife Fund. www.wwfcanada.org/hormone-disruptors/list.htm.

65. Westin, J.B. Carcinogens in Israeli milk: a study in regulatory failure. *Int J Health Serv*, 1993; 23(3):497-517.

66. Health Canada. Cancer incidence maps at the province/territory level. http://cythera.ic.gc.ca/dsol/cancer/m_prov_e.phtml?minx

67. Brophy, J.T et al. Occupational histories of cancer patients in a Canadian cancer treatment center and the generated hypothesis regarding breast cancer and farming. *Int J Occup Environ Health*, 2002 Oct-Dec; 8(4):346-53.

68. Soto, A.M. et al. The pesticides endosulphan, toxaphene and dieldrin have estrogenic effects on human estrogen-sensitive cells. EHP, 1994;102:380-83.

69. Rice, Bonnie (for Greenpeace). Polyvinyl Chloride (PVC) Plastic: Primary Contributor to the Global Dioxin Crisis. October 1995.

70. Mittelstaedt, Martin. Environmentalists urge testing of air near garbage dumps. *The Globe and Mail*, Nov. 28, 1998:A9.

71. This list is taken from a Greenpeace Report, Taking Back Our Stolen Future: Hormone disruption and PVC plastic, April 1996.

72. Greenpeace, Death in Small Doses: The Effects of Organochlorines on Aquatic Ecosystems. 1992.

73. Greenpeace, Taking Back Our Stolen Future. April, 1996:15.

74. Rier, S.E., D.C. Martin, J.L. Becker. Endometriosis in rhesus monkeys (Macaca mulatta) following chronic exposure to 2,3,7,8-tetrachlordibenzo-p-dioxin. *Fundamental and Applied Toxicology*. 1993;21:433-41.

75. Greenpeace. Poisoning the Future: Impact of Endocrine Disrupting Chemicals on Wildlife and Human Health. October 1997:23.

76. Isabella, Judith. Getting too close to seal level. *The Globe and Mail*, Oct.3, 1998:D5.

77. Isabella, Judith. Getting too close to seal level. *The Globe and Mail*, Oct.3, 1998:D5.

78. Colborn, Theo, D. Dumanoski, J. Peterson Myers. *Our Stolen Future*. New York, NY: Penguin, 1996:88.

79. Greenpeace. Taking Back Our Stolen Future: Hormone Disruption and PVC Plastic. 1996:15.

80. Greenpeace. Poisoning the Future: Impact of Endocrine Disrupting Chemicals on Wildlife and Human Health. October 1997:13.

81. Greenpeace. Poisoning the Future: Impact of Endocrine Disrupting Chemicals on Wildlife and Human Health. October 1997:23.

82. Paris-Pombo, A., K.J. Aronson, C.G. Woolcott, W.D. King. Dietary predictors of concentreations of polychlorinated biphenyl in breast adipose tissue of women living in Ontario, Canada *Arch Environ Health*, 2003 Jan; 58(1):48-54.

83. Steingraber, Sandra. *Living Downstream: An Ecologist Looks at Cancer and the Environment*. Addison-Wesley Publishing Co. Inc., Reading, Mass. 1997:52-53.

84. Leiss, J.K. & D. Savitz, Home pesticide use and childhood cancer: a case-controlled study. *AJPH*, 1993; 85:249-252.

85. Davis, J.R. et al. Family pesticide use and childhood brain cancer. *Archives of Environmental Contamination and Toxicity*, 1993;24:87-92.

86. Commission for Environmental Cooperation. *Taking Stock: North American Pollutant Releases and Transfers.* Montreal, QC: Communications and Public Outreach Department of the CEC Secretariat, 1999:67.

87. TCE: ATSDR. *Case Studies in Environmental Medicine: Trichloroethylene Toxicity.* Atlanta,GA.: ATSDR, 1992.

88. Commission for Environmental Cooperation. *Taking Stock: North American Pollutant Releases and Transfers.* Montreal, QC: Communications and Public Outreach Department of the CEC Secretariat, 1999:67.

89. Joseph, B. Breast health. *Vegetarian Times,* July 1997: 83-90.

90. Spears, Tom. Cancers may come out of the tap. *Owen Sound Sun Times,* Nov. 24, 1998:1.

91. GSE Report, Vol.1, Issue 1, Praxus, Inc., Novato, CA:6.

92. GSE Report, Vol.1, Issue 1, Praxus, Inc., Novato, CA:10.

93. Thanks to Joanne Leung from the Canadian College of Naturopathic Medicine for providing this information in her research paper on composting toilets. April 7, 1999.

94. Ema, M., R. Kurasoka, H. Amano, Y. Ogawa. Comparative developmental toxicity of n-butyl benzyl phthalate and di-n-butylphthalate in rats. *Arch Environ Contam Toxicol,* 1995;28:233.

95. Colon, I, et al. Identification of phthalate esters in the serum of young Puerto Rican girls with premature breast development. *Env Health Persp,* 2000 Sept; 108(9):895-900.

96. Colborn, Theo, D. Dumanoski, J. Peterson Myers. *Our Stolen Future.* New York, NY: Penguin, 1996:136.

97. Greenpeace.Which of these toys contain hazardous chemicals?

98. Miller, S. Hidden hazards health impacts of toxins in polymer clays. 2002 July. *Vermont Public Interest Research Group,* http://www.vpirg.org/downloads/hiddenhazards.pdf. accessed May 23, 2003.

99. Schantz, N. Biodegradation and bioaccumulation of phthalate esters. 1998. http://www.ecpi.org/technical papers. Accessed May 23, 2003.

100. National Toxicology Program Center for the evaluation of risks to human reproduction: Expert panel review of phthalates. http://www.mindfully.org/plastic/phthalates-reproduction-NTP14ju100.htm. Accessed May 23, 2003.

101. Cybulski, S. and Genne, Anne-Helene. Phthalates: An overview, route of elimination and estrogenic effects. Canadian College of Naturopathic Medicine 3rd year student paper. April 2, 2003.

102. Colborn, Theo, D. Dumanoski, J. Peterson Myers. *Our Stolen Future.* New York, NY: Penguin, 1996:134.

103. Davis, Devra Lee, H. Bradlow. Can environmental estrogens cause breast cancer? *Scientific American,* Oct. 1995:166-72.

104. Colborn, Theo, D. Dumanoski, J. Peterson Myers. *Our Stolen Future.* New York, NY: Penguin, 1996:107.

105. Waters, Jane. Taking back our stolen future. *International J. Alternative & Complementary Medicine,* 1996;14 (12);19, 22-23.

106. World Wildlife Fund. News release: Lab analysis reveals hormone-disrupting chemicals in everyday household soaps. Feb. 11, 1997; and personal communication with Julia Langar.

107. Wenning, R.J. Uncertainties and data needs in risk assessment of three commercial polybrominated diphenyl ethers: probabilitic exposure analysis and comparison with European Commission results. *Chemosphere,* 2002 Feb; 46(5):779-96.

108. Sarick, Lila. To spray or not to spray? D that is the question. *The Globe and Mail,* Aug. 29, 1998:A10.

Chapter 5: Detoxifying Our Bodies

1. Von Tempelhoff, G.F., F. Nieman, L. Heilmann, G. Hommel. Association between blood rheology, thrombosis and cancer survival in patients with gynecological malignancy. *Clin Hemorheol Microcirc,* 2000; Vol. 22(2):107-30.

2. Von Tempelhoff, G.F. et al. Association between blood rheopogy, thrombosis, and cancer survival in patients with gynecologic malignancy. *Clin hemorheal microcirc,* 2000; 22(2):107-30.

3. Hole, J.H. *Human Anatomy and Physiology.* Dubuque, Iowa: Wm. C. Brown Publishers, 1984:629..

4. Simpson-Haidaris, P.J., B. Rybarczyk. Tumors and fibrinogen. The role of fibrinogen as an extracellular matrix protein. *Ann N Y Acad Sci,* 2001; 936:406-425.

5. Guyton, A.C. *Textbook of Medical Physiology.* Toronto, ON: W.B. Saunders Co., 1981:97.

6. Dirix, L.Y. et al. Plasma fibrin D-dimer levels correlate with tumor volume, progression rate and survival in patients with metastatic breast cancer. *Br J Cancer,* 2002, Feb. 1; 86(3):389-95.

7. Miller, B., L. Heilmann. Hemorheologic parameters in patients with gynecological malignancies. *Gynecol Oncol,* 1989; 33(2):177-81.

8. Derham, R.J., P.C. Buchan. Haemorheological consequences of estrogen and progestogen therapy. *Eur J Obstet Gynecol Reprod Biol,* 1989 Aug; 32(2):109-14.

9. Bouix, D., et al. *Clin Hemorheol Microcirc,* 1998 Nov; 19(3):219-27.

10. Davis, E., H. Rozov. Xanthinol nicotinate in peripheral vascular disease. *Practitioner,* 1975 Dec.; 215(1290):793-98.

11. Rimpler, M. The action of proteases in malignant processes. *Journal of the American Holistic Veterinary Medical Association*; 1996 April 30; Vol 15(1):21-28.

12. Jain, R.K. Determinants of tumor blood flow: a review. *Cancer Res,* 1988 May 15; 48(10):2641-2658.

13. Murray, M., J. Pizzorno. *Encyclopedia of Natural Medicine.* Rocklin, CA: Prima Publishing, 1998:108-24.

14. Health Canada. Potential drug interactions with St. John's Wort. *Health Canada Information Backgrounder.* URI. www.hcsc.gc/english/archives/ warnings/2000/2000_36ebk.htm. Nov 12, 2000.

15. Thorne Research. Detox Program Handout. 2000 May: 7.

16. Murray, M., J. Pizzorno. *Encyclopedia of Natural Medicine.* Rocklin, CA: Prima Publishing, 1998:108-24.

17. Malhotra, S., Bailey, D.G., Paine, M.F., et al. Seville orange juice-felodipine interaction:comparison with dilute grapefruit juice and involvement of furocoumarins. *Clin Pharacol Ther,* http://www.vpirg.org/downloads/ hiddenhazards.pdf. accessed May 23, 2003.

18. Yee, G.C. et al. Effect of grapefruit juice on blood cyclosporin concentration. *Lancet,* 1995; 345:955-56.

19. Somasundaram, S., N.A. Edmund, D.T. Moore, et al. Dietary curcumin inhibits chemotherapy-induced apoptosis in models of human breast cancer. *Cancer Res,* 2002 Jul 1; 62(13):3868-75.

20. Edenharder, R., et al Protection by beverages, fruits, vegetables, herbs, and flavonoids against genotoxicity of 2-acetylaminofluorine and 2-amino-1-methyl-6-phenylimidazol[4,5-b]pyridine (PhIP) in metabolically competent V79 cells. *Mutat Res,* 2002 Nov 26; 521(1-2):57-72.

21. Matsen, John. *The Secrets to Great Health from Your Nine Liver Dwarves.* North Vancouver, BC: Goodwin Books, Ltd., 1998:282.

22. Collin, J. No, not snake oil, castor oil! *Townsend Letter for Doctors,* 1989 July:34.

23. Myers, Dennis. Urine and saliva testing. *Euro-American Health: A New Biology.* www.euroamericanhealth.com. May 29, 2003.

24. From a handout called Detoxify for All You're Worth, by Dr Leo Roy.

25. Vaupel, P. et al. Blood flow, oxygen and nutrient supply, and the metabolic microenvironment of human tumors: A review. *Cancer Research,* 1989;49(23):6449-65.

26. Lee, A.H., I.F. Tannock. Homogeneity of intracellular pH and of mechanisms that regulate intracellular pH in populations of cultured cells. *Cancer Research,* 1998;1(9):1901-08.

27. Myers, Dennis. Urine and saliva testing. *Euro-American Health: A New Biology.* www.euroamericanhealth.com. May 29, 2003.

28. From a handout called Detoxify for All You're Worth, by Dr Leo Roy.

29. Hobbs, C. *Foundations of Health: Healing with Herbs and Foods.* Capitola, CA: Botanica Press, 1992:158.

30. Rogers, S. *Wellness Against All Odds.* Syracuse, NY: Prestige Publishing, 1994.

31. Borriello, S.P., K. Setchell, M. Axelson, A.M. Lawson. Production and metabolism of lignans by the human faecal flora. *Journal of Applied Bacteriology*, 1985;58,37-43.

32. Cichoke, A. The effect of systemic enzyme therapy on cancer cells and the immune system. *Townsend Letter for Doctors and Patients.* Nov 1995:30-32.

33. Gignac, Tara. The use of digestive enzymes in cancer therapy. Toronto, ON: Canadian College of Naturopathic Medicine, April 2000:2.

34. Cichoke, A. The effect of systemic enzyme therapy on cancer cells and the immune system. *Townsend Letter for Doctors and Patients.* Nov 1995:31.

35. Moskvichyov, B.V., E.V. Komarov, G.P. Ivanova. Study of trypsin thermodenaturation process. *Enzyme Microb Technol,* 1986; 8:498-502.

36. Gotze, H., S.S. Rothman. Enteropancreatic circulation of digestive enzymes as a conservative mechanism. *Nature,* 1975; 257:607-09.

37. Liebow, C., S.S. Rothman. Enteropancreatic circulation of digestive enzymes. *Science,* 1975; 189:472-74.

38. Wald, M., T. Olejar, P. Pouckova, M. Zadinova. Proteinases reduce metastatic dissemination and increase survival time in C57BI6 mice with the Lewis lung carcinoma. *Life Sciences,* 1988a; 63(17):237-43.

39. Wald, M., T. Olejar, P. Pouckova, M. Zadinova. The influence of proteinases on in vivo blastic transformation in rat species SD/Ipcv with spontaneous lymphoblastic leukemia. *British*

Journal of Haematology, 1998b; 102(1):294.

40. Wald, M. et al. Mixture of trypsin, chymotrypsin, and papain reduces formation of metastases and extends survival time of C57Bl6 mice with syngeneic melanoma B16. *Cancer Chemother Pharmacol,* 2001; 47(Suppl):S16-S22.

41. Wald, M. et al. The influence of trypsin, chymotrypsin, and papin on the growth of human pancreatic adenocarcinoma transplanted to nu/nu mice. *European Journal of Cancer,* 1999; 35(4),no. 543:148.

42. Stauder, G., F. Beaufort, P. Streichhan. Radiotherapy side-effects in abdominal cancer patients and their reduction by hydrolytic enzyme preparations. *Dtsch Zschr Onkol,* 1991; 23(1):7-16.

43. Desser, L. et al. Concentrations of soluble tumour necrosis factor receptors, 2-microglobulin, IL-6 and TNF in serum of multiple myeloma patients after chemotherapy and after combined enzyme-therapy. *Int J Immunotherapy,* 1997; XIII(3/4):111-19.

44. Sakalova, A. et al. Survival analysis of an additional therapy with oral enzymes in patients with multiple myeloma. *British Journal of Haematology,* 1998; 102:353.

45. Perasalo, J. The traditional use of sauna for hygiene and health in Finland. *Annals of Clinical Research.* 1988:20(4):220-23.

46. Hubbard, L. R. *Clear Body, Clear Mind.* Copenhagen, Denmark: New Era Publications Int., 1990.

47. Roehm, D.C. Effect of a clearing program of sauna baths and megavitamins on adipose DDE and PCBs and on clearing of symptoms of Agent orange (dioxin) toxicity. *Clinical Research,* 1983:31:243.

48. Roehm, D.C. Effect of a clearing program of sauna baths and megavitamins on adipose DDE and PCBs and on clearing of symptoms of Agent orange (dioxin) toxicity. *Clinical Research,* 1983:31:243.

49. Kilburn, K.H., R.H. Warsaw, M.G. Shields. Neurobehavioral dysfunction in firemen exposed to polychlorinated biphenyls (PCBs): possible improvement after detoxification. *Arch Environ Health,* 1989, Nov-Dec;44(6):345-50.

50. Steinman, D. *Diet for a Poisoned Planet.* New York, NY: Crown Publishing, 1990:300-06.

51. Krop, J. Chemical sensitivity after intoxication at work with solvents: response to sauna therapy. *Journal of Alternative and Complementary Medicine,* 1998;4(1):77-86.

52. Ahuja, M., V. Comeau, M. Garieri, V. Lurie, C. Pustowka, K. Stauffert, B. Steels, C. Tibelius, S. Tripodi, F. Tutt. Sauna as a method of detoxification in the prevention and treatment of breast cancer. Toronto, ON: Canadian College of Naturopathic Medicine, April, 1999.

53. Steinman, D. *Diet for a Poisoned Planet.* New York, NY: Crown Publishing, 1990:300-06.

54. Bhajan, Yogi. *Sadhana Guidelines for Kundalini Yoga Daily Practise.* Los Angeles, CA: Kundalini Research Institute, 1996:30.

Chapter 6: Activating Our Lymphatic and Immune Systems

1. Singer, S. & S. Grismaijer. *Dressed to Kill: The Link Between Breast Cancer and Bras.* Garden City Park, NY: Avery Publishing Group, 1995.

2. Singer, S. & S. Grismaijer. *Dressed to Kill: The Link Between Breast Cancer and Bras.* Garden City Park, NY: Avery Publishing Group, 1995.

3. De Schepper, Luc. *Peak Immunity: How to Fight CEBV, Candida, Herpes Simplex Viruses and Other Immune-Suppressed Conditions and Win.* Van Nuys, CA: Le Fever Publications, 1989.

4. Zava, D., C. Dullbaum, M. Blen. Estrogen and progestin bioactivity of foods, herbs and spices. *Biol Med,* 1998;217(3):369-78.

5. Duke, J. Dr. Duke's Phytochemical and Ethnobotanical Databases. *Agricultural Research Service.* www.ars-grin.gov/cgi-bin/duke/chemical Accessed June 12, 2003.

6. Kloppenberg, R., et al. Heilpflanzen in der Krebsmedizin. Berlin, Germany: 1997.

7. Walters, R. *Options: The Alternative Cancer Therapy Book.* Garden City Park, NY: Avery Publishing Group, 1993.

8. Moss, R. *Cancer Therapy: The Independent Consumer's Guide to Non-Toxic Treatment and Prevention.* New York, NY: Equinox Press, 1992:322.

9. Hartwell, J. *Plants Used Against Cancer.* Lloydia; 32(2) June 1968, 33(1); March 1970.

10. Holmes, P. *The Energetics of Western Herbs.* Vol.II. 2nd ed. Berkeley, CA: NatTrop Publishing, 1993:574-76.

11. Zava, D., C. Dullbaum, M. Blen. Estrogen and progestin bioactivity of foods, herbs and spices. *Biol Med,* 1998;217(3):369-78.

12. Naiman, Ingrid. *Cancer Salves: A Botanical Approach to Treatment.* Santa Fe, NM: Seventh Ray Press, 1999.

13. Ahmad, Nihal et al. Green tea constituent epigallocatechin-3-gallate and induction of apoptosis and cell cycle arrest in human carcinoma

cells. *Journal of the National Cancer Institute*, 1997;89(24):1881-86.

14. Scientists learn how tea blocks cancer. *Toronto Star*, April 1, 1999:A14.

15. Brinker, F. The Hoxsey treatment: cancer quackery or effective physiological adjuvant? *Journal of Naturopathic Medicine*, 1997;6(1):9-23.

16. Brinker, F. The Hoxsey treatment: cancer quackery or effective physiological adjuvant? *Journal of Naturopathic Medicine*, 1997;6(1):9-23.

17. Walker, Morton. The anticancer components in Essiac. *Townsend Letter for Doctors and Patients*, Dec. 1997:76-82.

18. Bardon, S., K. Picard, P. Martel. Monoterpenes inhibit cell growth, cell cycle progression and cyclin D1 gene expression in human breast cancer cell lines. *Nutr Cancer*, 1998;32(1):1-7.

19. Hang, J., M. Gould. Mammary carcinoma regression induced by perillyl alcohol, a hydroxylated analog of limonene. *Cancer Chemother Pharmacol*, 1994;34(6):477-83.

20. Jones, C. Lovely lavender holds compelling anticancer potential. *Herbs for Health*, 1998;Jan/Feb:17.

21. Ziegler, J. Raloxifene, retinoids and lavender: 'me too' tamoxifen alternatives under study. *Jour Nat Canc Inst*, 1996;88(16):1100-02.

22. Essential Science Publishing. *People's Desk Reference for Essential Oils*. New York, NY: Essential Science Publishing, 1999:48

23. Nanba, H., Maitake D-fraction: Healing and preventative potential for cancer. *Journal of Orthomolecular Medicine*, 1997;12:43-49.

24. Nanba, H., Activity of Maitake D-fraction to inhibit carcinogenesis and metastasis. *Annals of the New York Academy of Sciences*, 1995;768:243-45.

25. Nanba, H., Anti-tumor activity of orally administered D-fraction from Maitake Mushroom. *J. Naturopathic Med*, 1993;41:10-15.

26. Yamada,Y., H. Nanba, H. Kuroda. Antitumor effect of orally administered extracts from the fruitbody of Grifola frondosa (Maitake). *Chemotherapy* (Tokyo), 1990;38(8):790-96.

27. Nanba, H., Maitake D-fraction: Healing and preventative potential for cancer. *Journal of Orthomolecular Medicine*, 1997;12:43-49.

28. Activity of maitake D-fraction to inhibit carcinogenesis and metastasis. *Annals of the New York Academy of Sciences*, 1995;768:243-245.

29. Mizuno, T., H. Saito, T. Nishitoba, & H. Kawagishi, Antitumor active substances from mushrooms. *Food Reviews International*, 1995;111:23-61.

30. Stamets, P. & C. Dusty Wu Yao. MycoMedicinals: Information on medicinal mushrooms. *Townsend Letter for Doctors and Patients*, 1998;179:152-62.

31. Wang, S.Y., M.L. Hsu, C.H.Tzeng, S.S. Le, M.S. Shiao & C.K. Ho, The anti-tumor effect of Ganoderma lucidum is mediated by cytokines released from activated macrophages and T-lymphocytes. *International Journal of Cancer*, 1997;70(6):669-705.

32. Yang, D.A., S. Li, & X. Li, Prophylactic effects of Zhu Ling and BGG on postoperative recurrence of bladder cancer. *Chung-Hua-Wai-Ko-Tsa-Chih*, June 29, 1994;(6):393-95,399.

33. Chang, H.M. & P.P. But. *Pharmacology and Applications of Chinese Materia Medica*. Vol.1. Singapore: World Scientific, 1986.

34. Ito, H., K. Shimura, H. Itoh, M. Kawade. Antitumor effects of a new polysaccharide-protein complex (ATOM) prepared from Agaricus blazei (Iwade strain 101) Himematsutake and its mechanisms in tumor-bearing mice. *Anticancer Research*, Jan-Feb 1997;17(1A):277-84.

35. Ebina, T. & K. Murata. Antitumor effect of intratumoral administration of a Coriolus preparation, PSK: inhibition of tumor invasion in vitro. *Gan To Kagaku Ryoho*, 1994;21:2241-43.

36. Sugimachi, K., Y. Maehara, M. Ogawa, T. Kakegawa and M. Tomita. Dose intensity of uracil and tegafur in postoperative chemotherapy for patients with poorly differentiated gastric cancer. *Cancer Chemotherapy and Pharmacology*, 1997;40(3):233-38.

37. Casura, L. 'Mr. Medicinal Mushroom': An interview with mycologist Paul Stamets. *Townsend Letter for Doctors and Patients*, June 1998;(179):11-17,151-269.

38. Ghoneum, M., A. Jewett. Production of tumor necrosis factor-alpha and interferon-gamma from human peripheral blood lymphocytes by MGN-3, modified arabinoxylan from rice bran, and its synergy with interleukin-2 in vitro. *Cancer Detect Prev*, 2000; 24(4):314-324.

Chapter 7: Eating Right for Breast Health

1. Asami, D.K., Y.J.Hong, D.M. Barrett, A.E. Mitchell. Comparison of the total phenolic and ascorbic acid content of freeze-dried and air-dried marionberry, strawberry and corn grown using conventional, organic, and sustainable agricultural practices. *Agric Food Chem*, 2003 Feb 26; 51(5):1237-1241.

2. Carbonaro, M., M. Mattera, S. Nicoli, P. Bergamo, M. Cappelloni. Modulation of antioxidant

compounds in organic vs conventional fruit. *J Agric Food Chem,* 2002 Sep 11; 50(19):5458-5462.

3. Worthington, V. Nutritional quality of organic versus conventional fruits, vegetables and grains. *J Altern Complement Med,* 2001 Apr; 7(2):161-173.

4. Mollison, B. *Introduction to Permaculture.* Tyalgum, NSW, Australia: Tagari Publications, 1991.

5. Steimetz, K.A., J.D. Potter. Vegetables, fruit and cancer prevention: a review. *J Am Diet Assoc,* 1996;96:1027-39.

6. Phillips, R.L., Cancer among Seventh Day Adventists. *Journal of Environmental Pathology and Toxicology,* 1980;3:157-69.

7. Sanches, A., et al. A hypothesis on the etiological role of diet on age of menarche. *Medical Hypothesis,* 1981;7:1339-45.

8. Weed, Susun. *Breast Cancer/Breast Health!* Woodstock, NY: Ash Tree Publishing, 1996:46-52.

9. Zimmerman, M. Phytochemicals and disease prevention. *Alternative and Complementary Therapies,* Apr/May 1995;1(3)154-57.

10. Holzman, D. Nutritional chemoprevention: using food to fight cancer. *Alternative and Complementary Medicine,* Mar/Apr, 1996;2(2), 65-67.

11. Wattenberg, L.W. & W.D. Loub. 1978. Inhibition of polycyclic aromatic hydrocarbon-induced neoplasia by naturally occurring indoles. *Cancer Research,* 1978;38:1410-13.

12. Michnovicz, J.J. *How to Reduce Your Risk of Breast Cancer.* New York, NY: Warner Books, 1994:103.

13. Wong, GYC et al. A dose-ranging study of indole-3-carbinol for breast cancer prevention. Strang Cancer Prevention Center. *Breast Cancer Research and Treatment,* 1997;46(1):81.

14. Fahey, J.W., Y. Zhang, & P. Talalay. Broccoli sprouts: An exceptionally rich source of inducers of enzymes that protect against chemical carcinogens. *Proc. Natl. Acad. Sci. USA.,* 1997; 94:10367-72.

15. Raloff, J. Anticancer agent sprouts up unexpectedly. *Science News,*1997;152:183.

16. Anonymous. Garlic fights nitrosamine formation … as do tomatoes and other produce. *Science News,* 1994;145.

17. Nakagawa, H., et al. Growth inhibitory effects of diallyl disulfide on human breast cancer cell lines. *Carcinogenesis,* 2001 Jun; 22(6):891-897.

18. Hirsch, K et al. Effect of purified allicin, the major ingredient of freshly crushed garlic, on cancer cell proliferation. *Nutr Cancer,* 2000; 38(2):245-254.

19. Nakagawa, H., et al. Growth inhibitory effects of diallyl disulfide on human breast cancer cell lines. *Carcinogenesis,* 2001 Jun; 22(6):891-897.

20. Teas, J. The consumption of seaweed as a protective factor in the etiology of breast cancer, *Medical Hypotheses,* 1981;7:(5)601-13.

21. Yamamoto, I., H. Maruyama, M. Morguchi. The effect of dietary seeweeds on 7,12-dimethylbenz[a} anthracance-induced mammary tumorigenesis in rats. *Cancer Lett,* 1987 May; 35(2):109-118.

22. Weed, S. *Breast Cancer? Breast Health.,* Woodstock, NY: Ash Tree Publishing, 1996:272.

23. Bensky, Dan, A. Gamble. *Chinese Herbal Medicine Materia Medica.* Seattle, WA. Eastland Press Inc., 1986:129.

24. Balch, J.F. The *Super Anti-oxidants: Why they will change the face of healthcare in the 21st Century.* New York, NY: M. Evans & Co.,1998:129.

25. Kantesky, P.A., et al. Dietary intake and blood levels of lycopene: association with cervical dysplasia among non-Hispanic, black women. *Nutrition and Cancer,* 1998;31;31-40.

26. Sharoni, Y., et al. Effects of lycopene-enriched tomato oleoresin on 7,12-dimethylbenz(a)anthracene-induced rat mammary tumors. *Cancer Detection and Prevention.* 1997;21(2):118-23.

27. Buckler, J., A.J. DeNault, V. Franc, T. Strukoff. Breast cancer treatment and prevention: limonene, lycopene and alpha-lipoic acid. Toronto, ON: Canadian College of Naturopathic Medicine, April, 1999.

28. Guthrie, N., K. Carroll. Inhibition of human breast cancer cell growth and metastasis in nude mice by citrus juices and their constituent flavonoids. In *Biological Oxidants and Antioxidants: Molecular Mechanisms and Health Effects.* Packer, L. and A. Ong, eds. Champaign, IL: AOCS Press, 1998:310-16.

29. Gould, M., et al. Limonene chemoprevention of mammary carcinoma induction following direct in situ transfer of v-Ha-ras. *Cancer Research,* 1994;54(13):3540-43.

30. Erasmus, Udo. *Fats that Heal, Fats that Kill.* Burnaby, BC: Alive Books, 1993:400.

31. Erasmus, Udo. *Fats that Heal, Fats that Kill.* Burnaby, BC: Alive Books, 1993:53.

32. Kohlmeier, L. Biomarkers of fatty acid exposure and breast cancer risk. *Am J Clin Nutr,* 1997;66(suppl): 1548S-56S.

33. Cave, W. Omega three PUFAs in rodent models

of breast cancer. *Breast Cancer Research and Treatment,* 1997:46:239-46.

34. Okuyama et al. Dietary fatty acids: The Omega 6/Omega 3 balance. *Progress in Lipid* 1997:41.

35. Takeda, S. et al. Lipid peroxidation in human breast cancer cells in response to gamma-linolenic acid and iron. *Anticancer Research.* 1992;12:329-34.

36. Bakker, N., P. Van't Veer and P. Zock. Adipose fatty acids and cancers of the breast, prostate and colon: An ecological study. *Breast Cancer,* 1997(72):587-91.

37. Fogg, J., D. Derbyshire, E. Bennett, M. Melanson. Essential fatty acids and their role in breast cancer prevention and treatment. Toronto, ON: Canadian College of Naturopathic Medicine, April, 1999.

38. Erasmus, Udo. *Fats that Heal, Fats that Kill.* Burnaby, BC: Alive Books, 1993:365.

39. Thompson, L. et al. Flaxseed and its lignan and oil components reduce mammary tumor growth at a late stage of carcinogenesis. *Carcinogenesis,* 1996:17(6):1373-76.

40. Abdi-Dezfuli, F. et al. Eicosapentaenoic acid and sulphur substituted fatty acid analogues inhibit the proliferation of human breast cancer cells in culture. *Breast Cancer Research and Treatment,* 1997;45:230.

41. Jiang, W., R. Bryce and R. Mansel. Gamma linolenic acid regulates gap junction communication in endothelial cells and their interaction with tumor cells. *Prostaglandins, Leukotrienes and Essential Fatty Acids,* 1997,56(4):307.

42. Hardman, W.E., C.P.R., Avula, G. Fernandes, I.L. Cameron. Three percent dietary fish oil concentrate increased efficacy of doxorubicin against MDA-MB 231 breast cancer xenografts. *Clin Can Res,* 2001; 7:2041-2049.

43. Rose, D.P., J.M. Connolly, X.H. Liu. Effects of linoleic acid and gamma –linolenic acid on the growth and metastases of a human breast cancer cell line in nude mice and on its growth and invaseive capacity in vitro. *Nutr Cancer,* 1995; 24(1):33-45.

44. Ip, Clement. Review of the effects of trans fatty acids, oleic acid, omega-3 polyunsaturated fatty acids. *Am J Clin Nut.* 1997:66(suppl):1523S-9S.

45. Bakker, N., P. Van't Veer, P. Zock. Adipose fatty acids and cancers of the breast, prostate and colon: an ecological study. *Breast Cancer,* 1997;72:587-91.

46. Simopoulos, A.P. The importance of the ratio of omega-6/omega-3 essential fatty acids. *Biomed Pharmacother,* 2002 Oct; 56(8):365-379.

47. Lipworth, L., et al. Olive oil and human cancer: An assessment of the evidence. *Preventive Medicine,* 1997;26:181-90.

48. Aziziyan, S., N. Rezvani, C. Radulovici, A. Nozari. Dietary fat and breast cancer prevention. Toronto, ON: Canadian College of Naturopathic Medicine, April, 1999.

49. Boyd, N. Nutrition and breast cancer. *Journal of the National Cancer Institute,* 1993;Jan.6;85(1):6-7.

50. Woods, M., et al. Hormone levels during dietary changes in pre-menopausal African-American women. *Journal of the National Cancer Institute.* 1996;Oct.2;88(19):1369-74.

51. Phillips, R.L., Role of life-style and dietary habits in risk of cancer among Seventh-Day Adventists. *Cancer Research,* 1975;35:3513.

52. McAndrew, Brian. Toxic chemical gets into fatty products. *Toronto Star,* July 1, 1998.

53. Jibrin, Janis. The ultra diet for healthy breasts. *Prevention,* Sept 1996:65-71,148.

54. Gerber, M. Fiber and breast cancer: another piece of the puzzle — but still an incomplete picture. *Journal of the National Cancer Institute,* 1996;88:13,857-58.

55. Gerber, M. Fiber and breast cancer: another piece of the puzzle - but still an incomplete picture. *Journal of the National Cancer Institute,* 1996;88:858.

56. Cohen, L.A., et al. Wheat bran and psyllium diets: effects on N-methylnitrosoura-induced mammary tumorigenesis in F344 rats. *J Natl Cancer Inst,* 1996;Jul;88(13):899-907.

57. Rohan, T.E. et al. Dietary fiber, vitamins A, C, and E and the risk of breast cancer: A cohort study. *Cancer Causes and Control,* 1993;4:29-37.

58. Simone, C. Nutritional Medicine Today 1997 Conference: Breast cancer nutritional and lifestyle modification to augment oncology care (audiotape). Richmond Hill, ON: Audio Archives of Canada, 1997.

59. Koch-Kattenstroth, S. and E. Shoyama. Fiber and breast cancer. Toronto, ON: Canadian College of Naturopathic Medicine, April, 1999.

60. Petrakis, N.L. & E.B. King. 1981. Cytological abnormalities in nipple aspirates of breast fluid from women with severe constipation. *Lancet,* 1981;ii:1203-05.

61. Rose, D.P., M. Goldman, J.M. Connolly & L.E. Strong. High fiber diet reduces serum oestrogen concentrations in pre-menopausal women. *American Journal of Clinical Nutrition,* 1991;54:520-25.

62. Rose, D.P., M. Lubin and J. Connolly. Effects of diet supplementation with wheat bran on

serum estrogen levels in the follicular and luteal phases of the menstrual cycle. *Nutrition*, 1997;13(6):535-39.

63. Carper, Jean. *The Food Pharmacy*. New York, NY: Bantam, 1988.

64. Kennedy, A. The evidence for soybean products as cancer preventive agents. *J Nutrition*, 1995;125:733.

65. Walker, Morton. Soybean isoflavones lower risk of degenerative diseases, *Townsend Letter for Doctors and Patients*, August/September, 1994.

66. Xu, X., A.M. Duncan, K.E. Wangen, M.S. Kurzer. Soy consumption alters endogenous estrogen metabolism in postmenopaual women. *Cancer Epidemiol Biomarkers Prev*, 2000 Aug; 9(8):781-86.

67. Constantinou, A., K. Kiguchi, E. Huberman. Induction of differentiation and DNA strand breakage in human HL-60 and K-562 leukemia cells by genistein. *Cancer Res*, 1990 May 1;50(9s):2618-24.

68. Ingram, D., K. Sanders, M. Kolybaba, D. Lopez. Case-control study of phytoestrogens and breast cancer. *Lancet*, 1997;350 Oct.4: 990-93.

69. Ingram, D., K. Sanders, M. Kolybaba, D. Lopez. Phyto-oestrogens and breast cancer. Int *Clin Nutr Rev*, 1998;18(1):35-36.

70. Adlercreutz, H., & W. Mazur. Phyto-oestrogens and western disease. *The Finnish Medical Society DUODECIM, Ann Med*, 1997;29,103.

71. Adlercreutz, H., & W. Mazur. Phyto-oestrogens and western disease. *The Finnish Medical Society DUODECIM*, Ann Med 29, 1997:95-120.

72. Zava, D., M. Blen, G. Duwe. Estrogenic activity of natural and synthetic estrogens in human breast cancer cells in culture. *Environmental Health Perspectives*, April 1997;105(Sup.3): 637-45.

73. Kaufman, P., et al. A comparative survey of leguminous plants as sources of the isoflavones, genistein and daidzen: implications for human nutrition and health. *Journal of Alternative and Complementary Medicine*, 1997;3(1):7-12.

74. Adlercreutz, H. Evolution, nutrition, intestinal microflora, and prevention of cancer: A hypothesis. *Proc Soc Exp Biol Med*, 1998;217(3):241-46.

75. Kaufman, P., et al. A comparative survey of leguminous plants as sources of the isoflavones, genistein and daidzen: implications for human nutrition and health. *Journal of Alternative and Complementary Medicine*, 1997;3(1):10-11.

76. Adlercreutz, H., & W. Mazur. Phyto-oestrogens and western disease. *The Finnish Medical Society DUODECIM, Ann Med*, 1997;29:95-120.

77. Wahlqvist, M. Phytoestrogens: Emerging multi-faceted plant compounds. *Medical Journal of Australia*, 1997;Aug.4;167:119-20.

78. Cassidy, A., S. Bingham, & K. Setchell. Biological effects of isoflavones in young women: importance of the chemical composition of soyabean products. *British Journal of Nutrition*, 1995;74:587-601.

79. Colditz, G.A., A. Frazier. Models of breast cancer show that risk is set by events of early life: prevention efforts must switch focus. *Cancer Epidem Biomarker Prevent*, 1995;4:567.

80. Setchell, K.D.R., et al. Exposure of infants to phyto-estrogens from soy-based infant formulas. *Lancet*, 1997;350:23-27.

81. High, C., K. Wolfe. Are soy products safe for infants and pregnant women? Toronto, ON: Canadian College of Naturopathic Medicine, April, 1999.

82. DeSimone, S., B. Finucan. Soy: Too good to be true. (Part 2 of 2). *Gerson Healing Newsletter Online*, March 11, 2000; http://gerson.org/healing/articles/nl_soytoogood.htm:3.

83. Divi, R.L., H.C. Chang, D.R. Doerge. Anti-thyroid isoflavones from soybean: isolation, characterization, and mechanisms of action. *Biochem Pharmacol*, 1997 Nov 15;54(10):1087-96.

84. Fort, P., N. Moses, M. Fasano, T. Goldberg, F. Lifshitz. Breast and soy-formula feedings in early infancy and the prevalence of autoimmune thyroid disease in children. *J Amer Coll Nutr*, 1990; Apr 9(2):164-67.

85. Setchell, K.D., L. Zimmer-Nechemias, J. Cai, J.E. Heubi. Isoflavone content of infant formulas and the metabolic fate of these phytoestrogens in early life. *Am J Clin Nutr*, 1998 Dec 68(6)Suppl:1453S-1461S.

86. Thompson, L. and M. Serraino. Lignans in flaxseed and breast carcinogenesis. Toronto, ON: Dept. of Nutritional Sciences, Univ. of Toronto, 1989.

87. Setchell, K.D.R., H. Adlerkreutz. Mammalian lignans and phyto-estrogens:recent studies on their formation, metabolism and biological role in health and disease. In Rowland, I.R., ed. *Role of the Gut Flora in Toxicity and Cancer*. London, UK: Academic Press, 1998:315-75.

88. Adlercreutz, H., et al. Excretion of the lignans enterolactone and enterodiol and of equol in omnivorous and vegetarian post-menopausal women and in women with breast cancer. *Lancet*, 1982;ii:1295-99.

89. Adlercreutz, H., et al. Determination of urinary lignans and phytoestrogen metabolites, potential antiestrogens and anticarcinogens, in urine

of women on various habitual diets. *J Steroid Biochem*, 1986;25:791-97.

90. Serraino, M., L. Thompson. The effect of flaxseed supplementation on the inhibition and promotional stages of mammary carcinogenesis. *Nutrition and Cancer*, 1992;17:153-59.

91. Thompson, Lilian. Antitumorigenic effect of a mammalian lignan precursor from flaxseed. *Nutrition and Cancer*, 1996;26(2):159-65.

92. Thompson, Lilian. Flaxseed and its lignan and oil components reduce mammary tumor growth at a late stage of carcinogenesis. *Carcinogenesis*, 1996;17(6):1373.

93. Dabrosin, C., J. Chen, L. Wang, L.U. Thompson. Flaxseed inhibits metastasis and decreases extracellular vascular endothelial growth factor in human breast cacner xenografts. *Cancer Letter*, 2002 Nov 8; 185(1):31-37.

94. Gerson, M. *A Cancer Therapy: Results of Fifty Cases*. Del Mar, CA: Totality Books, 1977:163-66.

95. Inagawa, H., T. Nishizawa, K. Noguchi et al. Anti-tumor effect of lipopolysaccharide by intradermal administration as a novel drug delivery system. *Anticancer Res*, 1997;17:2153-58.

96. Wong, G.Y.C., M. Katare, M.P. Osborne, N.T. Telang. Preventive efficacy of Lentinas elodes mycelium extract (LEM) in human mammary carcinogenesis (abstr. 321). In 19th Annual San Antonio Breast Cancer Symposium. [San Antonio, Texas] December 11-14, 1996, Program and Abstracts, 1996:265.

97. Nanba, H., K. Mori, T. Toyomasu, H. Kuroda. Antitumor action of shiitake (Lentinus elodes) fruit bodies orally administered to mice. *Chem Pharm Bull*, 1987;35:2453-58.

98. Jones, Kenneth. Shiitake: a major medicinal mushroom. *Alternative and Complementary Therapies*, Feb.,1998:55.

99. Sharma, O.P. *Biochem Pharmacol*, 1976;25:1811-12.

100. Bensky, D. & A. Gamble. *Chinese Herbal Medicine Materia Medica*. Seattle, WA: Eastland Press, 1986:390-91.

101. Thaloor, D., et al. Inhibition of angiogenic differentiation of human umbilical vein endothelial cells by curcumin. *Cell Growth and Differentiation*, 1998;9(4):305-12.

102. Hall, A. Curcuma longa: A therapeutic role in the fight against breast cancer. Toronto, ON: Canadian College of Naturopathic Medicine, April, 1999.

103. Mehta, K. et al. Antiproliferative effect of curcumin (diferuloylmethane) against human breast tumor cell lines. *Anti-Cancer Drugs*, 1997;8(5):470-81.

104. Choudhuri, T., S. Pal, M.L. Agwaral, T. Das, G. Sa. Curcumin induces apoptosis in human breast cancer cells through p53-dependent Bax induction. *FEBS Lett*, 2002 Feb 13; 512(1-3):334-340.

105. Arnold, S.F., D.M. Klotz, B.M. Collins, P.M. Vonier, L.J. Guillette Jr., & J.A.McLachlan. *Science*, 1996;272,1489-92.

106. Verma, S.P., E. Salamone & B. Goldin. Curcumin and genistein, plant natural products, show synergistic inhibitory effects on the growth of human breast cancer MCF-7 cells induced by estrogenic pesticides. *Biochem and Biophys Res Comm*, 1997;233:692-96.

107. Galland, L. Intestinal toxicity: New approaches to an old problem. *Alternative and Complementary Therapies*, Aug. 1997;3(4):288-95.

108. Zhu, B.T., D.P. Loder, M.X. Cai, C.T. Huang, A.H. Conney. Dietary administratio of an extract from rosemary leaves enhances the liver microsomal metabolism of endogenous estrogens and decreases their uterotropic action in CD-1 mice. *Carcinogenesis*, Oct. 1998;19(10):1821-27.

109. Brand Miller, J., K. Foster-Powell, S. Colagiuri. *The G.I. Factor: The Glycaemic Index Solution*. Sydney, Australia: Hodder Headline Australian Pty Ltd., 1996.

110. Clorfene-Casten, Liane. *Breast Cancer: Poisons, Profits and Prevention*. Monroe, ME: Common Courage Press, 1996:27.

111. Greenpeace. *Death in Small Doses: The Effects of Organochlorines on Aquatic Ecosystems*. London, England: Greenpeace Communications, 1992.

112. EPA (U.S. Environmental Protection Agency). *National Dioxin Study Tier 4-Combustion Sources: Engineering Analysis Report*. Washington, DC. U.S. EPA Office of Air Quality Planning and Standards, 1988.

113. Greenpeace. *Chlorine Chemicals in Cod Liver Oil*. London, England: Greenpeace Communications, 1995.

114. Kushi, Michio. *The Cancer Prevention Diet*. New York, NY: St Martin's Press, 1993:125.

115. Gaskill, S.P., et al. Breast cancer diet and mortality in the United States. *Cancer Research*, 39:3628-37.

116. Le, M. G. et al. Consumption of dairy produce and alcohol in a case-control study of breast cancer. *Journal of the National Cancer Institute*, 77:633-36.

117. Gilbert, Susan. Fears over milk, long dismissed, still simmer. *New York Times*, Jan.19, 1999:D7.

118. Pizzorno, J. & M. Murray. Sodium, potassium, calcium and phosphorus content of foods. *A Textbook of Natural Medicine*. Seattle, WA: John Bastyr College Publications, 1985: IV:ImmSup.3-4.

119. Janssens J.P., et al. Effects of soft drink and table beer consumption on insulin response in normal teenagers and carbohydrate drink in youngsters. *Eur J Cancer Prev*, 1999;Aug;8(4):289-95.

120. Alcohol and the breast, *Journal of the National Cancer Institute*, 1993;85:692, 722.

121. Yu, H., J. Berkel. Do insulin-like growth factors mediate the effect of alcohol on breast cancer risk? *Med Hypotheses*, 1999;Jun:52(6):491-96.

Chapter 8: Nutritional Supplements for Breast Health

1. Ching, S., D. Ingram, R. Hahnel, J. Beilby, E. Rossi. Serum levels of micronutrients, antioxidants and total antioxidant status predict risk of breast cancer in a case control study. *J Nutr*, 2002 Feb; 132(2):303-06.

2. Katsouyanni, K., et al. Diet and breast cancer: a case control study in Greece. *Int J Cancer*, 1986:38815-20.

3. Weed, Susun. *Breast Cancer/Breast Health!* Woodstock, NY: Ash Tree Publishing,1996:47.

4. Lamson, D., M. Brignall. Antioxidants and cancer therapy II: Quick reference guide. *Alter Med Rev*, 2000; 5(2):152-163.

5. Biskind, M.S., G.R. Biskind. Effect of vitamin B complex deficiency on inactivation of estrone in the liver. *Endocrinology*, 1942;31:109-14.

6. Inculet, R.I. et al. Water soluble vitamins in cancer patients on parenteral nutrition: a prospective study. *Journal of Parenteral Enteral Nutrition*, May-June 1987;11(3):243-49.

7. Jacobson, E.L. A biomarker for the assessment of niacin nutriture as a potential preventive factor in carcinogenesis. *Journal of Internal Medicine*, 1993;233:59-62.

8. Henning, S.M. et al. Male rats fed methyl — and folate- deficient diets with or without niacin develop hepatic carcinomas associated with decreased tissue NAD concentrations and altered poly (ADP-ribose) polymerase activity. *Journal of Nutrition*, Jan 1997;127(1):30-36.

9. Hageman, G.J., R.H. Stierum. Niacin, poly(ADP-ribose) polymerase-1 and genomic stability. *Mutat Res*, 2001 Apr 18;475(1-2):45-56.

10. Jacobson, E.L., et al. Niacin deficiency and cancer in women. *Journal of the American College of Nutrition*, 1993;12(4):412-16.

11. Kim, J. Use of vitamins as adjunct to conventional cancer therapy. 2nd Denver Conference on Nutrition and Cancer. Sept. 7-11, 1994.

12. Jacobson, M, E. Jacobsen. Niacin, nutrition, ADP-ribosylation and cancer. The 8th International Symposium on ADP-ribosylation, Texas College of Osteopathic Medicine, Fort Worth, TX, 1987.

13. Gerson, Max. *A Cancer Therapy: Results of Fifty Cases*. Del Mar, CA: Totality Books, 1958.

14. Davis, B.A., B.E. Cowing. Pyridoxal supplementationreduces cell proliferation and DNA synthesis in estrogen-dependent and independent mammary carcinoma cell lines. *Nutr Cancer*, 2000; 38(2):281-286.

15. Folkers, K. Relevance of the biosynthesis of coenzyme Q10 and the four bases of DNA as a rationale for the molecular causes of cancer and a therapy. *Biochem Biophys Res Comm*, 1996;224:358-61.

16. Zhang, S.M., et al Plasma folate, vitamin B6, vitamin B12, homocysteine, and risk of breast cancer. *J Natl Cancer Inst*, 2003 Mar 5; 95(5):373-80.

17. Choi, S.W. Vitamin B12 deficiency: a new risk for breast cancer? *Nutr Rev*, 1999;Aug;57(8):250-53.

18. Standish, L. *Breast Cancer Beyond Convention* New York, NY: Atria Books, 2002:278.

19. Standish, L. *Breast Cancer Beyond Convention* New York, NY: Atria Books, 2002:280.

20. Shamsuddin, A.M., G.Y. Yang, I. Vucenik. Novel anti-cancer functions of IP6: growth inhibition and differentiation of human mammary cancer cell lines in vitro. *Anticancer Res*, 1996 Nov-Dec;16(6A):3287-92.

21. Vucenik, I., G.Y. Yang, A.M. Shamsuddin. Comparison of pure inositol hexaphosphate and high-bran diet in the prevention of DMBA-induced rat mammary carcinogenesis. *Nutr Cancer*, 1997;28(1):7-13.

22. Saied, I.T., A.M. Shamsuddin. Up-regulation of the tumor suppressor gene p53 and WAF1 gene expression by IP6 in HT-29 human colon carcinoma cell line. *Anticancer Res*, 1998 May-June;18(3A):1479-84.

23. Zhang, S. et al. Dietary carotenoids and vitamins A, C, and E and risk of breast cancer. *J Natl Cancer Inst*, 1999, Mar 17:91(6):547-56.

24. Riordan, N.H., H.D. Riordan, X.L. Meng, Y. LI, J.A. Jackson. Intravenous ascorbate as a tumor cytotoxic chemotherapeutic agent. *Medical Hypotheses;* 1995; 44:207-213.

25. Riordan N., J.A. Jackson, H.D. Riordan.

Intravenous vitamin C in a terminal cancer patient. *Journal of Orthomolecular Medicine,* 1996; 11:80-82.

26. Jamison, J.M., J. Gilloteaux, H. Taper, J. Summers. Evaluation of the in vitro and in vivo antitumor activities of vitamin C and K-3 combinations against human prostate cancer. *Journal of Nutrition,* 2001; 131:158S-160S.

27. Calderon, P.B., et al. Potential therapeutic application of the association of vitamins C and k(3) in cancer treatment. *Curr Med Chem,* 2002 Dec; 9(24):2271-2285.

28. Gilloteaux, J., J.M. Jamison, M. Venugopal, D. Giammar, J.L. Summers. Scanning electron microscopy and transmission electron microscopy aspects of synergistic antitumor activity of vitamin C- vitamin K3 combinations against human prostatic carcinoma cells. *Scanning Microsc,* 1995 Mar; 9(1):159-173.

29. Wu, F.Y., W.C> Liao, H.M. Chang. Comparison of antitumor activity of vitamins K1, K2, and K3 on human tumor cells by two (MTT and SRB) cell viability assays. *Life Sci,* 1993; 52(22):1797-1804.

30. Lamson, D.W., M.S. Brignall. Antioxidants and Cancer III: Quercetin. *Altern Med Rev,* 2000; 5(3):196-208.

31. Ainsleigh, H.G. Beneficial effects of sun exposure on cancer mortality. *Prev Med,* 1993;22:132-40.

32. Colston, K.W., et al. Possible role for vitamin D in controlling breast cancer cell proliferation. *Lancet,* 1989;i:188-91.

33. Ambrosone, C.B. et al. Interaction of family history of breast cancer and dietary antioxidants with breast cancer risk. *Cancer Causes and Control,* Sept. 1995;6(5):407-15.

34. Guthrie, N. et al. Inhibition of proliferation of estrogen receptor-negative MDA-MB-435 and positive MCF-7 human breast cancer cells by palm oil tocotrienols and tamoxifen, alone and in combination. American Society for Nutritional Sciences, 1997.

35. Moss, R. *Cancer Therapy: The Independent Consumer's Guide to Non-Toxic Treatment and Prevention.* New York, NY: Equinox Press, 1992:78.

36. Gilloteaux, J., J.M. Jamison, M. Venugopal, D. Giammar, J.L. Summers. Scanning electron microscopy and transmission electron microscopy aspects of synergistic antitumor activity of vitamin C- vitamin K3 combinations against human prostatic carcinoma cells. *Scanning Microsc,* 1995 Mar; 9(1):159-73.

37. Jacobson E.A. et al. Effects of dietary fat, calcium, and vitamin D on growth and mammary tumorigeneis induced by 7,12-dimethylbenz(a)anthracene in female Sprague-Dawley rats. *Cancer Research,* 1989;49:6300-03.

38. Anonymous. Diet of teenage girls may increase their risk of breast cancer. *Primary Care and Cancer,* 1994;14(2):8.

39. Gerson, Max. *A Cancer Therapy: Results of Fifty Cases.* Del Mar, CA: Totality Books, 1958.

40. Ramesha A, et al. Chemoprevention of 7,12-dimethylbenz(a)anthracene-induced mammary carcinogenesis in rats by the combined actions of selenium, magnesium, ascorbic acid and retinyl acetate. *Jpn J Cancer Res,* 1990:1239-46.

41. Teas, J. et al. Dietary seaweed and mammary carcinogenesis in rats. *Cancer Research,* 1984;44:2758-61.

42. Moss, R. *Cancer Therapy: The Independent Consumer's Guide to Non-Toxic Treatment and Prevention.* New York, NY: Equinox Press, 1992:94.

43. Wei, H.J. et al. Effect of molybdenum and tungsten on mammary carcinogenesis in Sprague-Dawley rats. *Chung Hua Chung Liu Tsa Chih,* 1987;9:204-07.

44. Astrup, A. et al. Pharmacology of thermogenic drugs. *Am J Clin Nutr,* 1992;55(1 Supp):863-67.

45. Ladas, HD. The potential of selenium in the treatment of cancer. *Holistic Medicine.* 1989;4:145-56.

46. Ksrnjavi, H. and D. Beker. Selenium in serum as a possible parameter for assessment of breast disease. *Breast Cancer Research and Treatment,* 1990;16:57-61.

47. Moss, R. *Cancer Therapy: The Independent Consumer's Guide to Non-Toxic Treatment and Prevention.* New York, N.Y., Equinox Press, 1992:112.

48. Magalova, T., et al. Copper, zinc and superoxide dismutase in precancerous, benign diseases and gastric, colorectal and breast cancer. *Neoplasma,* 1999;46(2):100-04.

49. Magalova, T., et al. Zinc and copper in breast cancer. *Therapeutic Uses of Trace Elements,* 1996;65:373-75.

50. Haynes, J. Coenzyme Q10 and breast cancer. *Townsend Letter for Doctors and Patients.* Aug/Sept 1997:160-62.

51. Murray, M.T. *Coenzyme Q10.* Rocklin, CA: Prima Publishing, 1996:196-308.

52. Bagchi, D. A review of the clinical benefits of coenzyme Q10. *Journal of Advancement in Medicine,* 1997;10(2):139-48.

53. Takimoto, M. et al. Protective effects of CoQ10 administration on cardiac toxicity in FAC therapy. *Gan To Kogaku Rryoho,* 1982;9:1,116-21.

54. Lockwood, K., S. Moesgaard, T. Yamamoto, and

K. Folkers. Progress on therapy of breast cancer with vitamin Q10 and the regression of metastases. *Biochemical and Biophysical Research Communications*, 1995;212:1,172-77.

55. Gaby, A.R. The role of coenzyme Q10 in clinical medicine: Part 1. *Alternative Medicine Review*, 1996;1:1,11-13.

56. Jolliet, P. et al. Plasma coenzyme Q10 concentrations in breast cancer: prognosis and therapeutic consequences. *International Journal of Clinical Pharmacology and Therapeutics*, 1998;36(9):506-09.

57. Lockwood et al. Partial and complete regression of breast cancer in patients in relation to dosage of coenzyme Q10. *Biochemical and Biophysical Research Communications*, 1993:1504-08; 1994, Mar 30.

58. Choopra, R. Relative bioavailability of coenzyme Q10 formulations in human subjects. *International Journal of Vitamin and Nutrition Research*, 1998;68:109-13.

59. Lamson, D., M. Brignall. Antioxidants and cancer therapy II: Quick reference guide. *Alter Med Rev*, 2000; 5(2):152-163.

60. Lamson, D., M. Brignall. Antioxidants and cancer therapy II: Quick reference guide. *Alter Med Rev*, 2000; 5(2):152-163.

61. Colacci, A., et al. Inhibition of chemically induced cell transformation by lipoic acid. *Proceedings of the Annual Meeting of the American Association of Cancer Research*, 1997;38:A2419.

62. Berkson, B.M. Alpha lipoic acid (thioctic acid): My experience with this outstanding therapeutic agent. *Journal of Orthomolecular Medicine*, 1998;13(1):44-47.

63. Challam, J. Alpha-lipoic acid: A new antioxidant backed up by solid scientific research. *The Nutrition Reporter*, 1996;7(7):1.

64. Berkson, B.M. Alpha lipoic acid (thioctic acid): My experience with this outstanding therapeutic agent. *Journal of Orthomolecular Medicine*, 1998;13(1):44-47.

65. Buckler, J., A.J. DeNault, V. Franc, T. Strukoff. Breast cancer treatment and prevention: limonene, lycopene and alpha-lipoic acid. Toronto, ON: Canadian College of Naturopathic Medicine, April, 1999.

66. Natureworks. *Alpha Lipoic Acid Fact Book*. New York, NY: Abkit, Inc., 1996:18-19.

67. Murray, *M.T. Encyclopedia of Nutritional Supplements*. Rocklin, CA. Prima Publishing, 1996:343-46.

68. Ahn, D. et al. The effects of dietary ellagic acid on rat hepatic and esophageal mucosal cytochromes P450 and Phase II enzymes. *Carcinogenesis*, 1996 Apr; 17(4):821-828.

69. Smith, W.A., J.W. Freeman, R.C. Gupta. Effect of chemopreventive agents on DNA adduction induced by the potent mammary carcinogen dibenzo{a,1} pyrene in the human breast cells MCF-7. *Mutat Res*, Sept 1;480-481:97-108.

70. Smith, W.A., J.M. Arif, R.C. Gupta. Effect of cancer chemopreventive agents on microsome-mediated DNA adduction of the breast carcinogen Dibenzo{a,}pyrene. *Mutat Res*, 1998 Feb 13; 412(3):307-314.

71. Narayanan, B.A. et al p53/p21(WAF1/C1P1) expression and its possible role in G1 arrest and apoptosis in ellagic acid treated cancer cells. *Cancer Lett*, 1999 Mar 1; 136(2):215-221.

72. Saleem, A., et al. Inhibition of cancer growth by crude extract and the phenolics of Terminalia chebula retz fruit. *J Ethnopharmacol*, 2002 Aug; 81(3):327-336.

73. Eckert, K, E. Grabowski et al. Effects of oral bromelain administration on the impaired immunocytotoxicity of mononuclear cells from mammary tumor patients. *Oncol Rep*, 1999 Nov-Dec; 6(6):1191-1199.

74. Awad, A.B., A. Downie, C.S. Fink, U. Kim. Dietary phytosterol inhibits the growth and metastasis of MDA-MB-231 human breast cancer cells grown in SCID mice. *Anticancer Res*, 2000 Mar-Apr; 20(2A): 821-824.

75. Brignall, M.S. Prevention and treatment of cancer with indole-3-carbinol. *Alt Med Rev*, 2001; 6(6): 580-589.

76. Dwivedi, C., et al. Effect of calcium glucarate on beta-glucuronidase activity and glucarate content of certain vegetables and fruits. *Biochem Med Metab Biol*, 1990 Apr; 43(2):83-92.

77. Calcium-D-glucarate. *Alt Med Rev*, 2002 Aug; 7(4):336-339.

78. Eliaz, I. The role of modified citrus pectin in the prevention of cancer metastasis. *Townsend Letter for Doctors and Patients*, 1999;July;192:64-65.

79. Blask, D., S. Wilson, F. Zalatan. Physiological melatonin inhibition of human breast cancer cell growth in vitro: Evidence for a glutathione-mediated pathway. *Cancer Res*, 1997;57:1909-14.

80. Tamarkin, L., C.J. Baird, O. Almeida. Melatonin: A coordinating signal for mammalian reproduction? *Science*, 1985;227:714-20.

81. Lissoni, P., S. Barni, S. Meregalli et al. Modulation of cancer endocrine therapy by melatonin: A phase II study of tamoxifen plus melatonin in metastatic breast cancer patients progression under tamoxifen alone. *Br. J. Cancer*, 1995;71:854-56.

82. Lissoni, P., S. Crispino, S. Barni et al. Pineal gland and tumor cell kinetics: serum labelling rate in breast cancer. *Oncology*, 1990;47:3:275-77.

83. Bartsch, H., C. Bartsch. Effect of melatonin on experimental tumors under different photoperiods and times of administration. *J. Neural. Transm*, 1981;52:269-79.

Chapter 9: Psychological and Spiritual Means for Preventing Breast Cancer

1. Hamer, R.G. *The New Medicine: Questions and Answers*, handout.

2. Achterberg, J. *Imagery in Healing*. Boston, MA: Shambhala, 1985:189.

3. Psychosomatic Dimensions of Cancer Therapy. Dr. Bernard Greenwood. *Consumer Health Newsletter*, Jan./Feb. 1987; 8(1).

4. LeShan, Lawrence. *Cancer as a Turning Point: A Handbook for People with Cancer, Their Families and Health Professionals.* New York: Penguin, 1994:21

5. LeShan, Lawrence. *Cancer as a Turning Point: A Handbook for People with Cancer, Their Families and Health Professionals.* New York: Penguin, 1994:72-73.

6. Frankl, Viktor. *Man's Search for Meaning: An Introduction to Logotherapy*. Translated by Ilse Lasch. New York, NY: Pocket Books, 1963:115.

7. Jayne, Walter Addison. *The Healing Gods of Ancient Civilizations*. New Hyde Park, NY: University Books Inc., 1962:240-303.

8. Ingerman, Sandra. *Welcome Home: Life After Healing*. San Francisco, CA: Harper-San Francisco, 1993.

9. Johnson, Robert. *Inner Work*. New York, NY: Harper and Row, 1986.

10. I heard this idea first in a lecture by Yogi Bhajan and have since read it in Jean Shinoda Bolen's book, Close to the Bone. New York, NY: Touchstone - Simon and Schuster, 1996:71.

11. Dossey, Larry. *Healing Words: The Power of Prayer and the Practice of Medicine*. New York, NY: HarperCollins, 1993:28.

12. Koenig-Bricker, Woodene. *Prayers of the Saints: An Inspired Collection of Holy Wisdom*. New York, NY: HarperCollins, 1996.

Chapter 10: Breast Disease Treatments

1. Love, S. *Dr. Susan Love's Breast Book*. Cambridge, MA: Perseus Publishing, 2000:381.

2. Cooper, L.S. et al. survival of premenopausal breast carcinoma patients in relation to menstrual timing of surgery and estrogen receptor/progesterone receptor status of the primary tumor. *Cancer*, 1999 Nov 15; 86(10):2053-58.

3. My thanks goes to my friend and colleague, Jen Green, N.D. of Toronto for compiling this information and sharing it with me.

4. Naiman, I. *Cancer Salves: A Botanical Approach to Treatment*. Santa Fe, NM: Seventh Ray Press. 1999:203-05.

5. Mock V; Pickett M; Ropka ME; Lin EM; Stewart KJ; Rhodes VA; McDaniel R; Grimm PM; Krumm S; McCorkle R. Fatigue and quality of life outcomes of exercise during cancer treatment. *Cancer Practice: A Multidisciplinary Journal of Cancer Care*, 2001 May-Jun; 9(3): 119-27 (35 ref).

6. Petrella RJ. Best of the literature. Exercise reduces chemotherapy fatigue in breast cancer patients. *Physician and Sportsmedicine*, 2001 Nov; 29(11): 5.

7. Pinto BM; Clark MM; Maruyama NC; Feder SI. Psychological and fitness changes associated with exercise participation among women with breast cancer. *Psycho-oncology*, 2003 Mar-Apr; 12 (2):118-26.

8. Jones, C. Allies in the breast cancer battle: herbs for prevention, treatment and healing. *Herbs for Health*, 1998, Jan/Feb:29-33.

9. Xia YS, Wang JH, Shan L J. Acupuncture plus ear point press in preventing vomiting induced by chemotherapy with Cisplatin. *International Journal of Clinical Acupuncture*, Jan 1 200: 11(2): 145-48.

10. Dibble SL, Chapman J, et al. Acupuncture for nausea: results of a pilot study. *Oncology Nursing Forum*. 2000 Jan-Feb; 27 (1):41-47.

11. Mayer DJ. Acupuncture: an evidence-based review of clinical literature. *Annual Review of Medicine*. 2000;51:49-63.

12. Anderson, P.M., et al. Oral glutamine reduces the duration and severity of stomatitis after cytotoxic cancer chemotherapy. *Cancer*, 1998; 83:1433-39.

13. Skubitz KM; Anderson PM. Oral glutamine to prevent chemotherapy induced stomatitis: a pilot study. *Journal of Laboratory and Clinical Medicine*, 1996 Feb; 127(2): 223-28.

14. Muscaritoli, M, Micozzi, A, Conversano, L, Martino, P, Petti, MC, et al.: Oral glutamine in the prevention of chemotherapy-induced gastrointestinal toxicity. *Eur J Cancer*, 1997;33:319-320.

15. Wadleigh, RG, Redman, RS, Graham, ML, Krasnow, SH, Anderson, A, et al: Vitamin E in the treatment of chemotherapy-induced

mucositis. *Am J Med,* 1992;92:481-84.

16. Standish, L. *Breast Cancer Beyond Convention.* Tagliaferri, M., I. Cohen, D. Tripathy eds. New York, NY: Atria Books, nd:280.

17. Cohen, I. *Breast Cancer Beyond Convention.* Tagliaferri, M., I. Cohen, D. Tripathy eds. New York, NY: Atria Books, 2003:77-78.

18. Wei, Z. Clinical observation on therapeutic effect of acupuncture at St 36 for leucopenia. J TCM, 1998; 18:94-95.

19. Zhou, J., Z. Li, P. Jin. A clinical study on acupuncture for prevention and treatment of toxic side effects during radiotherapy and chemotherapy. *J TCM,* 1999;19:16-21.

20. Lissoni, P. et al. Chemoneuroendocrine therapy of metastatic breast cancer with persistent thrombocytopenia with weekly low-dose epirubicin plus melatonin: a phase 2 study. *J Pineal Res,* 1999 Apr; 26(3):169-173.

21. Cohen, I. *Breast Cancer Beyond Convention.* Tagliaferri, M., I. Cohen, D. Tripathy eds. New York, N.Y. Atria Books, 2003:72.

22. Cohen, I. *Breast Cancer Beyond Convention.* Tagliaferri, M., I. Cohen, D. Tripathy eds. New York, N.Y. Atria Books, 2003:65-66.

23. Love, S. *Dr. Susan Love's Breast Book.* Cambridge, MA: Perseus Publishing, 2000:534-35.

24. Folkers, K, and Wolaniuk, A: Research on coenzyme Q_{10} in clinical medicine and in immunomodulation. *Drugs Exp Clin Res, 1985:*11:539-45.

25. Okamoto, K, and Ogura, R: Effects of vitamins on lipid peroxidation and suppression of DNA synthesis induced by adriamycin in Ehrlich cells, *J Nutr Sci Vitamino,* 1985;31, 129-37.

26. Shaeffer, J, El-Mahdi, AM, and Nichols, RK: Coenzyme Q_{10} and adriamycin toxicity in mice. *Res Commun Chem Pathol Pharmacol,* 1980:29:309-15, 1980.

27. Domae, N, Sawada, H, Matsuyama, E, Konishi, T, and Uchino, H: Cardiomyopathy and other chronic toxic effects induced in rabbits by doxorubicin and possible prevention by coenzyme Q_{10}. *Cancer Treat Rep,* 1981:65:79-91.

28. Stoll, B.A. N-3 fatty acids and lipid peroxidation in breast cancer inhibition. *Br J Nutr,* 2002 Mar; 87(3):193-198.

29. Hardman WE; Avula CP; Fernandes G; Cameron IL. Three percent dietary fish oil concentrate increased efficacy of doxorubicin against MDA-MB 231 breast cancer xenografts. *Clinical Cancer Research,* 2001 Jul;7 (7): 2041-49.

30. Ogilvie GK; Fettman MJ; Mallinckrodt CH; Walton JA et al. Effect of fish oil, arginine, and doxorubicin chemotherapy on remission and survival time for dogs with lymphoma: a double-blind, randomized placebo-controlled study. *Cancer,* 2000;Apr 15; 88 (8):1916-28.

31. Shao Y; Pardini L; Pardini RS. Intervention of transplantable human mammary carcinoma MX-1 chemotherapy with dietary menhaden oil in athymic mice: increased therapeutic effects and decreased toxicity of cyclophosphamide. *Nutrition and cancer,* 1997; 28 (1):63-73.

32. Olson, R.D., W.E. Stroo, R.C. Boerth. Influence of N-acetylcysteine on the anti-tumor activity of doxorubicin. *Semin Oncol,* 1983; 10:29-34.

33. Teicher, B.A. et al. In vivo modulation of several anticancer agents by beta-carotene. *Cancer Chemother Pharmacol,* 1994; 34:235-41.

34. Bracke, M.E. et al. Influence of tangeretin on tamoxifen's therapeutic benefit in mammary cancer. *JNCI,* 1999; 91:354-59.

35. Lamson, D.W., M. Brignall. Antioxidants and cancer therapy II: Quick reference guide. *Alt Med Rev,* 2000; 5(2):152-63.

36. Jacobson, E.L. A biomarker for the assessment of niacin nutriture as a potential preventive factor in carcinogenesis. *Journal of Internal Medicine*, 1993;233:59-62.

37. Kim, J. Use of vitamins as adjunct to conventional cancer therapy. *2nd Denver Conference on Nutrition and Cancer.* Sept 7-11, 1994.

38. Tanaka, Y. et al. Application of algal polysaccharides as in vivo binders of metal pollutants. *Proc Seventh Int Seaweed Symp,* 1972.

39. Tanaka, Y. et al. Studies on inhibition of intestinal absorption of radioactive strontium. *Can Med Assoc J,* 1968;99:169-75.

40. Inano, H., M. Onoda. Radioprotective action of curcumin estracted from Curcuma longa LINN:inhibitory effect on formation of urinary 8-hydroxy-2-deoxyguanosine, tumorigenesis, but not mortality, induced by gamma-ray irradiation. *Int J Radiat Oncol Biol Phys,* 2002 Jul 1; 53(3):735-43.

41. Kapitanov, A.B., et al. Radiation-protective effectiveness of lycopene. *Radiats Biol Radioecol,* 1994 May-June; 34(3):439-445.

42. Gorshkov, A.I., Comparative evaluation of radiation protective efficiency of regimens with various contents of calcium, potassium and iron. *Gig Sanit,* 1994 Jun;(6):18-20.

43. Perepelkin, S.R., N.D. Egorova. Prophylactic and therapeutic role of the B group vitamin, mesoinositol, in radiation sckness against a background of the use of a milk and egg diet. *Radiobiologiia,* 1980 Jan-Feb; 20(1):137-39.

44. Green J. Clinical experience of Naturopathic Doctor relayed to me personally. Toronto, ON: May, 2003.

45. Mendecki, J, Friedenthal, E, Dawson, H, and Seifter, E: beta-Carotene reduces toxicity and carcinogenicity of cyclophosphamide in control and tumor-bearing mice (abstr). *Adv Exp Med Biol,* 1994;364:177.

46. Mendecki, J, Friedenthal, E, Dawson, H, and Seifter, E: beta-Carotene reduces toxicity and carcinogenicity of cyclophosphamide in control and tumor-bearing mice (abstr). *Adv Exp Med Biol,* 1994;364:177; and Salvadori, DMF, Ribeiro, LR, Oliveira, MDM, Pereira, CAB, and Becak, W: The protective effect of beta-carotene on genotoxicity induced by cyclophosphamide. *Mutat Res,* 1992;265:237-44.

47. Kurbacher, CM, Wagner, U, Kolster, B, Andreotti, PE, Krebs, D, et al. Ascorbic acid (vitamin C) improves the antineoplastic activity of doxorubicin, cisplatin, and paclitaxel in human breast carcinoma cells in vitro. *Cancer Lett,* 1996;103:183-89.

48. Chiang, CD, Song, EJ, Yang, VC, and Chao, CCK: Ascorbic acid increases drug accumulation and reverses vincristine resistance of human non-small-cell lung cancer cells. *Biochem J,* 1994;301, 759-64.

49. Prasad, KN, Sinha, PK, Ramanujam, M, and Sakamoto, A: Sodium ascorbate potentiates the growth inhibitory effect of certain agents on neuroblastoma cells in culture. *Proc Natl Acad Sci USA,* 1979;76:829-32..

50. Taper, HS, de Gerlache, J, Lans, M, and Roberfroid, M: Non-toxic potentiation of cancer chemotherapy by combined C and K3 vitamin pre-treatment. *Int J Cancer,* 1987;40:575-79.

51. Moore, C, Chu, M, Tibbetts, L, and Calabresi, P: Potentiation of BCNU by vitamin C in a murine model of CNS leukemia (abstr). *Pharmacologist,* 1979;21:233.

52. Shimpo, K, Nagatsu, T, Yamada, K, Sato, T, Niimi, H, et al.: Ascorbic acid and adriamycin toxicity. Am J Clin Nutr, 1991;54:1298S-1301S; and Fujita, K, Shimpo, K, Yamada, K, Sato, T, Niimi, H, et al.: Reduction of adriamycin toxicity by ascorbate in mice and guinea pigs. *Cancer Res,* 1982;42:309-16.

53. Waxman, S, and Bruckner, H: The enhancement of 5-fluorouracil antimetabolic activity by Leucovorin, menadione, and alpha-tocopherol. *Eur J Cancer Clin Oncol* 1982:18:685-92.

54. Chinery, R, Brockman, JA, Peeler, MO, Shyr, Y, Beauchamp, RD, et al.: Antioxidants enhance the cytotoxicity of chemotherapeutic agents in colorectal cancer: a p53-independent induction of p21 WAF1/CIP1 via C/EBPbeta. *Nature Med,* 1997;3:1233-41.

55. Perez-Ripoll, EA, Rama, BN, and Webber, MM: Vitamin E enhances the chemotherapeutic effects of adriamycin on human prostatic carcinoma cells in vitro. *J Urol,* 1986;136:529-31.

56. Guthrie, N, Gapor, A, Chambers, AF, and Carroll, KK: Inhibition of proliferation of estrogen receptor-negative MDA-MB-435 and -positive MCF-7 human breast cancer cells by palm oil tocotrienols and tamoxifen, alone and in combination. *J Nutr,* 1997;127:544S-548S.

57. Chinery, R, Brockman, JA, Peeler, MO, Shyr, Y, Beauchamp, RD, et al. Antioxidants enhance the cytotoxicity of chemotherapeutic agents in colorectal cancer: a p53-independent induction of p21WAF1/C1P1 via C/EBPbeta. *Nat Med,* 1997 Nov; 3(11):1233-1241.

58. Myers, CE, McGuire, WP, Liss, RH, Ifrim, I, Grotzinger, K, et al. Adriamycin: the role of lipid peroxidation in cardiac toxicity and tumor response. *Science,* 1997;197:165-67; Sonneveld, P: Effect of alpha-tocopherol on the cardiotoxicity of adriamycin in the rat. *Cancer Treat Rep,* 1978:62:1033-36.

59. Legha, SS, Wang, YM, Mackay, B, Ewer, M, Hortobagyi, GN, et al. Clinical and pharmacologic investigation of the effects of alpha-tocopherol on adriamycin cardiotoxicity. *Ann NY Acad Sci,* 1982;393:411-18.

60. Perez, JE, Macchiavelli, M, Leone, BA, Romero, A, Rabinovich, MG, et al. High-dose alpha-tocopherol as a preventive of doxorubicin-induced alopecia. *Cancer Treat Rep,*1986:70:1213-14.

61. Yu, W, Simmons-Menchaca, M, Gapor, A, Sanders, BG, and Kline, K: Induction of apoptosis in human breast cancer cells by tocopherols and tocotrienols. *Nutr Cancer,* 1999;33:26-32; and Guthrie, N, Gapor, A, Chambers, AF, and Carroll, KK: Effect of palm oil tocotrienols on epidermal growth factor receptor protein tyrosine kinase activity in human breast cancer cells (abstr). *FASEB J,* 1998:12:A657.

62. Hermansen, K, K. Wassermann. The effect of vitamin E and selenium on doxorubicin-induced delayed toxicity in mice. *Acta Pharamacol Toxico,*1986:58:31-37.

63. Okamoto, K, and Ogura, R: Effects of vitamins on lipid peroxidation and suppression of DNA synthesis induced by adriamycin in Ehrlich cells, *J Nutr Sci Vitaminol,* 1985:31:129-37.

64. Shaeffer, J, El-Mahdi, AM, and Nichols, RK: Coenzyme Q_{10} and adriamycin toxicity in mice. *Res Commun Chem Pathol Pharmacol,* 1980:29:309-15.

65. Domae, N, Sawada, H, Matsuyama, E, Konishi, T, and Uchino, H: Cardiomyopathy and other chronic toxic effects induced in rabbits by doxorubicin and possible prevention by coenzyme

Q_{10}. *Cancer Treat Rep,* 1981;65:79-91.

66. Folkers, K, Choe, JY, and Combs, AB: Rescue by coenzyme Q_{10} from electrocardiographic abnormalities caused by the toxicity of adriamycin in the rat. *Proc Natl Acad Sci USA,* 1978;75:5178-80; Combs, AB, Choe, JY, Truong, DH, and Folkers, K: Reduction by coenzyme Q_{10} of the acute toxicity of adriamycin in mice. *Res Commun Chem Pathol Pharmacol,* 1977;18:565-68; Shaeffer, J, El-Mahdi, AM, and Nichols, RK: Coenzyme Q_{10} and adriamycin toxicity in mice. *Res Commun Chem Pathol Pharmaco,* 1980:29:309-15; Ohara, H, Kanaide, H, and Nakamura, M: A protective effect of coenzyme Q_{10} on the adriamycin-induced cardiotoxicity in the isolated perfused rat heart. *J Mol Cell Cardiol,* 1981;13:741-52; Shinozawa, S, Etowo, K, Araki, Y, and Oda, T: Effect of coenzyme Q_{10} on the survival time and lipid peroxidation of adriamycin (doxorubicin)-treated mice. *Acta Med Okayama,* 1983;38:57-63.

67. Domae, N, Sawada, H, Matsuyama, E, Konishi, T, and Uchino, H: Cardiomyopathy and other chronic toxic effects induced in rabbits by doxorubicin and possible prevention by coenzyme Q_{10}. *Cancer Treat Rep,* 1981:65:79-91; and Shaeffer, J, El-Mahdi, AM, and Nichols, RK: Coenzyme Q_{10} and adriamycin toxicity in mice. *Res Commun Chem Pathol Pharmacol,* 1980:29:309-15.

68. Folkers, K, and Wolaniuk, A: Research on coenzyme Q_{10} in clinical medicine and in immunomodulation. *Drugs Exp Clin Res,* 1985:11:539-45.

69. Scambia, G, Ranelletti, FO, Benedetti-Panici, P, De Vincenzo, R, Bonanno, G, et al.: Quercetin potentiates the effect of adriamycin in a multidrug-resistant MCF-7 human breast-cancer cell line: P-glycoprotein as a possible target. *Cancer Chemother Pharmacol,*1994;34:459-64.

70. Scambia, G, Ranelletti, FO, Benedetti-Panici, P, Piantelli, M, Bonanno, G, et al.: Inhibitory effect of quercetin on primary ovarian and endometrial cancers and synergistic activity with cis-diamminedichloroplatinum(II). *Gynecol Oncol,* 1992;45:13-19.

71. Logvinova, A.V. et al. Soy-derived antiapoptotic fractions protect gastrointestinal epithelium from damage caused by methotrexate treatment in the rat. *Nutr Cancer,* 1999;33:33-39.

72. Morgan, L.R. The control of ifosamide-induced hematuria with N-acetylcysteine in patients with advanced carcinoma of the lung. *Semin Oncol,* 1982; 9(suppl):71-74.

73. Oriana, S. et al. A preliminary clinical experience with reduced glutathione as protector

against cisplatin toxicity. *Tumori,* 1987;73:337-40.

74. Conklin, K.A. Dietary antioxidants during cancer chemotherapy: Impact on chemotherapeutic effectiveness and development of side effects. *Nutrition and Cancer,* 2000;37(1):1-18.

75. Garcia, J.J. et al Melatonin enhances Tamoxifen's ability to prevent the reduction in microsomal membrane fluidity induced by lipid peroxidation. *J MembrBiol,* 1998, Mar 1; 162(1):59-65.

76. Cover, C.M., et al Indole-3-carbinol and tamoxifen cooperate to arrest the cell cycle of MCF-7 human breast cancer cells. *Cancer Res,* 1999, Mar 15;59(6):1244-51.

77. Lee, J., D. Zava,, V, Hopkins. *What Your Doctor May Not Tell You About Breast Cancer.* New York, NY: Warner Books, 2002:152.

78. Messina, M.J. Legumes and soybeans:overview of their nutritional profiles and health effects. *Am J Clin Nutr,* 1999 Sep; 70(3 Supp):439S-450S.

79. Iwasaki, T., M. Mukai. Ipriflavone inhibits osteolytic bone metastases of human breast cancer cells in a nude mouse model. *Int J Cancer,* 2002 Aug.

80. Hirsch, K., M. Danilenko, J. Giat, et al. Effect of purified allicin, the major ingredient of freshly crushed garlic, on cancer cell proliferation. *Nutr Cancer,* 2000;38(2):245-54.

81. Kachhap, S.K., P.P. Dange, R.H. Santani, S.S. Sawant, S.N. Gosh. Effect of omega-3 fatty acid (docosahexanoic acid) on BRCA gene expression and growth in MCF-7 cell line. *Cancer Biother Radiopharm,* 2001 Jun; 16(3):257-63.

82. Narayanan, B.A., O. Geoffroy, M.C. Willingham, G.G. Re, D.W. Nixon. P53/p21(WAF1/CIP1) expression and its possible role in G1 arrest and apoptosis in ellagic acid treated cancer cells. *Cancer Lett,* 1999 Mar 1;136(2):215-21.

83. El-Sherbiny, Y.M., M.C. Cox, Z.A. Ismail, A.M. Shamsuddin, I Vucenik. *Anticancer Res,* 2001 Jul-Aug;21(4A): 2393-2403.

84. Cover, C.M., et al. Indole-3-carbinol inhibits the expression of cyclin-dependent kinase-6 and induces a G1 cell cycle arrest of human breast cancer cells independent of estrogen receptor signaling. *J Biol Chem,* 1998 Feb13;273(7):3838-3847.

85. Shi, w., M.N. Gould. Induction of cytostasis in mammary carcinoma cells treated with the anticancer agent perillyl alcohol. *Carcinogenesis,* 2002 Jan;23(1):131-42.

86. Bardon, S., K. Picard, P. martel. Monoterpenes inhibit cell growth, cell cycle progression, and cyclin D1 gene expression in human breast can-

cer cell lines. *Nutr Cancer*, 1998;32(1):1-7.

87. Liberto, M., D. Cobrinik. Growth factor-dependent induction of p21(C1P1) by the green tea polyphenol, epigallocatechin gallate. *Cancer Lett*, 2000 Jun 30;154(2):151-61.

88. Jacobson, E.L., W.M. Shieh, A.C. Huang. Mapping the role of NAD metabolism in prevention and treatment of carcinogenesis. *Mol Cell Biochem*, 1999 Mar;193(1-2):69-74.

89. Hu, H., N.S. Ahn. X. Yang, Y.S. Lee, K.S. Kang. Ganoderma lucidum estract induces cell cycle arrest and apoptosis in MCF-7 human breast cancer cell. *Int J Cancer*, 2002 Nov 20; 102(3):250-53.

90. Mediavilla, M.D., S. Cos, E.J. Sanchez-Barcelo. Melatonin increases p53 and p21WAF1 expression in MCF-7 breast cancer cells. *Life Sci*, 1999;65(4):42-25.

91. Cos, S., M.D. Mediavilla et al. Does melatonin induce apoptosis in MCF-7 human breast cancer cells in vitro? *J Pineal Res*, 2002 Mar;32(2):90-96.

92. Mehta, K., P. Pantazis, T. McQueen, B.B. Aggarwal. Antiproliferative effect of curcumin against human breast cancer cell lines. *Anti-Cancer Drugs*, 1997;8(5):470-81.

93. Li, Z., Y. Wang, B. Mo. The effects of carotenoids on the proliferation of human breast cancer cell and gene expression of bcl-2. *Zhonghua Yu Fang Yi Xue Za Zhi*, 2002 Jul;36(4):254-57.

94. Awad, A.B., H. Williams, C.S. Fink. Phytosterols reduce in vitro metastatic ability of MDA-MB-231 human breast cancer cells, *Nutr Cancer*,2001;40(2):157-64.

95. Shi, w., M.N. Gould. Induction of cytostasis in mammary carcinoma cells treated with the anti-cancer agent perillyl alcohol. *Carcinogenesis*, 2002 Jan;23(1):131-42.

96. Simon, A., et al. Inhibitory effect of curcuminoids on MCF-7 cell proliferation and structure-activity relationships. *Cancer Letter*, 1998;129(1):111-16.

97. Choi, J.A. et al. Induction of cell cycle arrest and apoptosis in human breast cancer cells by quercetin. *Int J Oncol*, 2001 Oct;19(4):837-44.

98. Hewitt, A.L., K.W. Singletary. Soy extract inhibits mammary adenocarcinoma growth in a syngeneic mouse model. *Cancer Letter*, 2003 Mar 31;192(2):133-43.

99. Li, X.K., M. Motwani, W. Tong, W. Bornmann, G.K. Schwartz. Huanglian, a Chinese herbal extract, inhibits cell growth by suppressing the expression of cyclin B1 and inhibiting CDC2 kinase activity in human cancer cells. *Mol Pharmacol*, 2000 Dec;58(6):1287-93.

100. Hirsch, K., M. Danilenko, J. Giat, et al. Effect of purified allicin, the major ingredient of freshly crushed garlic, on cancer cell proliferation. *Nutr Cancer*, 2000;38(2):245-54.

101. Simon, A., et al. Inhibitory effect of curcuminoids on MCF-7 cell proliferation and structure-activity relationships. *Cancer Letter*, 1998;129(1):111-16.

102. Holy, J.M. Curcumin disrupts mitotic spindle structure and induces micronucleation in MCF-7 breast cancer cells. *Mutat Res*, 2002, Jun 27;518(1):71-84.

103. Zhang, G.L. Treatment of breast proliferation disease with modified xiao yao san and er chen decoction. *Zhong Xi Yi Jie He Za Zhi*, 1991 Jul;11(7):400-22, 388.

Further Reading

Achterberg, Jeanne. *Imagery in Healing: Shamanism and Modern Medicine.* Boston, MA: Shambhala, 1985.

Achterberg, Jeanne, Barbara Dossey, Leslie Kolkmeier. *Rituals in Healing.* Toronto, ON: Bantam Books, 1994.

Arnot, Bob. *The Breast Cancer Prevention Diet.* New York, NY: Little, Brown and Co., 1998.

Austin, S. and Cathy Hitchcock. *Breast Cancer: What You Should Know (But May Not Be Told) About Prevention, Diagnosis and Treatment.* Rocklin, CA: Prima Publishing, 1994.

Barks, Coleman. *The Illuminated Rumi.* New York, NY: Broadway Books, 1997.

Berthold-Bond, Annie. *Clean & Green: The Complete Guide to Non-Toxic and Environmentally Safe Housekeeping.* Woodstock, NY: Ceres Press, 1994.

Bhajan, Yogi. *Kundalini Yoga for Youth and Joy.* Eugene, OR: 3HO Transcripts, 1983.

Bhajan, Yogi. *Healing through Kundalini: Specific Applications.* Compiled by Vikram K. Khalsa and Alice Clagett. Eugene, OR: 3HO Transcripts, 1987.

Bhajan, Yogi. *Owner's Manual for the Human Body.* Los Angeles, CA: 3HO Foundation and Kundalini Research Institute, 1993.

Bhajan, Yogi. *Sadhana Guidelines for Kundalini Yoga Daily Practise.* Los Angeles, CA: Kundalini Research Institute, 1996.

Bhajan, Yogi. *Survival Kit: Meditations and Exercises for Stress and Pressure of the Times.* Compiled by S.S. Vikram K. Khalsa and Dharm Darshan K. Khalsa. San Diego,

CA: Kundalini Research Institute, 1980.

Bhajan, Yogi. *The Kundalini Yoga Manual.* Claremont, CA: KRI Publications, 1976.

Bensky, D. & A. Gamble. *Chinese Herbal Medicine Materia Medica.* Seattle, WA: Eastland Press, 1986.

Boericke, W. *Homeopathic Materia Medica and Repertory.* Delhi, India: B. Jain Publishers Pvt. Ltd., 1996.

Bolen, Jean Shinoda. *Close to the Bone.* New York, NY: Touchstone - Simon and Schuster, 1996.

Boyle, W. & A. Saine. *Lectures in Naturopathic Hydrotherapy.* East Palestine, OH: Buckeye Naturopathic Press, 1988.

Braverman, Eric. *The Healing Nutrients Within.* New Canaan, CT: Keats Publishing, 1987.

Brinker, F. *An Introduction to the Toxicology of Common Botanical Substances.* CITY, STATE: National College of Naturopathic Medicine, 1983.

Canfield, Jack et al. *Chicken Soup for the Surviving Soul.* Deerfield Beach, FL: Health Communications, Inc., 1996.

Clark, Hulga. *The Cure for All Diseases.* San Diego, CA: ProMotion Publishing, 1995.

Clorfene-Casten, Liane. *Breast Cancer: Poisons, Profits and Prevention.* Monroe, ME: Common Courage Press, 1996.

Colborn, Theo, D. Dumanoski, J. Peterson Myers. *Our Stolen Future.* New York, NY: Penguin, 1996.

Commission for Environmental Cooperation. *Taking Stock: North American Pollutant Releases and Transfers 1995*. Montreal, QC: CEC, 1998.

Dadd, Debra Lynn. *The Nontoxic Home: Protecting Yourself and Your Family from Everyday Toxics and Health Hazards*. Los Angeles, CA: J.P. Tharcher, 1986.

Davis, R. et al. *The Relaxation and Stress Reduction Workbook*. 3rd ed. New York: New Harbinger Publications, 1988.

Day, Charlene. *The Immune System Handbook*. North York, ON: Potentials Within, 1991.

De Schepper, Luc. *Peak Immunity: How to Fight CEBV, Candida, Herpes Simplex Viruses and Other Immune-Suppressed Conditions and Win*. Van Nuys, CA: Le Fever Publications, 1989.

Dharmananda, Subhuti. *A Bag of Pearls*. Portland, OR: Institute for Traditional Medicine and Preventive Health Care, 1990.

Dharmananda, Subhuti. *Chinese Herbology*. Portland, OR: Institute for Traditional Medicine and Preventive Health Care, 1989.

Dossey, Larry. *Healing Words: The Power of Prayer and the Practice of Medicine*. New York, NY: HarperCollins, 1993.

Dunford, Randy. *Clean Your House Safely & Effectively Without Harmful Chemicals*. McKinney, TX: Magni Group, Inc., 1993.

Epstein, S. and D. Steinman. *The Breast Cancer Prevention Program*. New York, NY: Macmillan, 1997.

Erasmus, Udo. *Fats that Heal, Fats that Kill*. Burnaby, BC: Alive Books, 1993.

Falcone, Ron. *Natural Medicine for Breast Cancer*. New York, NY: Dell Publishing, 1996.

Frankl, Viktor. *Man's Search for Meaning: An Introduction to Logotherapy*. Translated by Ilse Lasch. New York, NY: Pocket Books, 1963.

Gerson, Max. *A Cancer Therapy: Results of Fifty Cases*. Del Mar, CA: Totality Books, 1977.

Guernsey, H. *The Application of the Principles and Practice of Homoeopathy to Obstetrics*. New Delhi, India: B. Jain Publishers Pvt. Ltd., 1988.

Gittleman, Ann Louise. *Guess What Came for Dinner?* Garden City Park, NY: Avery, 1993.

Gofman, John. *Preventing Breast Cancer: The Story of a Major, Proven, Preventable Cause of This Disease*. 2nd. ed. San Francisco, CA: Committee for Nuclear Responsibility, 1996.

Gupta, D., R. Attanasio & R. Reiter, eds. *The Pineal Gland and Cancer*. Tubingen, Germany: Muller and Bass, 1988.

Hobbs, C. *Foundations of Health: Healing with Herbs and Foods*. Capitola, CA: Botanica Press, 1992.

Hole, J. *Human Anatomy and Physiology*. Dubuque, IA: Wm. C. Brown Publishers, 1984.

Holmes, P. *The Energetics of Western Herbs*. Vol. I and II. 2nd ed. Berkeley, CA: NatTrop Publishing, 1993.

Hubbard, L. R. *Clear Body, Clear Mind*. Copenhagen, Denmark: New Era Publications Int., 1990.

Ingerman, Sandra. *Welcome Home: Life After Healing*. San Francisco, CA: Harper-San Francisco, 1993.

Johnson, Robert. *Inner Work*. New York, NY: Harper and Row, 1986.

Joseph, Barbara. *My Healing from Breast Cancer*. New Canaan, CT: Keats Publishing, Inc., 1996.

Kaur, Sardarni Premka. *Peace Lagoon*. Pomona, CA: K.R.I. Publications, 1984.

Kent, James Tyler. *Lectures on Homeopathic Materia Medica*. New Delhi, India: Jain Publishing Co., 1983.

Keuneke, Robin. *Total Breast Health*. New York, NY: Kensington Books, 1998.

Khalsa, Gururattan K. *Transitions to a Heart-Centered World through the Kundalini Yoga and Meditations of Yogi Bhajan*. San Diego, CA: Yoga Technology Press, 1988.

Koenig-Bricker, Woodene. *Prayers of the Saints: An Inspired Collection of Holy Wisdom*. New York, NY: HarperCollins, 1996.

Kroeger, Hanna. *Parasites: The Enemy Within*. Boulder, CO: Hannah Kroeger Publications, 1991.

Krohn, Jacqueline, Frances Taylor, MA, and Jinger Prosser, LMT. *Natural Detoxification: The Complete Guide to Clearing Your Body of Toxins*. Point Roberts, WA: Hartley and Marks Publishers Inc., 1996.

Kushi, Michio. *The Cancer Prevention Diet*. New York, NY: St Martin's Press, 1993.

Lad, V. & D. Frawley. *The Yoga of Herbs*. Santa Fe, NM: Lotus Press, 1986.

Lawless, Gary. *First Sight of Land*. Nobleton, ME: Blackberry Books, 1990.

Lee, John R. *What Your Doctor May Not Tell You About Menopause*. New York, NY: Warner Books Inc., 1996.

LeShan, Lawrence. *Cancer as a Turning Point: A Handbook for People with Cancer, their Families and Health Professionals*. New York, NY: Penguin, 1994.

Lilienthal, S. *Homeopathic Therapeutics*. New Delhi, India: Indian Books and Periodicals Syndicate, 1890.

Love, S. *Susan Love's Breast Book*. Cambridge, MA: Perseus Publishing.

Mascaro, Juan. *The Upanishads*. Toronto, ON: Penguin, 1965.

Matson, John. *The Secrets to Great Health From Your Nine Liver Dwarves.* North Vancouver, BC: Goodwin Books, 1998.

Michnovicz, J. *How to Reduce Your Risk of Breast Cancer*. New York, NY: Warner Books, 1994.

Mollison, B. *Introduction to Permaculture*. Tyalgum, NSW, Australia: Tagari Publications, 1991.

Moss, R. *Cancer Therapy: The Independent Consumer's Guide to Non-Toxic Treatment and Prevention*. New York, NY: Equinox Press, 1992.

Murphy, Robin. *Homeopathic Medical Repertory*. Pagosa Springs, CO: Hahnemann Academy of North America, 1993.

Ontario Breast Cancer Information Exchange Project. *A Guide to Unconventional Cancer Therapies*. Toronto, ON 1994.

Naiman, Ingrid. *Cancer Salves: A Botanical Approach to Treatment*. Santa Fe, NM: Seventh Ray Press, 1999.

Pizzorno, J. & M. Murray. *A Textbook of Natural Medicine*. Seattle, WA: John Bastyr College Publications, 1985.

Radhakrishan, Sarvepalli and Charles A. Moore. *A Sourcebook in Indian Philosophy*. Princeton, NJ: Princeton University Press, 1957.

Rogers, S. *Wellness Against All Odds*. Syracuse, NY: Prestige Publishing, 1994.

Rossi, Ernest. *The Psychobiology of Mind-Body Healing*. New York, NY: W.W. Norton, 1986.

Rossi, Ernest. *The 20 Minute Break*. Los Angeles, CA: Jeremy P. Tarcher Inc., 1991.

Roy, Rob. *The Sauna*. White River Junction, VT: Chelsea Green Publishing Company, 1996.

Santillo, Humbart. *Food Enzymes: the Missing Link to Radiant Health*. Prescott, AZ: Hohm Press, 1993.

Santillo, Humbart. *Intuitive Eating*. Prescott, AZ: Hohm Press, 1993.

Siegel, Bernie. *Love, Medicine and Miracles: Lessons Learned About Self-Healing from a Surgeon's Experience with Exceptional Patients*. New York, NY: Harper and Row, 1986.

Siegel, Bernie. *Peace, Love and Healing*. New York: Harper and Row, 1989.

Simonton, O. C., S. Simonton, and J. Creighton. *Getting Well Again*. Los Angeles, CA: Tarcher, 1978.

Singer, S. & S. Grismaijer. *Dressed to Kill: The Link Between Breast Cancer and Bras*. Garden City Park, NY: Avery Publishing Group, 1995.

Singh, R. *Self-Healing: Powerful Techniques*. London, ON: Health Psychology Associates, 1997.

Stamets, Paul. *The Mushroom Cultivator: A Practical Guide to Growing Mushrooms at Home*. Olympia, WA: Agarikon Press, 1983.

Stamets, Paul. *Growing Gourmet and Medicinal Mushrooms*. Berkeley, CA: Ten Speed Press, 1993.

Stamets, Paul. *MycoMedicinals: An Informational Booklet on Medicinal Mushrooms*. Olympia, WA: MycoMedia Publications, 1998.

Steinman, D. *Diet for a Poisoned Planet*. New York, NY: Crown Publishing, 1990.

Steingraber, Sandra. *Living Downstream: An Ecologist Looks at Cancer and the Environment*. Reading, MA: Addison-Wesley Publishing Co. Ltd., 1997.

Tagliaferra, M., I. Cohen, D. Tripathy, eds. *Breast Cancer Beyond Convention*. New York, NY: Atria Books, 2003.

Tierra, M. *Planetary Herbology*. Santa Fe, NM, Lotus Press. 1988.

Weed, S. *Breast Cancer? Breast Health!* Woodstock, NY: Ash Tree Publishing, 1996.

Wigmore, Ann. *The Hippocrates Diet and Health Program*. Garden City Park, NY: Avery, 1983.

Wigmore, A. *The Sprouting Bible*. Wayne, NJ. Avery Publishing Group, 1986.

Acknowledgments

I have been supported by several communities in writing this book, and it is the offspring of that support. Firstly, my naturopathic colleagues who are working with me in creating solutions to breast cancer: my thanks goes to Kathleen Finlay N.D. in Owen Sound for your superb suggestions to improve Chapters 3 and 5 and for collaborating with me in teaching breast health; to Jen Green N.D. for your very important work on inflammation and antioxidants; to Michelle Stapleton N.D. for adding to our experience using the cancer salves; to Anthony Godfrey N.D. for your support and understanding of the spiritual dimensions of breast cancer; to Verna Hunt N.D. for your contribution on thermography and for making this diagnostic tool available to Canadians; to Stephen Tripodi N.D. for being there as a sounding board and for collaborating on a sauna protocol; to Ingrid Pincott N.D. in B.C. for promoting Rachel Carson Day to the Canadian naturopathic community; to Tom Francesscott N.D. in New York for teaching the Healthy Breast Program in your community; and to the many other naturopathic doctors in Canada and the U.S. who have shared the first edition of this book with their patients and used it as a teaching tool. I am also indebted to Dr. Mary Danylak for your conference presentations on intravenous vitamin C and dental toxicity. My thanks goes to Jan Palko and Mary Kovacs for sharing your experience using Darkfield Microscopy with me and stressing the importance of biological terrain. Thankyou to Sarah Cowley and Pam Hammond for the breast massage guidelines.

A special thanks to Dr George Gillson of Rocky Mountain Analytical in Calgary for reviewing the chapter on hormones and for your many valuable suggestions. Thank you also for making saliva hormone testing available in Canada and for educating women about alternatives to traditional hormone replacement therapy.

I would like to thank the people who have invited me to teach the Healthy Breast Program in their communities and who continue to educate women in breast health: Kristina Lindstrom in Madrid, Spain; Parmatma Kaur Leviton in Ottawa, Canada; Gurunater Kaur Khalsa in Herndon, Virginia; Kerry Koenig-Little in Orillia, Ontario; Helen Gaidatsis and Madeline Montpool in Newmarket, Ontario; Hope Nemiroff in Kingston, New York; Janet Jacks at Goodness Me! Natural Foods in Hamilton; Kathleen Mercer and Harmony Whole Foods in Orangeville, Ontario; Satya Singh Khalsa at the Yoga Festival in France; and the many dedicated women at the Breast Cancer Research and Education Fund in St. Catharines, Ontario.

I deeply appreciate the staff and students at

the Canadian College of Naturopathic medicine for providing me with the opportunity to teach breast health. Special thanks to Cheryl Proctor N.D., Janet Patterson, and Melissa Clements for their ongoing support and organizational skills. To the third year students at CCNM I thank you for your research papers which have made it much easier for me to put the pieces together in the breast cancer puzzle, so we all may benefit.

Thank you to the many participants in the Healthy Breast Teacher Training Program — please continue to spread the word. Special thanks to Suzie Schmidt, Sherry Leblanc, Janet Miller, and Veronica Wolff for your enthusiasm and support, which has given me strength.

I am indebted to members of my Owen Sound community who have nurtured me through this intensive writing schedule – especially to Elinor Renny, for being with me on Fridays to do whatever needs to be done, for organizing my sometimes chaotic office, and for offering unconditional support. I am truly and deeply grateful. Thank you to MaryAnn Thomas of the Ginger Press, who has been a sounding board and early morning yoga partner throughout the writing of this edition and who I appreciate immensely. Thank you to Susan Gibson and Allan Stone for your many clippings on breast health and for your wisdom and support, and to Mark Vacheresse at Parker Pharmacy for your help with the biochemistry of estrogen metabolism.

I am profoundly grateful to my patients – remarkable women confronting a serious disease – thank you for following through with difficult life changes and for trusting in the process of healing. We are learning how to manage this disease together, and each of you adds to my knowledge base.

My deepest gratitude to my husband, Har-Prakash, for your tremendous support and encouragement and for caring for our three children while I have been typing on my perch at the clinic. Thank you for giving me space. And I thank my children for their understanding and resilience in allowing me to do this important work.

This book would not be here were it not for the dedication of my editor, Bob Hilderley, who has shepherded it from its previous incarnation to its present form, and whose organizational expertise has made it a much better book. Thank you for seeing its merit and adopting it as your own from the beginning. I am very thankful to have worked on it twice with you. My gratitude also extends to Bob Dees at Robert Rose Inc for delivering the book to a wider audience and for telling me you wanted "more information in fewer pages." I hope I have satisfied your request.

Finally I would like to acknowledge the Great Spirit who fed and nurtured me continuously throughout this remarkable project and brought me the resources I needed, when I needed them. It has been a privilege to listen and obey.

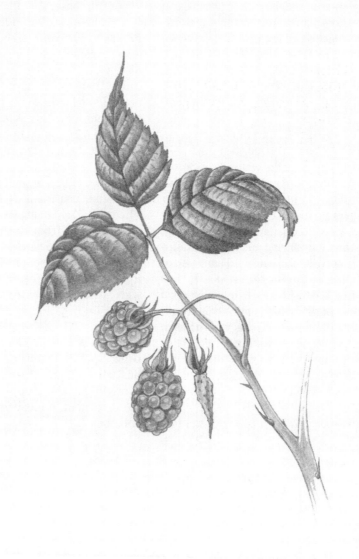

Index

Please note: this index sorts numbers before letters.

complexion, 17

conjugation reactions, 139-140

constipation, 25, 81, 166, 178, 184, 217. *See also* bowel, colon, enemas

cortisol, 27, 67, 75, 76, 89

culture, 285

cystein, 84, 220, 226
  N-acetyl- (NAC), 69, 100

D

dairy, 15, 79, 83, 231-234, 249

dandelion, 144, 191, 195, 208

Day, Rachel Carson, 5, 122

DDE, 113

DDT, 113

depression, 132, 240, 269, 311, 314. *See also* dopamine

DES (diethyl stilbestrol), 73-74

detergents, 107, 119-120

detoxification, 7, 8, 11, 12, 21, 24, 39, 61, 68, 85, 95, 97, 130-147, 157-170, 178, 182, 184, 189, 204, 206, 208, 225, 227, 230, 243-248, 252, 257, 258, 282, 296, 305, 320, 324, 328, 330-335, 356

dieldrin, 109, 113

diet, 6-19, 22-27, 30-39, 45, 47, 50, 59, 64, 67, 69-74, 77, 79, 83-88, 93-101, 105, 106, 115, 130, 136, 139-156, 160-167, 170, 197, 201-257, 282, 296, 299, 306, 311-316, 321- 373

diethyl stilbestrol. *See* DES

digestive organs, 38, 133, 134, 146

DIM, 257, 262, 265

dioxins, 113-116

docosohexanoic acid, 312

DNA, 10, 19, 21, 47, 64-68, 149, 206, 219, 244-246, 250, 253, 257, 311-312

dopamine, 43, 78-79, 83

dreams, 266, 285, 288, 290, 294

drugs
  fertility, 26
  prescription, 22-23, 30. *See also* birth control pill

dry brush massage, 175-176

E

electricity and electromagnetic fields, 105-106

ellagic acid, 47, 68, 142

endocrine system, 27, 38

endometriosis, 115

enemas, 7, 156-159. *See also* bowel, colon, constipation

environment, 9-21, 26-39, 47, 61-79, 84, 99-130, 134, 148, 149, 153, 160-169, 172-180, 190, 199, 203-213, 221, 231, 240, 249, 251, 256, 258, 278, 294, 300, 326, 328, 332-338, 341-347, 351-358, 360, 361, 370-373

enzymes, 24, 30, 48, 68, 81, 131-151, 161-164, 170, 186, 196, 203-207, 217-219, 229, 233, 236, 237, 243, 244, 250, 254, 257, 258, 260-265, 282, 314, 328, 330, 355, 356, 358, 364, 373

essential fatty acids, 210-213

estradiol (E2), 62

estriol (E3), 62

estrogen, 7, 11, 14, 18, 20, 22, 37, 43, 45-47, 60-80, 86-87, 91, 95, 98, 217-218

estrone (E1), 62

evening primrose oil, 24, 212

exercise, physical, 8, 19, 22, 45, 164, 273, 315, 324, 331

F

fat, 203-240
  to avoid, 210-215

fertility drugs, 26

fiber, 15, 22, 34, 45, 70, 130, 156, 216-218, 230

fibroadenomas, 46, 56

fibrocystic breast disease, 11, 45-46, 144, 184, 186-187, 212, 252, 315

flaxseed, 11, 24, 25, 33, 39, 47, 51, 63-79, 85, 87, 96, 97, 100, 136, 142-146, 151, 156, 159, 167, 202, 205, 208-226, 230, 231, 237, 239, 240, 249, 256, 257, 261-263, 314-316, 327, 330, 348, 359-361

formaldehyde, 46, 102, 106-107

stress, 24, 43, 47, 67, 75-79, 89-90, 94

sugar, 21, 43, 76, 86, 93, 138, 150, 156, 212, 230, 234, 240

sulfation, 95, 140, 144

sulphur-containing compounds, 142-143

supplements, 242-265

sweat. *See* saunas

T

TCE (trichloroethylene), 116

T cells, 12, 115, 174, 181, 210

testes, 108-109

testosterone, 66-67, 75, 79, 86, 89, 97

thermography, 6, 55, 74, 78

thymus gland, 92, 135, 173-174, 181, 243, 253, 255, 281-282

thyroid, 80, 118-119, 223, 252

tonsils, 37, 174

toxaphene, 109

toxins, 133-170. *See also* pollution, sewage

TRH (thyrotropin-releasing hormone), 80

trichloroethylene. *See* TCE

tumor markers, 56

U

ultradian rhythms, 92, 94

ultrasound, 6, 23, 40, 53, 56-58, 83

V

vagina, 66, 73, 153, 314

vegetarian diet, 203-209

visualization, 303-306

vitamins, 243-249

W

waist-to-hip ratio, 19-29

water, 8, 153, 157

white blood cells. *See under* blood

X

xenoestrogens, 62, 64, 68, 74, 84, 95-100, 326

Y

yeast, 143, 240, 244, 245, 246, 251, 253, 254, 256. *See also* candidiasis

yoga, 7, 10, 11, 17, 28, 33, 149, 151, 155, 165, 174, 267, 273, 282, 287, 290, 304, 332, 333, 340, 356, 370-375

Z

Zava, David, 77, 81

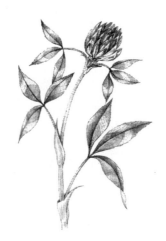